Palliative Care Consultant

A reference guide for palliative care

Guidelines for Effective Management of Symptoms

Fourth Edition

Bridget McCrate Protus, PharmD, MLIS, CGP, CDP
Director of Drug Information, HospiScript Services

Jason M. Kimbrel, PharmD, BCPS
Vice President of Operations & Clinical Services, HospiScript Services

Phyllis A. Grauer, PharmD, CGP, CPE
Clinical Consultant, HospiScript Services

HospiScript, a Catamaran Company
4525 Executive Park Drive
Montgomery, AL 36166
Tel: 866-970-7500
www.hospiscript.com

Cover design: Scott J. McClusky

ISBN-13: 978-0-9889558-4-4
ISBN-10: 0988955849

Editors

Bridget McCrate Protus, RPh, PharmD, MLIS, CGP, CDP
Director of Drug Information, HospiScript Services
Assistance Professor- Practice, The Ohio State University College of Pharmacy, Columbus, Ohio

Jason M. Kimbrel, RPh, PharmD, BCPS
Vice President of Operations & Clinical Services, HospiScript Services
Associate Professor of Pharmacy Practice, Ohio Northern University College of Pharmacy, Ada, Ohio

Phyllis A. Grauer, RPh, PharmD, CGP, CPE
Clinical Consultant, HospiScript Services
Assistance Professor- Practice, The Ohio State University College of Pharmacy, Columbus, Ohio

Author/Reviewers

Kyna Setsor Collier, RN, BSN, CHPN
Clinical Nurse Educator, HospiScript Services

Jessica Geiger-Hayes, RPh, PharmD, BCPS
Clinical Pharmacist, HospiScript Services

Michael R. Lux, RPh, PharmD
Clinical Pharmacist, HospiScript Services

Kelly Reilly Kroustos, RPh, PharmD, CGP, CDP
Clinical Pharmacist, HospiScript Services
Associate Professor of Pharmacy Practice,
Ohio Northern University College of Pharmacy, Ada, Ohio

Julie Vandaveer, RPh, PharmD, CGP
Clinical Pharmacist, HospiScript Services

Allison M. Webb, RPh, PharmD, CGP, CDP
Clinical Pharmacist, HospiScript Services

Lacey A. Davis, RPh, PharmD, BCPS
Clinical Pharmacist, Aultman Hospital, North Canton, Ohio

Maureen Jones, RPh, PharmD, CGP, CDP
Clinical Pharmacist, HospiScript Services

Candice N. Tavares, RPh, PharmD
Clinical Pharmacist, Specialty Pain Management and
Palliative Care, CenterLight Healthcare, Bronx, NY

Heidi Trautwein, RPh, PharmD, CGP, FASCP
Clinical Pharmacist, HospiScript Services

Becky Wagner, RPh, PharmD, CDP
Clinical Pharmacist, HospiScript Services

Contributors

Jennalie Blackwood, RPh, PharmD
Clinical Editor, Wolters Kluwer, St. Louis, MO

Marliese Gibson, RPh, PharmD
Clinical Pharmacist, HospiScript Services

Ashraf Kittaneh, RPh, PharmD
PGY1 Pharmacy Practice Resident, Riverside Methodist Hospital, Columbus, Ohio

Melissa O'Neill Hunt, RPh, PharmD
Pediatric Clinical Pharmacist, HospiScript Services

Laura Warren, RPh, PharmD
Clinical Pharmacist, Clinical Apothecaries Inc, Medina, Ohio

Kristy Montoya
Pre-pharmacy program, The Ohio State University

Acknowledgements

The 4th edition of the *Palliative Care Consultant (PCC)* was produced through a collaborative relationship with the Midwest Care Alliance and HospiScript Services. This edition combines the work of the previous *PCC* editions with an industry leader known for implementing and managing symptoms in an economical, efficient manner using effective care pathways. HospiScript Services would like to extend our gratitude to the Midwest Care Alliance for their expertise, flexibility, and desire to help meet an industry need.

To the staff of HospiScript Services:

The authors wish to thank all of our colleagues for their assistance in the creation of this resource. Without their generous support this work would not have been possible. Their compassionate commitment to improving end of life care for all individuals is an inspiration.

Special Recognition:

Jennalie Blackwood and Marliese Gibson for their assistance in copyediting the text.
Ashraf Kittaneh, Laura Warren, and Kristy Montoya for their assistance in developing the drug information tables.
Melissa O'Neill Hunt for her dedication and persistence in creating the GEMS algorithms and putting up with Phyllis, Jason, and Bridget during countless algorithm review and revisions.
Scott McClusky for creating the beautiful cover art, design, and layout.

Additional books from HospiScript Services
available from HospiBooks.com or Amazon.com

Pediatric Palliative Care Consultant: Guidelines for Effective Management of Symptoms
Melissa O'Neill Hunt, Bridget McCrate Protus, Janine Penfield Winters, Diane C. Parker
Retail: $79.99
ISBN-10: 0988955830
ISBN-13: 978-0988955837

Wound Care at End of Life: A Guide for Hospice Professionals
Kyna Setsor Collier, Bridget McCrate Protus, Connie L. Bohn, Jason M. Kimbrel
Retail: $24.99
ISBN-10: 0988955822
ISBN-13: 978-0988955820

Dedication

This work is dedicated to all healthcare professionals, families, and caregivers and the loved ones to whom they provide comfort and peace.

To my husband, Seth, and my son, Zane, for their love, patience, and support; in honor and memory of my mom, Carolyn McCrate, for her love, encouragement, guidance, and inspiration; and in memory of my father-in-law, Herb Protus, who provided guidance on my professional path, sparked my love of pharmacy, and modeled the best of patient care in some of the most challenging of times. –BMP

I dedicate this text to my wife Jennifer, daughter Hanna, as well as my extended family and friends. Their tireless support and encouragement has enabled my pursuit of patient care within the hospice community that has improved the lives of so many people. To my colleagues, your dedication to our shared calling to advance end of life care is amazing and I am honored to have walked on this journey with each of you. – JMK

I dedicate this project to all the incredibly knowledgeable and compassionate pharmacists as well as the other members of the interdisciplinary team who use their skills to provide comfort and care to patients as they approach the end of their lives. It has been an honor and privilege to work side by side and learn from all of you. –PAG

You matter because you are you, and you matter to the end of your life. We will do all we can not only to help you die peacefully, but also to live until you die.

Dame Cicely Saunders

Foreword

The field of palliative care has undergone a remarkable evolution since entering its modern period several decades ago. Prior to that time, palliative care was only medicalized in the sense of providing morphine for pain relief, with most palliative care being entrusted to non-clinicians who provided social, emotional, and spiritual support. When in 1982, the Medicare Hospice Benefit codified how hospice would be delivered in our country, it purposefully melded the psychosocial and spiritual aspects of care with the medical. This created a major challenge, since this seemingly reinforced palliative care as being on the fringe of an increasingly specialized healthcare system that was geared only towards the medical side of care.

Remarkably, Hospice and Palliative Medicine has, in a relatively short period of time, come to be recognized as a specialty field of mainstream medicine within the US. It has achieved this status while coaxing the rest of the medical establishment to value the non-medical tenets of palliative care. However, remembering these roots has proven a challenge as palliative care is increasingly provided across a variety of settings, many of which are highly medicalized. Hospice remains the venue for the largest provision of palliative care in the US, and does so while holding true to the necessity of interdisciplinary team involvement.

Accompanying the modernization of palliative care, there have also been rapid advances in research, particularly in the realms of pharmacology and prescribing. Those who have been palliative care practitioners for some time, remember when prescribing was empiric, relying on personal experiences and word-of-mouth traditions. With the growing evidence-base for scientific prescribing, such clinicians have struggled to adapt when findings invalidated traditional practices. At the other extreme are those clinicians who are newly entering palliative care from other healthcare backgrounds. Their experiences result in similar difficulties of adapting, but in this situation it is to the utilization of not necessarily new medications, but new and sometimes novel ways of using seemingly familiar agents. These challenges apply to clinicians of all backgrounds, whether physician, nurse, or pharmacist.

The ultimate goal of advancing the evidence-base for palliative care is to enhance and improve patient experiences and care. I've found that my own role within the interdisciplinary team is best described as helping get the symptoms under control so other, often more important matters can be addressed by other team members. In order to accomplish this effectively, the latest information must be readily available for both teaching and reference by those caring for patients. Hence the necessity of periodically updating reference guides such as the Palliative Care Consultant (PCC).

This fourth edition of the PCC is a compilation of clinical information representing the current state of the art within hospice and palliative medicine. But the PCC goes a step beyond. It is a not only a useful guide describing the medications that work for a given set of symptoms, but it also helps frame the critical thinking necessary for clinicians to determine the etiology of symptoms. This is mandatory in providing the best management of the myriad palliative care situations encountered in this second decade of the 21st century. Incorporating this information with other reference material that is useful to the hospice and palliative care clinician makes the new edition of the Palliative Care Consultant a crucial tool in optimizing palliative care for our patients.

Ronald J Crossno, MD FAAFP FAAHPM
Senior National Medical Director for Gentiva Health Services
Past President for the American Academy of Hospice & Palliative Medicine
1904 Sager Rd, Rockdale, TX 76567

Disclaimer: This foreword represents the personal opinions of Dr. Crossno, which are not necessarily those of either Gentiva or AAHPM.

I. Introduction

II. Guidelines for Effective Management of Symptoms (GEMS™)

III. Disease State Management

IV. Appendices

Section I:

Introduction

- Introduction to Hospice and Palliative Care
- Concepts in Palliative Care
- Developing Communication Skills
- Hospice Regulatory Information
- CMS Guidelines for Medication Use in Long Term Care
- Compounded Medications in Palliative Care
- Medical Abbreviations

Introduction to Hospice and Palliative Care

Defining Palliative Care[1]
The definition of palliative care used to characterize palliative care in the United States described by both the U.S. Department of Health and Human Services (HHS) Centers for Medicare & Medicaid Services (CMS) and the National Quality Forum (NQF) states:

> *Palliative care means patient and family-centered care that optimizes quality of life by anticipating, preventing, and treating suffering. Palliative care throughout the continuum of illness involves addressing physical, intellectual, emotional, social, and spiritual needs and to facilitate patient autonomy, access to information, and choice.*

The following features characterize palliative care philosophy and delivery:
- Care is provided and services are coordinated by an interdisciplinary team.
- Patients, families, palliative and non-palliative health care providers collaborate and communicate about care needs.
- Services are available concurrently with or independent of curative or life-prolonging care.
- Patient and family hopes for peace and dignity are supported throughout the course of illness, during the dying process, and after death.

Domains of Palliative Care (*Adapted from National Consensus Project's Clinical Practice Guidelines*)[1]
- *Structure and process of care*: palliative care is provided across the health care spectrum necessitating the involvement of an interdisciplinary team to support the physical, psychological, social, and spiritual needs of the patient and family; best practices include quality assessment and performance improvement processes and respect for the patient and family values and preferences.
- *Physical aspects of care*: physical comfort, including pain and symptom management is a central feature of palliative care; physical comfort enables the promotion of psychological, spiritual, and social quality of life.
- *Psychological and psychiatric aspects of care*: psychological and psychiatric screening and assessments are provided; services offered are appropriate to patient and family needs, goals, and culture; grief and bereavement are fundamental to palliative care service.
- *Socials aspects of care*: interventions support the unique social structure of each family unit; specialists in social aspects of care and pediatric populations are provided.
- *Spiritual, religious, and existential aspects of care*: recognition that spiritual, religious, and existential care are fundamental to quality of life for patients and families; inclusive spiritual healing environment is provided.
- *Cultural aspects of care*: beliefs and values of the patient and family are supported according to individual cultural identification including race, ethnicity, socioeconomic class, and gender expression or sexual orientation; respects cultural practices and rituals.
- *Care of the patient at end of life*: interdisciplinary team provides care that supports the patient and family wishes for peaceful, dignified, and respectful death.
- *Ethical and legal aspects of care*: central ethical principles are understood by the interdisciplinary team within the context of each disciplines professional practice; care is provided in accordance with professional, state and federal laws, regulations, and current standards of care.

Defining Hospice Care[2,3]
Hospice is a special type of care in which medical, psychological, and spiritual support are provided to patients and families when medical therapies can no longer control the disease. Hospice care focuses on controlling pain and other symptoms of illness so patients can remain as comfortable as possible near the end of life. Hospice focuses on caring, not curing. The goal is to neither hasten nor postpone death. If the patient's condition improves or the cancer goes into remission, hospice care can be discontinued and active treatment may resume. Hospice services include doctor or nursing care, medical supplies and equipment, home health aide services, short-term respite services for caregivers, drugs to help manage pain and other symptoms, spiritual support and counseling, and social work services. Patients' families are also an important focus of hospice care, and services are designed to give them assistance and support. Hospice care most often takes place at home. However, hospice care can also be delivered in special in-patient facilities, hospitals, and nursing homes.

- The Medicare Hospice Benefit requires that a terminally-ill patient have a prognosis of 6 months or less; however, there is no 6-month limit to hospice care services.
- A patient in the final phase of life may receive hospice care for as long as necessary when a physician certifies that he or she continues to meet eligibility requirements.
- Under the Medicare Hospice Benefit, two 90-day periods of care (a total of six months) are followed by an unlimited number of 60-day periods.

Hospice Standards of Care *(Adapted from NHPCO Standards of Practice for Hospice Programs)*[4]

- *Patient and family centered care:* providing care and services to the patient and family as a unit of care, developing an individualized, patient-centered plan of care.
- *Ethical behavior and consumer rights:* highest standards of ethical conduct are upheld; the hospice respects, honors, and advocates for the rights of each patient and family.
- *Clinical excellence and safety:* interdisciplinary care team identifies and respects the desires of the patient and family to facilitate care outcomes of safe and comfortable dying through treatment, prevention, and promotion of excellent clinical care through continuous assessment of patient-family needs.
- *Inclusion and access:* all people have equal access to care regardless of race, ethnicity, religion, disability, gender, sexual orientation, age, or disease.
- *Organizational excellence:* a culture of quality and accountability is established; collaboration and communication within the organization are valued.
- *Workforce excellence:* a collaborative, interdisciplinary environment is promoted through professional development and support for all staff and volunteers.
- *Standards:* NHPCO's Standards of Practice for Hospice Programs and/or the National Consensus Project's Clinical Practice Guidelines for Quality Palliative Care serve as a foundation of service in the organization.
- *Compliance with laws and regulations:* compliance with all applicable laws, regulations, and standards of professional practice are ensured; systems are implemented to prevent fraud and abuse.
- *Stewardship and accountability:* fiscal and managerial oversight is provided by well-qualified organizational leadership.
- Performance measurement: Collecting, analyzing, and actively using performance metrics to encourage quality assessment and performance improvement in all areas of hospice care processes.

References

1. National Consensus Project for Quality Palliative Care. *Clinical Practice Guidelines for Quality Palliative Care.* 3rd ed. Pittsburgh, PA: National Consensus Project for Quality Palliative Care; 2013. Available at http://nationalconsensusproject.org.
2. National Hospice & Palliative Care Organization (NHPCO). NHPCO's facts and figures: hospice care in America. 2014 edition. Alexandria, VA; NHPCO, October 2014. Available at http://www.nhpco.org/sites/default/files/public/Statistics_Research/2014_Facts_Figures.pdf.
3. National Cancer Institute. Hospice Care. Bethesda, MD: National Cancer Institute; October 2012. Available at http://www.cancer.gov/cancertopics/factsheet/support/hospice.
4. National Hospice and Palliative Care Organization (NHPCO). Standards of Practice for Hospice Programs. Alexandria, VA: NHPCO; 2010. Available at http://www.nhpco.org/nhpco-standards-practice.

Figure 1. Palliative Care: World Health Organization Model

Palliative Care
World Health Organization Model

Disease therapy with curative or restorative intent

Disease progression

Terminal phase

H O S P I C E

D E A T H

B E R E A V E M E N T

PALLIATIVE CARE
Diagnosis through life span

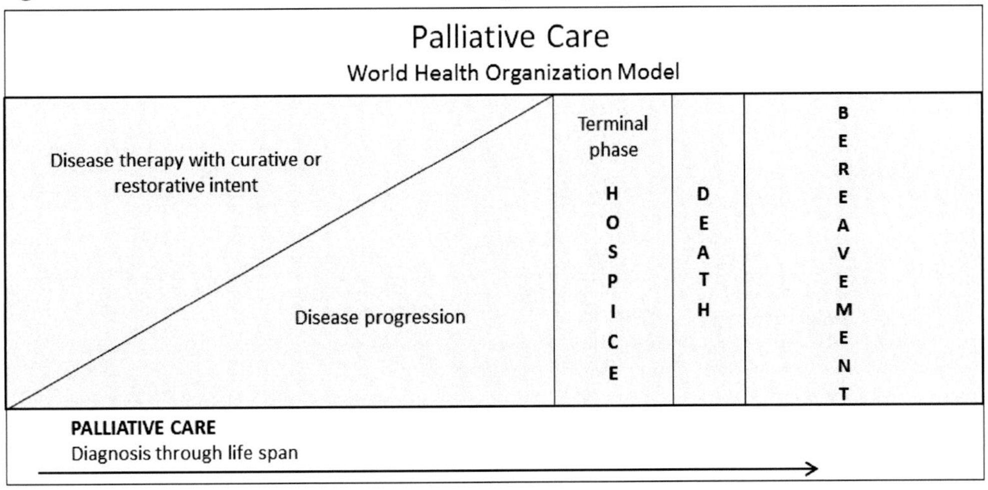

Figure 2. Vision of the Palliative Care Continuum

Vision of Palliative Care Continuum

Living with risk factors

Life Limiting Disease
Focus: curative/restorative treatment

Palliative Care
Focus: symptom management/whole person care

Life closure

Imminent death

Death & bereavement

Hospice Care
< 6 month prognosis

Figure 3. Interdisciplinary Team Model[2]

The interdisciplinary team is a hallmark of hospice and palliative care. The collaborative and patient-centered care approach enables individualized, holistic support to the patient and family.

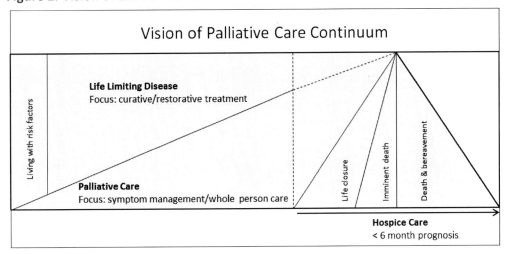

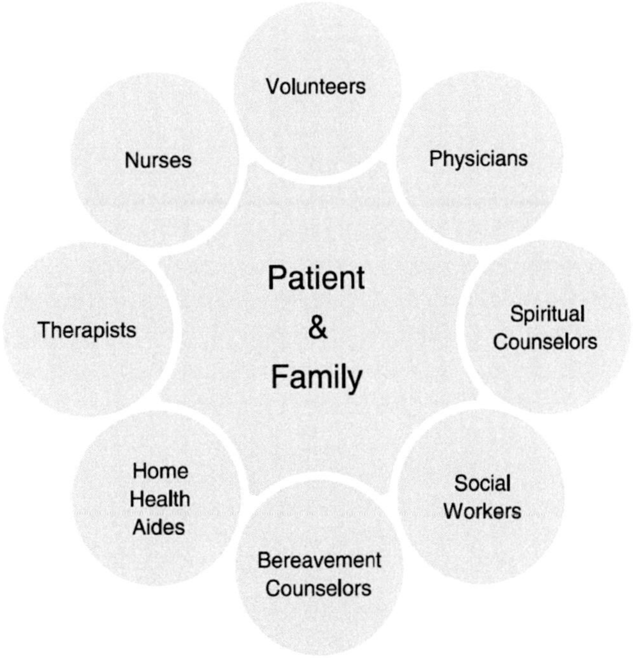

Volunteers

Nurses

Physicians

Therapists

Patient & Family

Spiritual Counselors

Home Health Aides

Bereavement Counselors

Social Workers

Figure 4. Models of Disease Trajectory[3-6]

Trajectory 1
Individual retains function and comfort for an extended period until the malignancy becomes overwhelming followed by relatively rapid decline and death.

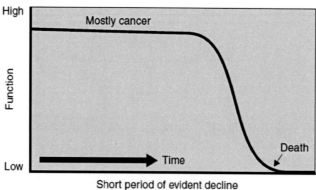

Trajectory 2
Individual retains most function for an extended period of time interrupted with episodic exacerbation of illness; sudden death during an exacerbation is probable.

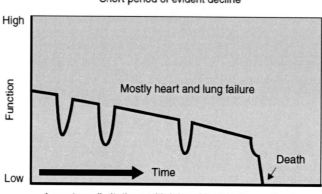

Trajectory 3
Individual experiences a slow, progressive decline in old age; presence of frailty and neurological disease often with cognitive impairment; death may be delayed with interventions, but suffering may be increased.

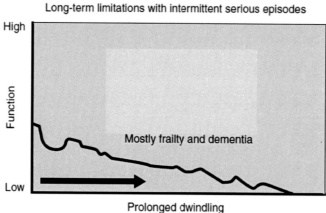

References

1. National Consensus Project for Quality Palliative Care. *Clinical Practice Guidelines for Quality Palliative Care*. 3rd ed. Pittsburgh, PA: National Consensus Project for Quality Palliative Care; 2013. Available at http://nationalconsensusproject.org.
2. National Hospice & Palliative Care Organization (NHPCO). NHPCO's facts and figures: hospice care in America. 2014 edition. Alexandria, VA; NHPCO, October 2014. Available at http://www.nhpco.org/sites/default/files/public/Statistics_Research/2014_Facts_Figures.pdf.
3. Lynn J, Adamson DM. *Living Well at the End of Life: Adapting Health Care to Serious Chronic Illness in Old Age*. Santa Monica, CA: Rand Health; 2003. Available at http://www.rand.org/pubs/white_papers/WP137.html.
4. Lynn, J. Living long in fragile health: the new demographics shape end of life care. *Improving End of Life Care: Why Has It Been So Difficult? Hastings Center Report Special Report*. 2005;35(6): S14-S18.
5. Murray SA, Kendall M, Boyd K, Sheikh A. Illness trajectories and palliative care. *BMJ*. 2005;330:1007-1011.
6. Stabenau HF, Morrison LJ, Gahbauer EA, et al. Functional trajectories in the year before hospice. *Ann Fam Med*. 2015; 13(1):33-40. Available at http://www.annfammed.org/content/13/1/33.long.

Developing Communication Skills

Communication skills are critical in hospice and palliative care; however, knowing when and how to approach difficult conversations can be challenging even for experienced clinicians. Communication models can provide a systematic approach to facilitate these conversations. Communication models can be used as guides to ensure key components of conversations are not missed, or as training tools to assist clinicians in developing patient-family discussion skills. All models require adaptation to effectively meet the needs of each unique patient and family situation. The BUILD model is presented below as an example of a holistic approach to communication that elicits information and understanding, develops trust and respect, enables collaboration in the plan of care, and supports a shared decision-making process. [1-4]

First impressions are lasting ones. The admission visit and end-of-life discussions establish the foundation of trust. These conversations are not one-time occurrences. Patients and families are often physically and emotionally overwhelmed and therefore able to take in only limited amounts of information. Important topics may need to be revisited several times. Discussions regarding interventions that have worked in the past but may no longer work are essential. Place emphasis on hospice's dedication to quality of life and comfort rather than curative care. The BUILD model can be used to discuss medication appropriateness, discontinuation of non-essential medications, and provides a framework for conversations about the use of medical interventions [e.g. feeding tubes, artificial hydration, implantable cardioverter defibrillators (ICD)]. [1-4]

BUILD™ Model of Communication with Patients and Families[1,4]

Component	Description	EXAMPLE Phrases & Conversation Points
BUILD the foundation	Build trust and respect	• "Thank you for talking with me today." • "Are you ready to talk about this?" • "Who needs to be present for this discussion?" • "This must be very difficult for you."
UNDERSTAND the patient and caregiver	Identify care priorities and quality of life	• Learn what the patient and family know regarding the topic at hand • "I want to make sure we are on the same page." • "Help me understand what you'd like to see happen." • "How do you think this illness affects your loved one?" • "What symptoms are of greatest concern to you?"
INFORM the patient and caregiver	Provide information on treatments, interventions, and expected outcomes	• Discuss evidence based information in a neutral manner • Bridge medical terminology and reasoning • Use print materials with illustrations and language appropriate to the patient and family's health literacy level. • "What worked before may not work now."
LISTEN to the patient and caregiver	Use active listening techniques	• Learn what is important to the patient and family • "If you had three wishes, what would you wish for?" • "What does quality of life look like to you?" • "We can't reverse the disease, but we can provide comfort."
DEVELOP a plan with the patient and caregiver	Acknowledge where the patient and caregiver are in the process	• Acknowledge the patient and family as decision-makers • Provide choices and work together as a team to develop a plan • Revisit the topic on an ongoing basis; make adjustments as necessary • "I'll bring what we've discussed to our hospice team tomorrow so everyone understands your concerns."

References

1. Collier KS, Protus BM. Facilitating difficult conversations about discontinuing medications or interventions. *HospiScript News*. 2014;10(1):1-3.
2. Malloy P, Virani R, Kelly K, Munevar C. Beyond bad news: communication skills of nurses in palliative care. *J Hosp Palliat Nurs*. 2010;12(3):166-174.
3. Wittenberg-Lyles E, Goldsmith J, Ragan S. The COMFORT initiative: palliative nursing and the centrality of communication. *J Hosp Palliat Nurs*. 2010;12(5):282-292.
4. Collier KS, Kimbrel JM, Protus BM. Medication Appropriateness at End of Life: A New Tool for Balancing Medicine and Communication for Optimal Outcomes- the BUILD Model. *Home Healthcare Nurse* 2013;31(9):518-524.

Hospice Regulatory Information

Hospice care in the United States is estimated to serve 1.5-1.6 million patients yearly. Hospice care, commonly referred to as the Medicare Hospice Benefit, is regulated as such primarily because 87.2% of the patients receive healthcare coverage though Medicare. Regulatory oversight to hospices comes from the federal statute known as the Hospice Conditions of Participation (CoPs). The last update to the CoPs was in 2008 and focused on multiple subparts including: Definitions; Eligibility, Election and Duration of Benefits; Patient Care; Core Services; Non-Core Services; Covered Services; Organizational Environment; and Payment. Updates to the CoPs occur each year with the release the Hospice Wage Index, which provides changes to the Payment section of the CoPs, as well as serves as a forum for other section updates. In addition to the annual Wage Index, Medicare may release transmittals throughout the year focusing on clarifications and defining expectations of the intended benefit.[1,2]

Hospice Regulations Affecting Medications[1-4]

Medication Therapy Management for hospice was first introduced in regulation in the 2008 Hospice CoPs. As defined in CoP section 418.106-a1, the hospice organization should utilize the skills of a drug expert, such as a pharmacist, to complete a drug profile review upon admission and subsequently at intervals thereafter to meet the needs of the patient. The drug profile review is a component of the comprehensive patient assessment and therefore must be completed within 5 days from admission and ongoing at least every 15 days.

Medication therapy management, often referred to as MTM, is not specific to the hospice industry. MTM is a term that describes services driven by pharmacists' surrounding the appropriate use of medications. Officially adopted by a consensus within the pharmacy profession in 2004, medication therapy management is defined as:

"...a service or group of services that optimize therapeutic outcomes for individual patients. Medication therapy management services include medication therapy reviews, pharmacotherapy consults, anticoagulation management, immunizations, health and wellness programs and many other clinical services. Pharmacists provide medication therapy management to help patients get the best benefits from their medications by actively managing drug therapy and by identifying, preventing and resolving medication-related problems." - Consensus definition of MTM[3]

Under the hospice CoP section 418.54-b6, MTM services should contain an evaluation of the drug profile, including the patient's prescription and over-the-counter medications, herbal remedies, and any other complementary or alternative therapy that could affect drug therapy. At a *minimum,* these 5 key components must be considered:
1. Effectiveness of drug therapy
2. Drug side effects
3. Duplicate drug therapy
4. Actual or potential drug interactions
5. Drug therapy currently associated with laboratory monitoring

Hospice agencies caring for patients under the Medicare Hospice Benefit should utilize the interdisciplinary team to help manage various drug related problems.

Medicare Claims Processing

Medicare Claims Processing Change Request (CR) 8358 was first published in 2013 and implemented in April 2014. A focus of this CR was to move the hospice industry towards reporting of meaningful data surrounding medication expenses onto their claim submissions for evaluation. A byproduct of the Affordable Care Act, hospice payment reform has been a lingering topic within the hospice space for quite some time. Displacement of the current bundled payment model, which began in 1983, has been expected since the Medicare Payment Advisory Committee (MedPAC) suggested changed in 2012. Change Request 8358 now requires that hospice agencies provide detailed line item of all medications and intravenous pumps purchased for patients under the hospice service upon billing Medicare for services rendered.

Revenue Codes were assigned to establish common billing practices

0250	Non-injectable prescription medications
0636	Injectable prescription medications
0294/029X	Infusion prescription medications/Infusion pumps

*Over-the-Counter medications were to be excluded from line item reporting

The use of the concept "Terminal Diagnosis" came into question in late 2013 as it relates to coverage of medications for hospice patients. The Centers of Medicare and Medicaid Services (CMS), upon evaluation of prescription billing practices mostly reflective of Medicare Part D, commented that hospice should be responsible for the "Terminal Prognosis" vs the "Terminal Diagnosis". The definition of terminal prognosis has yet to be officially defined by CMS, however has been established within the industry as those diagnoses in which impact the overall life expectancy of the patient and/or are diagnoses, conditions, or symptoms that are impact the terminal or related diagnoses. NHPCO developed an educational tool to aid in determining relatedness in December 2014 (Figure 1).[1]

The responsibility of payment for medications within hospice is directly related to the relationship in which the medication is considered to be related to the terminal prognosis. In addition to the relatedness determination, hospice must also consider the appropriateness and/or the ability of the medication to palliation. Hospice agencies have to demonstrate the ability to be fiscally responsible with the funds provided by payers, such as CMS. The use of a formulary is allowed and encouraged by hospice agencies; however the lack of a specific medication on a formulary doesn't preclude a hospice from having to provide medications needed by each patient.[2]

Medication Payment Responsibility	Medication Relatedness to Terminal Prognosis	
	Related	**Not Related**
Hospice	Yes	
Patient	Yes*	Yes*
Other Payer (e.g. Medicare Part D, Medicaid, etc)		Yes

Patient provided since deemed not medically necessary and part of the plan of care

Resources for Hospice Regulatory and Compliance Information

Federal and state legislative activity affecting hospice care is ongoing. In the coming months, CMS is expected to continue to overhaul the reimbursement structure and reporting practices for the Medicare Hospice Benefit. Private insurance providers tend to model their policies and practices after the structure of the Medicare Hospice Benefit. Hospice administration and management must remain well-informed and up-to-date about these regulatory changes. The following resources should be your first stops for this information. All three sites allow the user to subscribe to periodic email updates and breaking news.

Centers for Medicare & Medicaid Services (CMS) Hospice Center
- Official U.S. federal government information center for hospice-related rules, regulations, and guidance documents for hospice providers, including notification of public comment periods for proposed draft legislation.
- http://www.cms.gov/Center/Provider-Type/Hospice-Center.html

National Hospice and Palliative Care Organization (NHPCO) Regulatory and Compliance Center
- NHPCO is the largest nonprofit membership organization representing hospice and palliative care programs and professionals in the United States. NHPCO's Regulatory and Compliance Center provides a consolidated resource for regulatory alerts, compliance issues, quality initiatives, position statements, and state specific resources.
- http://www.nhpco.org/regulatory

National Association for Home Care& Hospice (NAHC) Legislative Action Center
- NAHC is a major nonprofit organization representing home care and hospice organizations in the United States, providing advocacy for home care and hospice staff and caregivers providing in-home patient care services. NAHC's Legislative Action Center integrates regulatory information for home care organizations, hospice organizations, guidance documents, and position statements.
- http://www.nahc.org/advocacy-policy/regulatory-issues/

Figure 1. Determining Relatedness to the Terminal Prognosis Process Flow

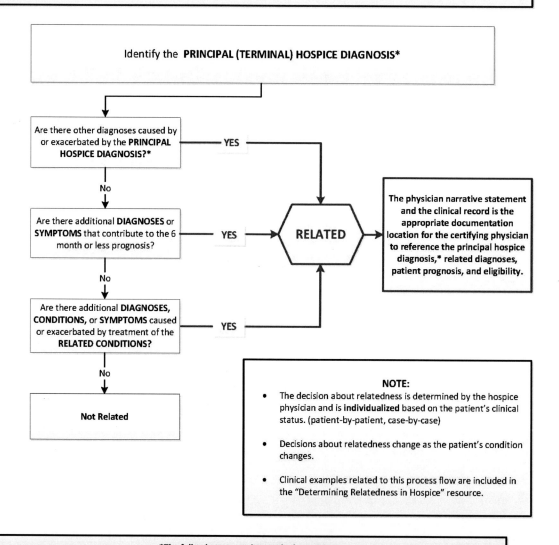

References

1. National Hospice and Palliative Care Organization (NHPCO). Regulatory & Compliance Center. Alexandria, VA; NHPCO. Available at http://www.nhpco.org/regulatory. Accessed December 29, 2014.
2. Centers of Medicare and Medicaid Services (CMS) Hospice Center. Baltimore, MD; CMS. Available at http://www.cms.gov/Center/Provider-Type/Hospice-Center.html. Accessed December 29, 2014.
3. American Pharmacists Association (APhA). APhA MTM Central. Washington, DC; APhA. Accessed December 29, 2014.
4. Gibbons P, Grauer P. Using the pharmacist's skills: a mandate and a benefit. *NHPCO Newsline* 2009;20(3): 31-32.

CMS Guidelines for Medication Use in Long Term Care Facilities

The Centers for Medicare & Medicaid Services (CMS) long term care facilities survey guidelines of the State Operations Manual (SOM), defines the criteria for use of psychopharmacologic medications, the rationale for tapering doses, the necessary documentation to explain medication use outside the guidelines, and the reasons a gradual dose reduction (GDR) that may be considered contraindicated. Although these guidelines generally emphasize the older adult resident, adverse consequences can occur in anyone at any age; therefore, these requirements apply to residents of all ages. The regulations present challenges for the palliative care team, long term care staff, and surveyors alike because medications appropriately prescribed for palliation of symptoms at the end of life may appear to violate the intent of the guidelines. The ultimate goal of the regulations and the accompanying interpretive guidelines are to assure that medication use maintains or improves the function or wellbeing of the patient. Note that the guidelines *do not* absolutely prohibit the use of any medication or class of medications. Prior to using medications and throughout the course of therapy however, the patient must be thoroughly assessed to ensure that medications are clinically indicated to treat a documented symptom or condition (this includes the use of "as needed" or "PRN" medications) and monitored for medication effectiveness and safety. The regulation pertaining to the appropriate use of medications is Tag F329 §483.25(l) Unnecessary Drugs.

F329. §483.25(l) Unnecessary Drugs
1. General. Each resident's drug regimen must be free from unnecessary drugs. An unnecessary drug is any drug when used in any of the following conditions:
      (i) In excessive dose (including duplicate therapy)
      (ii) For excessive duration
      (iii) Without adequate monitoring
      (iv) Without adequate indications for its use
      (v) In the presence of adverse consequences which indicate the dose should be reduced or discontinued
      (vi) Any combinations of the reasons above
2. Antipsychotic Drugs. Based on a comprehensive assessment of a resident, the facility must ensure that:
      (i) Residents who have not used antipsychotic drugs are not given these drugs unless antipsychotic drug therapy is necessary to treat a specific condition as diagnosed and documented in the clinical record; and
      (ii) Residents who use antipsychotic drugs receive gradual dose reductions, and behavioral interventions, unless clinically contraindicated, in an effort to discontinue these drugs.
In addition, follow the additional guidance in Appendix PP, Tag F329 for determination of unnecessary medications and guidance on managing patients with dementia.

Medication Management is a key concept in the regulations and includes the following sub-sets.
- Indications for use of medication (including initiation or continued use of antipsychotic medication). *Under this section, the need for end of life or palliative care is recognized.*
- Monitoring for efficacy and adverse consequences
- Dose (including duplicate therapy)
- Duration
- Tapering of a medication dose/gradual dose reduction for antipsychotic medications
- Prevention, identification, and response to adverse consequences

Indications for Use of Medication *(including initiation or continued use of an antipsychotic medication)*:
An evaluation of the resident helps to identify his/her needs, comorbid conditions, and prognosis to determine factors that are affecting signs, symptoms, and test results. This evaluation process is important when making initial medication/intervention selections and when deciding whether to modify or discontinue a current medication. Regarding "as needed" medications: evaluate and document the indication(s), specific circumstance(s) for use, and the desired frequency of administration. As part of the evaluation, gathering and analyzing information helps define clinical indications and provide baseline data for subsequent monitoring.

The evaluation clarifies whether:
- Other causes for the symptoms (including behavioral distress that could mimic a psychiatric disorder) have been ruled out
- The signs, symptoms, or related causes are persistent or clinically significant enough (e.g., causing functional decline) to warrant the initiation or continuation of medication therapy
- Non-pharmacological interventions are considered
- A particular medication is clinically indicated to manage the symptom or condition
- The intended or actual benefit is sufficient to justify the potential risk(s) or adverse consequences associated with the selected medication, dose, and duration.

The content and extent of evaluation may vary and may include, but are not limited to, the following:
- An appropriately detailed evaluation of mental, physical, psychosocial, and functional status, including comorbid conditions and pertinent psychiatric symptoms and diagnoses and a description of resident complaints, symptoms and signs (including the onset, frequency, scope, intensity, precipitating factors, and other important features)
- Each resident's goals and preferences
- Allergies to medications and foods and potential for medication interactions
- A history of prior and current medications and non-pharmacological interventions
- Recognition of the need for end-of-life or palliative care
- The refusal of care and treatment, including the basis for declining it, and the identification of pertinent alternatives.

The regulation addressing the use of antipsychotic medications identifies the process of tapering as a *"gradual dose reduction (GDR)"* and requires a GDR, *unless clinically contraindicated.*
- Within the first year in which a resident is admitted on an antipsychotic medication or after the facility has initiated an antipsychotic medication, the facility must attempt a GDR in two separate quarters (with at least one month between the attempts), *unless clinically contraindicated.*
- After the first year, a GDR must be attempted annually, *unless clinically contraindicated.*
- For an individual who is receiving antipsychotics to treat behavioral symptoms related to dementia the GDR may be clinically contraindicated if:
  - The resident's target symptoms returned or worsened after the most recent attempt at a GDR within the facility; and
  - The physician has documented the clinical rationale for why any additional attempted dose reduction at that time would be likely to impair the resident's function or increase distressed behavior.

For any individual who is receiving an antipsychotic medication to treat a psychiatric disorder *other than behavioral symptoms related to dementia* (for example, schizophrenia), the GDR may be considered contraindicated, if:
- The continued use is in accordance with relevant current standards of practice and the physician has documented the clinical rationale for why any attempted dose reduction would be likely to impair the resident's function or cause psychiatric instability by exacerbating an underlying psychiatric disorder;
  OR
- The resident's target symptoms returned or worsened after the most recent attempt at a GDR within the facility and the physician has documented the clinical rationale for why any additional attempted dose reduction at that time would be likely to impair the resident's function or cause psychiatric instability by exacerbating an underlying medical or psychiatric disorder.

Note that diagnoses alone do not warrant the use of an antipsychotic unless the following criteria are also met:
- The behavioral symptoms present a danger to the resident or others

AND one or both of the following:
- The symptoms are identified as being due to mania or psychosis (e.g., auditory, visual, or other hallucinations; delusions, paranoia or grandiosity)
- Behavioral interventions have been attempted and included in the plan of care, except in an emergency.

Inadequate Indications

Antipsychotic medications in persons with dementia *should not be used if the only indication is one or more of the following:*

- Wandering
- Impaired memory
- Nervousness
- Uncooperativeness (e.g. refusal of, or difficulty receiving care)
- Poor self-care
- Mild anxiety
- Sadness or crying alone that is not related to depression or other psychiatric disorders
- Restlessness
- Insomnia
- Fidgeting
- Inattention or indifference to surroundings

See current regulations for considerations specific to psychopharmacological medications other than antipsychotics (e.g. Sedatives/Hypnotics, Anxiolytics)

When antipsychotic medications are used without an adequate rationale, or for the sole purpose of limiting or controlling behavior of an unidentified cause, there is little chance that they will be effective, and they may cause complications such as movement disorders, falls, hip fractures, cerebrovascular adverse events and increased risk of death. If the resident expresses distress, staff should specifically describe the behavior (including potential underlying causes, onset, duration, intensity, precipitating events or environmental triggers, etc.) and related factors (such as appearance and alertness) in the medical record with enough detail of the actual situation to permit cause identification and individualized interventions. For example, noting that the resident is generally "violent," "agitated" or "aggressive" does not identify the specific behavior exhibited by the resident.

Of Particular Note in End-of-Life Care

There are specific rules regarding antipsychotic medications that may be problematic in end-of-life care because these medications are often used for symptoms not related to the medication's primary indications (e.g. haloperidol for nausea and vomiting, not a psychiatric diagnosis). The interpretive guidelines recognize the need to consider end-of-life care, but hospice and palliative care teams must be prepared to provide documentation of established protocols and standards of medication use if concerns arise. Proper assessment, documentation, monitoring and follow up that establish that medications are used in the patient's best interest will clear the way for quality pharmaceutical care at the end of life.

References

1. Center for Medicare & Medicaid Services (CMS). State Operations Manual. Publication 100-07. Baltimore, MD; CMS. Available at http://www.cms.gov/Regulations-and-Guidance/Guidance/Manuals/Internet-Only-Manuals-IOMs-Items/CMS1201984.html
2. Center for Medicare & Medicaid Services (CMS). State Operations Manual. Appendix PP – Guidance to Surveyors for Long Term Care Facilities. Rev 133. 02-06-2015. Available at http://www.cms.gov/Regulations-and-Guidance/Guidance/Manuals/Downloads/som107ap_pp_guidelines_ltcf.pdf

Compounded Medications in Hospice & Palliative Care

When the need arises for medications in dosage forms that are not commercially available, pharmacists may be able to prepare or "compound" those products.[1] However, not all compounded products are necessary or effective, and because of the time, labor, and materials involved, compounded products can be costly. The Food and Drug Administration (FDA) regulates the practice of pharmacy compounding with the support of the individual state Boards of Pharmacy, however, compounded drugs are not considered FDA-approved.

FDA Actions on Compounding Pharmacies

FDA continues proactive and for-cause inspections of compounding pharmacies. FDA plans to take enforcement actions as appropriate to protect the public health. Since 2012, when the fungal meningitis outbreak from contaminated injectable compounded medications began, FDA has been conducting inspections of compounding pharmacies in response to serious adverse event and quality issue reports and to identify pharmacies with deficient sterile compounding practices.[2] The current list of compounding facilities with recalls or other regulatory action in place is available on the FDA's website: www.fda.gov/Drugs/GuidanceComplianceRegulatoryInformation/

Historically, FDA provided pharmacy compounding guidelines in an attempt to regulate the pharmacy practice of compounding of medications. These guidelines arose from both a need to reign in some overzealous compounding pharmacies from manufacturing drug products and out of concerns for patient safety. FDA reports that compounded drug products are at risk for contamination and often may have potency less than the stated value, based on product assays. The pharmacy compounding guidelines also outlined basic information on reasonable compounding practice.[3]

In 2013, FDA announced the *withdrawal* of these guidelines, and began implementation of the new Compounding Quality Act. This new law distinguishes 2 categories of compounding facilities, registered outsourcing facilities (503B entities) and traditional compounding pharmacies (503A entities). A registered 503B outsourcing facility may compound sterile drugs and all drugs must be compounded in compliance with Current Good Manufacturing Practices (CGMP) or under the direct supervision of a licensed pharmacist in a registered facility. The outsourcing facility must also report specific information about the products that it compounds, including a list of all of the products it compounded during the previous 6 months, and information about the compounded products, such as the source of the ingredients used to compound. In addition, the outsourcing facility must meet other conditions described in the new law, including reporting adverse events and labeling its compounded products with certain information. Drugs produced by compounders that are not registered as outsourcing facilities must meet the conditions of section 503A of the law. For example, a compounded drug cannot be contaminated or made under insanitary conditions.[2]

For the traditional compounding pharmacies (503A), the FDA's current draft guidance includes components related to the individual compounder, safety and effectiveness of the compounded drug product, the source of bulk drug substances and excipients, and quantities and prescription requirements of compounded drug products. For example, drugs may be compounded for identified, individual patients based on a valid prescription order and the compounding of the drug is performed by a licensed pharmacist or physician. These compounded drug products must be based on an individual prescription order or in small quantities in anticipation of historically received orders when there is an established relationship between the pharmacist or physician and the patient. The compounded drug products cannot be essentially copies of commercially available drug products.[4]

Evaluating Use of Compounded Medications

In addition to any FDA guidance, the health care provider must consider pharmaceutics, bioavailability, and appropriateness of compounded drug products.

- Will the medication be adequately absorbed through the non-standard route?
- Is the added expense of compounding the product justified?
- Is there bioavailability data or other research supporting efficacy of the compound?
- Are all components of the compounded product necessary to its effectiveness?
- Does the compounding pharmacy maintain and promote safe compounding practices?

Topical preparations of medications that would usually be given orally or parenterally are frequently compounded when the patient has difficulty swallowing or refuses medications. Often these medications are combinations of anxiolytics, anti-emetics, neuroleptics, and anti-histamines. Multiple drug products are combined into one topical cream or gel to be applied for symptom management. Available published literature on systemic bioavailability of these topical-transdermal products demonstrates no measurable absorption suggesting no viable benefit.[5-7] Very high doses are compounded into concentrated topical gels in an attempt to ensure some level of bioavailability, resulting in potential skin irritation and considerable expense to the patient. Variability in skin type and surface area of application make absorption unpredictable and inconsistent, especially in cachectic and debilitated patients.

Compounding of rectal suppositories may be unnecessary and also adds additional expense. For example, ABHR [**A**tivan® (LORazepam), **B**enadryl®(diphenhydrAMINE), **H**aldol®‚ (haloperidol), **R**eglan®(metoclopramide)] suppositories are a common drug product used for nausea and vomiting in hospice patients. Often patients who receive these multi-drug preparations are already receiving one or more of the medications, resulting in duplication of therapy and potential toxicity and adverse effects. Additionally, the individual commercially available tablet or liquid drug formulations are generally effective when administered sublingually or per rectum without the time or expense required for compounding.

Still, some compounded products are very useful for symptom management. Pharmacists can add flavoring agents to make liquid medications more palatable. Compounded liquid formulations facilitate medication administration when the patient is unable swallow tablets.[1] Additionally, patient-specific dosing requirements may require higher or lower concentrations than are commercially available as oral liquid formulations. For example, magic mouthwash (Maalox®, Benadryl®, Lidocaine®) is used as an oral rinse for painful stomatitis. ChlorproMAZINE may be compounded into an oral concentrate (100 mg/mL) and used sublingually for management of agitation, hiccups, or nausea and vomiting. Medications, such as opioids, may be compounded into liquid concentrations higher than the commercially available product for sublingual use when volume is a factor.

When considering the use of compounded medications:

- Determine if all commercially available drugs, dosages, and routes have failed or are inappropriate.
- Request evidence-based, supportive literature including bioavailability data, if available.
- Always request written information on formulations including ingredients, dosages, beyond-use (expiration) dates, potential side effects, and rationale or indication for use.

References

1. McNulty JP, Muller G. Compounded drugs of value in outpatient hospice and palliative care. *Int J Pharm Compd.* 2014;18(3):190-200.
2. U.S. Food & Drug Administration (FDA). Guidance, Compliance & Regulatory Information. FDA implementation of the Compounding Quality Act. January 13, 2014. Available at http://www.fda.gov/Drugs/GuidanceComplianceRegulatoryInformation/PharmacyCompounding/ucm375804.htm. Accessed January 24, 2014.
3. U.S. Food & Drug Administration (FDA). Office of Regulatory Affairs. Compliance Policy Guide on Chapter 4 Human Drugs. Sec. 460.200 Pharmacy Compounding (withdrawn December 4, 2013). May 29, 2002.

4. U.S. Food & Drug Administration (FDA). Pharmacy compounding of human drug products under section 503A of the Federal Food, Drug, and Cosmetic Act (draft guidance). December 2013. Available at http://www.fda.gov/downloads/Drugs/GuidanceComplianceRegulatoryInformation/Guidances/UCM3770 52.pdf. Accessed January 24, 2014.

5. Fletcher DS, Coyne PJ, Dodson PW, et al. Randomized controlled trial of the effectiveness of topical "ABH Gel" (Ativan®, Benadryl®, Haldol®) vs placebo in cancer patients with nausea. *J Pain Symptom Manage*. 2014;48(5): 797-803.

6. Weiland AM, Protus BM, Kimbrel JM, Grauer PA, Hirsh J. Chlorpromazine bioavailability from a topical gel formulation in volunteers. *J Support Oncol*. 2013;11(3):144-148.

7. Sylvester RK, Schauer C, Thomas J, et al. Evaluation of methadone absorption after topical administration to hospice patients. *J Pain Symptom Manage*. 2011;41(5):828-835.

Medical Abbreviations

Abbreviations, symbols, and dose designations are frequently used as shorthand in healthcare settings. Unfortunately, lack of standardization and risk of misinterpretation can lead to medication errors and patient harm. Error-prone abbreviations should never be used when communicating medical information whether by verbal, handwritten, computer-generated labels, medication administration records, or computer order entry screens. A complete list of error-prone abbreviations is freely available from the Institute for Safe Medication Practices (ismp.org). The official "Do Not Use" list following The Joint Commission's National Patient Safety Goals, now integrated into the Information Management standards (IM.02.02.01) is included below in Table 1.[1,2]

If abbreviations are to be used within any healthcare organization, an approach to standardizing abbreviations, acronyms, and symbols should be developed. A list of standardized abbreviations developed by the organization using a published reference source is acceptable. The organization is responsible for eliminating any ambiguity related to the use of multiple abbreviations, symbols, or acronyms for the same term. An organizational list should not include any abbreviation or symbol from the error-prone or unacceptable list. A sample list is provided in Table 3.[3] Additionally, a list of "look-alike, sound-alike" confused drug names and a "do not crush or chew" list are included in the Appendix of this book.

Table 1. The Joint Commission Official "Do Not Use" List*[1,2]

Do Not Use	Potential Problem	Use Instead
U (unit)	Mistaken for "0" (zero) the number "4" (four) or "cc"	"unit"
IU (International Unit)	Mistaken for IV (intravenous) or the number 10 (ten)	"International Unit"
Q.D., QD, q.d., qd (daily) Q.O.D., QOD, q.o.d. qod (every other day)	Mistaken for each other Period after the Q mistaken for "I" and the "O" mistaken for "I"	"daily" "every other day"
Trailing zero (X.0 mg)* Leading zero missing (0.Xmg)	Decimal point missed	X mg 0.X mg
MS, MSO$_4$, MgSO$_4$	Can mean morphine sulfate or magnesium sulfate Confused for one another	"morphine sulfate" "magnesium sulfate"

*Applies to all orders and all medication-related documentation that is handwritten (including free-test computer entry) or on pre-printed forms. **Exception:** A "trailing zero" may be used only where required to demonstrate the level of precision of the value being reported, such as for laboratory results, imaging studies that report size of lesions, or catheter/tube sizes. It may not be used in medication orders or other medication-related documentation.

Table 2. Additional Error-Prone Abbreviations, Acronyms and Symbols

Do Not Use	Potential Problem	Use Instead
> (greater than) < (less than)	Misinterpreted as the number "7" or the letter "L" Confused for one another	"greater than" "less than"
Abbreviations for drug names	Misinterpreted due to similar abbreviations for multiple drugs	Full drug names
Apothecary units	Unfamiliar to many practitioners Confused with metric units	metric units
@	Mistaken for the number "2" (two)	"at"
cc	Mistaken for U (units) when poorly written	"mL" or "milliliters"
μg	Mistaken for mg (milligrams) resulting in 1,000-fold overdose	"mcg" or "micrograms"

Table 3. Drug Administration Abbreviations

Abbreviation	Definition	Abbreviation	Definition
AC	before meals	PO	by mouth
Amp	ampule	PR	per rectum
ATC	around-the-clock	PRN	as needed
BID	twice daily	Q	every
BTP	breakthrough pain	Qam	every morning
Cap	capsule	QID	four times a day
Conc	concentration	Qpm	every night
CIVI	continuous intravenous infusion	q 2 h	every two hours
CSCI	continuous subcutaneous infusion	q 3 h	every three hours
D/C	discontinue	q 4 h	every four hours
EC	enteric coated tablet	q 6 h	every six hours
El	elixir	q 8 h	every eight hours
GTT	drop	q 12 h	every twelve hours
HS	at bedtime	SC or SQ	subcutaneous
IM	intramuscular	SL	sublingual
INH	inhalation	Sol	solution
INJ	injection	SR	sustained release
IT	intrathecal	STAT	immediately
IV	intravenous	Supp	suppository
Liq	liquid	Susp	suspension
Loz	lozenge	Syr	syrup
NEB	nebulizer	t ½	terminal half-life
NPO	nothing by mouth	Tab	tablet
NR	normal release	TID	three times a day
OD	overdose	Top	topical
PC	after meals	Vag	vaginal

References

1. Institute for Safe Medication Practices (ISMP). ISMP's list of error-prone abbreviations, symbols and dose designations. ISMP 2013. Available at http://ismp.org/Tools/errorproneabbreviations.pdf Accessed January 24, 2014.
2. The Joint Commission (TJC). Facts about the official "Do Not Use" list. TJC 2013. Available at http://www.jointcommission.org/standards_information/npsgs.aspx Accessed January 24, 2014.
3. The Joint Commission (TJC). Standards FAQ details: acceptable abbreviations list. [Internet]. November 24, 2008. Available at http://www.jointcommission.org/standards_information/jcfaqdetails.aspx Accessed January 24, 2014.

Section II: GEMS

Guidelines for Effective Management of Symptoms

- Agitation & Delirium
- Anorexia & Cachexia
- Anxiety
- Ascites & Edema
- Bowel Obstruction
- Constipation
- Cough
- Depression
- Diarrhea
- Dysphagia
- Dyspnea
- Fatigue
- Fever
- Hiccups
- Infections
- Insomnia
- Muscle Spasms
- Nausea & Vomiting
- Pain
- Pruritus
- Secretions
- Seizures
- Xerostomia

Agitation and Delirium

Introduction and Background[1-4]
- Delirium is a disturbance in consciousness with reduced ability to focus, sustain, or shift attention.
- Delirium typically develops abruptly, over several hours to days, and has a fluctuating course.
- The etiology of delirium is usually multi-factorial. Although patients with dementia can develop delirium, pre-existing dementia does not account for changes in cognition and behavior.
- Treatment of delirium should focus on removing the causative factor, if possible.
- Patients may present with agitation without delirium (i.e., without disturbances of consciousness).
- Agitation can consist of excessive movement or verbal activity, irritability, uncooperativeness, threatening gestures, and, possibly, assault.

Prevalence[1,2]
- The incidence of delirium ranges from 28-88% depending on the stage of the terminal illness. Delirium is more prevalent at the end of life; 32-45% of patients develop delirium in the week prior to death.
- Agitation is a component in delirium in up 46% of patients.
- An etiology is discovered in fewer than 50% of terminally ill patients with delirium.

Causes [1, 3-8]
- Multiple causes of delirium are likely to coexist affecting the metabolic environment of the whole brain.
- Neurotransmitter imbalances in acetylcholine, dopamine, and gamma aminobutyric acid (GABA) can trigger delirium, especially drug-induced delirium.
- Patients with multiple risk factors (Table 1) are more likely to develop delirium. Awareness of risk factors may allow prevention of delirium or faster recognition of signs and symptoms.

Table 1. Risk Factors

• Advanced age	• Hearing loss	• Impending death
• Limitations on physical mobility	• Polypharmacy	• Reduced vision
• Severity of illness	• Social isolation	• Family conflict and stress
• Pre-existing cognitive impairment	• Renal failure	• Liver failure

Table 2. Potential Causes of Agitation or Delirium

Cause	Examples
Cerebral disease	Cancer – primary tumors or metastases, stroke, whole brain radiation
Discomfort	Constipation, fecal impaction, sleep deprivation, uncontrolled pain, urinary retention
Environmental change	Excessive temperatures or noise, moving place of residence, physical restraints
Infections	Pneumonia, sepsis, urinary tract infections
Metabolic disturbances	Alterations in blood glucose, dehydration, hyperammonemia, hypercalcemia, hypernatremia, hyponatremia
Organ failure	Liver (altered metabolism), kidneys (altered clearance), lungs (hypoxia)
Psychosocial	Anxiety, emotional or spiritual distress, fear, vision or hearing impairment
Substance withdrawal	Alcohol, benzodiazepines, illicit drugs, medications (Table 3), nicotine

Table 3. Medications That May Cause Agitation or Delirium

Class	Comments
Anticholinergics	Effects on cognition; increases risk of urinary retention & constipation; blurred vision. See Appendix for *Medications Associated with Anticholinergic Side Effects.*
Antipsychotics	Due to akathisia, restlessness, drug interactions with other psychoactive medications.
Benzodiazepines	Prolonged half-life, especially in elderly patients; increased confusion
Chemotherapy	Neurotoxic side effects (e.g. methotrexate, cytarabine, ifosfamide, interleukin-2)
Corticosteroids	Dose-related psychiatric adverse effects, agitation, mood changes
Dopamine agonists	Excessive levels of dopamine can cause agitation, confusion, dyskinesia, hallucinations
Opioids	Accumulation of neurotoxic metabolites, especially in patients with renal insufficiency; dose-related effects in opioid naïve patients

Clinical Characteristics [1-3, 6,9]

- General symptoms of delirium include: alterations in sleep-wake cycles, memory deficits (short and long term), delusions, hallucinations, incoherent speech, and emotional lability.
- Symptoms can continue more than 3 months after onset in up to 45% of patients.
- Delirium is classified into 3 sub-types: hypoactive, hyperactive, and mixed (Table 4).

Table 4. Types of Delirium

Type	Characteristics
Hypoactive	• Withdrawn, flat affect, lethargy, sedation, and reduced awareness of surroundings • Can be mistaken for depression • Difficult to differentiate from sedation due to opioids or the dying process • Most common sub-type in palliative care • May be more resistant to pharmacological treatment
Hyperactive	• Restlessness, agitation, emotional instability, hallucinations, and delusions • Patients may have fast or loud speech, anger, wandering, and combative behaviors • Associated with drug withdrawal, drug intoxication, or medication side effects
Mixed	• Alternating features of both hyperactive and hypoactive delirium • Can be difficult to diagnose due to the changing presentation of the patient

- Delirium is often underdiagnosed; base diagnosis on clinical assessment.
- The Confusion Assessment Method (CAM) diagnosis algorithm is one tool that may help diagnose delirium quickly and accurately. CAM examines 4 key features of delirium. Diagnosis of delirium by CAM requires the presence of features 1 and 2, and either 3 or 4:
    1. Acute change in mental status and fluctuations in status
    2. Inattention
    3. Disorganized thinking
    4. Abnormal level of consciousness

Non-Pharmacological Treatment [2,3,6,10,12]

- Provide caregiver education to minimize distress
- Avoid room and bed changes; reorient the patient frequently
- Place familiar objects in the room (family photographs, favorite blankets)
- Minimize indwelling catheters, intravenous lines, and physical restraints
- Provide a clock and calendar that are visible to the patient
- Adopt healthy sleep-wake cycles; minimize noise, and create a calm environment
- Promote staff continuity
- Ensure eyeglasses and hearing aids are available, if required
- Monitor bowel and bladder functioning

Pharmacotherapy [1,2,5,7,11-12]

- There are no approved medications for the treatment of delirium. There is little data evaluating the management of delirium, and few trials to compare regimens in controlled studies.
- Review medications for potential causative agents; minimize polypharmacy.
- Antipsychotics are commonly used in all care settings; haloperidol is most commonly used.
- Atypical antipsychotics have not been shown to be superior to haloperidol in clinical trials, but may have a lower incidence of extrapyramidal side effects (EPS) when higher doses are required.
- Avoid polypharmacy. Co-administration of two or more antipsychotics does not generally improve clinical response and increases the risk for adverse effects.
- Atypical antipsychotics (e.g., quetiapine) are the drugs of choice in patients with Parkinson's disease, Lewy Body Dementia, or patients with a history of EPS from conventional antipsychotics.
- Chlorpromazine can be used in place of haloperidol for terminally ill patients with severe agitation due to its sedating properties.
- Haloperidol and chlorpromazine have been shown to be equally effective at managing both hypoactive and hyperactive delirium. However, one study showed poorer responses when olanzapine is used for

hypoactive delirium. Other studies have shown that risperidone and aripiprazole may have better results when used in hypoactive delirium; consider as second line agents after haloperidol.

- Impaired cholinergic function has been hypothesized to be a cause of delirium. However, there is no evidence that cholinesterase inhibitors (donepezil, rivastigmine, galantamine) are effective in treating delirium.
- Benzodiazepines are associated with delirium, but are the drug of choice for delirium due to alcohol or benzodiazepine withdrawal.
- Agitation and delirium due to dehydration may respond to intravenous or subcutaneous hydration. Reserve this intervention for higher functioning patients with minimal fluid retention.
- Palliative sedation may be considered to manage irreversible and terminal agitation or delirium (refractory terminal restlessness). See also *Palliative Sedation* chapter.
  - o Only implement when consensus exists among patient, family, and hospice staff about the appropriateness of therapy.
  - o Benzodiazepines (e.g. midazolam, lorazepam) or barbiturates are generally used for palliative sedation, either alone, or in combination with antipsychotics.

Clinical Pearls [2,6,7]

- Agitation in patients with cognitive impairment or dementia is frequently due to the patient's inability to communicate an unmet need (pain, hunger, toileting). Always assess these basic components of patient care prior using any chemical (e.g. antipsychotics, benzodiazepines, sedatives) or physical restraints.
- Determining the etiology of delirium in palliative care may not always be feasible (e.g., imaging studies to rule out brain metastases, blood work to identify metabolic abnormalities). Clinicians should take an individualized approach to such testing, depending on the goals of care.
- Plan of care may depend on whether the potential etiology of delirium is reversible or irreversible. For example, agitation/delirium caused by pain, constipation, hypoxia, infection, dehydration, or medications may be reversible. However, agitation/delirium caused by sepsis or organ failure is irreversible, in most cases.
- If agitation or delirium is opioid-induced, dose reduction in an attempt to reverse the delirium may cause the return of unacceptable levels of pain. Consider opioid rotation in this case.
- Depending on patient and family goals of care, treatment of delirium may be withheld in patients who have a lethargic, somnolent delirium, or are having comforting hallucinations.
- *In June 2008, the FDA notified healthcare professionals that both conventional and atypical antipsychotics are associated with an increased risk of mortality in elderly patients treated for dementia-related psychosis. No antipsychotics have FDA-approved indications for treatment of dementia-related psychosis or behavioral and psychological symptoms of dementia.*

Pharmacological Management of Agitation & Delirium

Generic Name (Trade Name)	Adult Starting Dose	Routes	Common Strengths and Formulations	Comments
Antipsychotics: *Conventional*				
Chlorpromazine (Thorazine®)	10-25 mg Q8h PRN or ATC	PO SL PR IM	**Tablets:** 10 mg, 25 mg, 50 mg, 100 mg, 200 mg **Injection:** 25 mg/mL	• More sedating than haloperidol. • Use with caution in ambulatory patients due to risk of orthostatic hypotension. • Concentrated oral solution (100mg/mL) may be compounded for sublingual administration. • Associated with prolongation of QT interval. • Avoid use in patients with Lewy Body Dementia or Parkinson's disease.

Continued

Generic Name (Trade Name)	Adult Starting Dose	Routes	Common Strengths and Formulations	Comments
Antipsychotics: *Conventional, continued*				
Haloperidol (Haldol®)	0.5-1 mg BID PRN or ATC	PO SL PR SC IV IM	**Tablets:** 0.5 mg, 1 mg, 2 mg, 5 mg, 10 mg, 20 mg **Oral solution:** 2 mg/mL **Injection:** 5 mg/mL	• Oral solution and tablets can be given PO, SL, or PR. • Low doses have few side effects, but monitor for EPS, including akathisia (which can mimic agitation); abnormal movements. • Associated with prolongation of QT interval. • Avoid use in patients with Lewy Body Dementia or Parkinson's disease.
Antipsychotics: *Atypical*				
Aripiprazole (Abilify®)	5-10 mg Daily	PO	**Tablets:** 2 mg, 5 mg, 10 mg, 15 mg, 20 mg, 30 mg **Oral solution:** 1 mg/mL **Oral disintegrating tablets:** 10 mg, 15 mg	• Expensive with no generic equivalents. • Generally, no benefit over haloperidol or chlorpromazine. • Delayed onset of action and long half-life make aripiprazole less appropriate for elderly patients.
Olanzapine (Zyprexa®)	2.5-5 mg Daily	PO	**Tablets:** 2.5 mg, 5 mg, 7.5 mg, 10 mg, 15 mg, 20 mg **Oral disintegrating tablets:** 5 mg, 10 mg, 15 mg, 20 mg	• Generally, no benefit over haloperidol or chlorpromazine. • Associated with hyperglycemia and metabolic syndrome. • Monitor for EPS, including akathisia, or other abnormal movements. • Useful if unable to tolerate conventional antipsychotics.
Quetiapine (Seroquel®)	25 mg BID	PO	**Tablets:** 25 mg, 50 mg, 100 mg, 200 mg, 300 mg, 400 mg **ER tablets:** 50 mg, 150 mg, 200 mg, 300 mg, 400 mg	• ER tablets are expensive. • Antipsychotic of choice in patients with Parkinson's disease or Lewy Body Dementia. • May increase blood glucose levels. • Most sedating of the atypical antipsychotics.
Risperidone (Risperdal®)	0.25 mg-0.5 mg BID	PO	**Tablets:** 0.25 mg, 0.5 mg, 1 mg, 2 mg, 3 mg, 4 mg **Oral solution:** 1 mg/mL **Oral disintegrating tablets:** 0.25 mg, 0.5 mg, 1 mg, 2 mg, 3 mg, 4 mg	• Generally, no benefit over haloperidol or chlorpromazine. • Can increase blood glucose levels. • Orally disintegrating tablets more expensive than conventional tablets. • Oral solution may be mixed with coffee, milk, orange juice, water; incompatible with tea or cola.
Ziprasidone (Geodon®)	20 mg BID	PO	**Capsules:** 20 mg, 40 mg, 60 mg, 80 mg	• Generally, no benefit over haloperidol or chlorpromazine. • Administer capsules with food to reduce GI upset and nausea. • May increase blood glucose levels.

See Drug Dosing for Liver and Renal Disease for additional drug information.

References

1. LeGrand S. Delirium in palliative medicine: a review. *J Pain Symptom Manage*. 2012;44(4):583-94.
2. Breitbart W, Alici Y. Agitation and delirium at the end of life. *JAMA*. 2008;300(24):2898-2910.
3. Bush S, Bruera E. The assessment and management of delirium in cancer patients. *The Oncologist*. 2009;14:1039-49.
4. Zeller S, Rhoades R. Systematic reviews of assessment measures and pharmacologic treatments for agitation. *Clin Ther*. 2010;32:403-25.
5. Quijada E, Billings JA. Pharmacologic management of delirium; update on newer agents, 2nd edition. Fast Facts and Concepts #060. Available at: http://www.eperc.mcw.edu/EPERC/FastFactsIndex/ff_060.htm. April 2009. Accessed: January 3, 2014.
6. Marcantonio ER. In the clinic. Delirium. *Ann Intern Med*. 201;154(11):ITC6-2-ITC6-15.
7. Shuster JL. Confusion, agitation, and delirium at the end of life. *J Palliat Med*. 1998;1:177-186.
8. Alagiakrishnan K, Wiens C. An approach to drug-induced delirium in the elderly. *Postgrad Med J*. 2004;80(945):388-393.
9. Close J, Long C. Delirium. Opportunity for comfort in palliative care. *J Hosp Palliat Nurs*. 2012;14(6):386-96.
10. Breitbart W, Alici Y. Evidence-based treatment of delirium in patients with cancer. *J Clin Oncol*. 2012;30(11):1206-14.
11. Olsen M, Swetz K, Mueller P. Ethical decision making with end-of-life care: Palliative sedation and withholding or withdrawing life-sustaining treatments. *Mayo Clin Proc*. 2010;85(10):949-954.
12. Moyer D. Terminal delirium in geriatric patients with cancer at end of life. *Am J Hosp Palliat Med*. 2011;28(1)44-51.

Treatment Algorithm for Agitation & Delirium

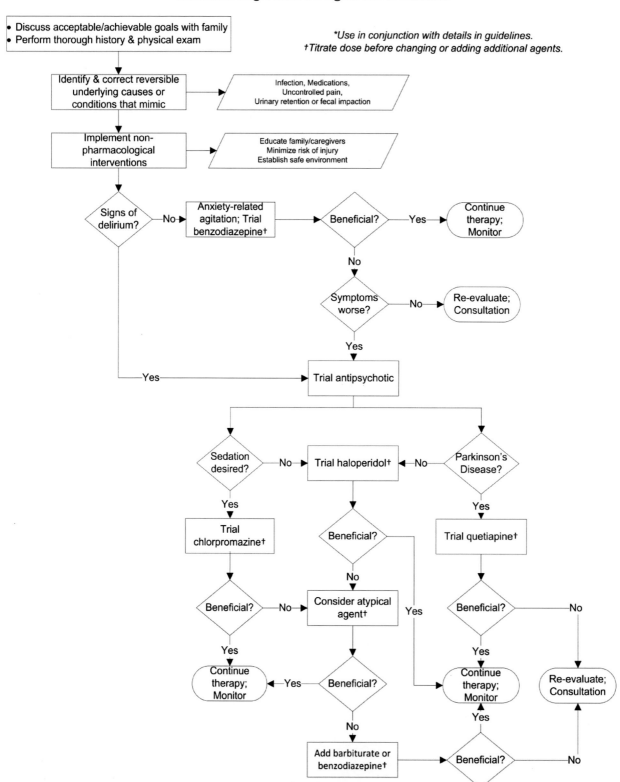

Anorexia and Cachexia

Introduction and Background[1-2]

- Anorexia is reduced appetite or loss of appetite, generally based on patient report.
- Cachexia is more complex and multifactorial, characterized by severe loss of body weight, muscle and fat loss, and increased protein catabolism due to an underlying disease.
- A third condition, sarcopenia, refers to loss of muscle mass and muscle strength. Age-related sarcopenia is seen in older patients. Cachexia and sarcopenia can overlap and may be impossible to distinguish.
- Anorexia-cachexia syndrome can lead to weakness, debilitation, compromised immune function, and decreased morale.
- Weight loss and lack of appetite can be very distressing to family members who often link weight and a healthy appetite with well-being and overall quality of caregiving.
- The goals for managing anorexia and cachexia are to improve the patient's quality of life as much as possible, to improve family and patient understanding of the symptoms and treatment limitations, relieving nausea and other identifiable causes.

Prevalence[3,4]

- Anorexia and cachexia are experienced by most terminally ill patients and are part of the dying process.
- Although commonly associated with late stage cancer, reported prevalence of anorexia ranges from 25% to over 90% in patients receiving palliative and end of life care with heart disease, kidney disease, AIDS, and COPD.

Causes[5,6]

- Anorexia-cachexia syndrome is a complex process occurring in late stage chronic inflammatory diseases and cancer.
- Reversible causes of anorexia should be identified and treated, if possible.

Table 1. Causes of Anorexia and Cachexia

Causes	Examples
Dietary	Altered taste, food presentation, odors
Disease process	Organ failure, liver metastases, slow gastric emptying rate, gastroparesis
Gastrointestinal	Gastritis, nausea & vomiting, constipation, bowel obstruction, decreased peristalsis
Iatrogenic	Chemotherapy, radiation, medications, opioid-induced constipation
Oral	Mucositis, dry mouth, dysphagia
Unrelieved symptoms	Pain
Psychosocial	Anxiety, depression

Clinical Characteristics[2,5,7,8]

- Anorexia-cachexia is a multifactorial catabolic process characterized by an increase in skeletal muscle and adipose tissue breakdown and decreased protein rebuilding process.
- Cachexia induced from chronic disease is independent of starvation and appropriate nutrition cannot reverse cachexia.

In patients diagnosed with cancer:

- Malnutrition in cancer patients is not the only factor responsible for weight loss; nutritional correction or supplementation is unlikely to reverse this condition.
- In cancer-associated *anorexia*, the two most important mediating factors are:
    o Reduced intake due to alterations in perception of food, nausea, vomiting, pain, and dysphagia.
    o Physiologic and metabolic alteration induced by tumors and tumor burden.
- In cancer-associated *cachexia*, basal metabolism is increased by as much as 50% leading to increased energy expenditure, resulting in fatigue, apathy, and depression.

Non-Pharmacological Treatment[6]

- Provide family education:
  - Patients generally lose their appetite and reduce food intake long before they reach the last hours of their lives.
  - Patients can live comfortably for a long time on very little food and water.
  - Wasting of the body is not a reflection of poor or inadequate caretaking or nutrition.
  - Patients are not starving to death. Forced feeding usually does not prolong life. Forced feeding can cause discomfort, nausea, vomiting as gut function diminishes.
  - Cachexia is a normal part of the end-of-life process.
- Regarding foods and meal planning, consider the following:
  - Involve the patient in meal planning.
  - Offer small portions of the patient's favorite foods and allow the patient to eat at their own rate and until they are satisfied.
  - Avoid foods with a strong odor, unless the patient requests them.
  - Offer easy-to-swallow foods, such as pudding, gelatin, etc.
  - Keep the patient company while he or she eats.
  - Serve meals in a room other than where the patient sleeps.
  - Consult a dietician experienced in end-of-life care to assist with family acceptance or for a second opinion if symptoms do not align well with disease progression, or if considering enteral or parenteral nutrition.
- Remember to enlist the support of the hospice social worker and spiritual care counselors:
  - Help the family find alternatives to sharing time together other than eating (e.g. listening to music, looking at pictures, reading aloud).
  - Suggest alternatives for family members as they may feel a strong obligation to feed the patient. For example, caregivers can alleviate symptoms and nurture their instinct to "do something" by moistening the patient's lips and mouth with a sponge.
  - Assess cultural and religious issues that may interfere with understanding and acceptance of the patient's lack of appetite and weight loss.
  - Consider enlisting pastoral care from hospice or patient's own belief system.

Pharmacotherapy[4-6,8-11]

- Medications are often prescribed in end-of-life care in an attempt to improve the patient's appetite, improve sense of well-being, and promote weight gain.
- All medications to improve appetite have limited benefit and are associated with adverse effects. Evaluate risk versus benefits of medications with patient and family as part of the goals of care discussion.
- Medications should only be considered as adjuncts to non-pharmacological approaches. Discontinue medication if no benefit is reported within 2 to 6 weeks of treatment.
- Weight gain is typically adipose tissue and not an increase in protein utilization or muscle mass.
- American Geriatrics Society recommends avoidance of megestrol acetate (Megace) use in elderly patients due to the increased risk of thromboembolic events and death while providing minimal effects on weight.
- Corticosteroids are used to increase appetite, improve mood and fatigue, reduce nausea, and manage inflammatory pain. Dexamethasone is most commonly used, but other corticosteroids, such as prednisone or methylprednisolone are also effective.

Clinical Pearls[5,8,12,13]

- If patient has feeling of fullness, early satiety, or "squashed stomach syndrome", metoclopramide (Reglan) may be beneficial to increase gastric motility and the gastric emptying rate.

- Practitioners should be prepared to discuss the benefits and burdens of enteral (tube) feeding with patients and families. The effectiveness of enteral or parenteral feedings in patients with anorexia-cachexia syndrome has not been supported in clinical literature.
- Thalidomide (Thalomid) 100–200 mg daily has limited evidence demonstrating weight increases in patients with cachexia but no improvement of anorexia over placebo. Thalidomide is extremely expensive (approximately $10,000/month) and is highly teratogenic. There is insufficient evidence to recommend use of thalidomide for anorexia-cachexia syndrome.
- Studies show anabolic agents such as oxandrolone (Oxandrin) may increase muscle mass in patients with cirrhosis, COPD, AIDS and neuromuscular disorders but are associated with edema, hypercalcemia, glucose intolerance, and prostatic hyperplasia. Oxandrolone is an androgen; avoid use in patients with breast or prostate cancer or history of hypercalcemia.
- Mirtazapine (Remeron) as an appetite stimulant may work well for some patients, especially those with comorbid depression and/or insomnia.

Pharmacological Management of Anorexia

Generic Name (Trade Name)	Adult Starting Dose	Routes	Common Strengths and Formulations	Comments
Antidepressants				
Mirtazapine (Remeron®)	7.5 mg QHS	PO	**Tablets**: 7.5 mg, 15 mg, 30 mg, 45 mg **Oral disintegrating tablets**: 15 mg, 30 mg, 45 mg	• Useful in patients with comorbid depression or insomnia; titrate dose. • Associated with dry mouth and constipation.
Corticosteroids				
Dexamethasone (Decadron®)	2 mg QAM	PO	**Tablets**: 1 mg, 2 mg, 4mg, 6 mg **Oral solution**: 1 mg/mL	• Useful in patients that might benefit from corticosteroid for pain or dyspnea; titrate dose.
Prednisone (Deltasone®)	10mg QAM	PO	**Tablets**: 5 mg, 10 mg, 20 mg **Oral solution**: 5 mg/mL	• Useful in patients that might benefit from corticosteroid for pain or dyspnea; titrate dose.
Hormonal Agents				
Megestrol (Megace®)	400mg Daily	PO	**Tablets**: 20 mg, 40 mg **Oral suspension**: 40 mg/mL, (ES) 125 mg/mL	• May take up to 8 weeks to see benefit. • Risk of thromboembolism in elderly and those with limited mobility. • ES suspension is expensive.
Oxandrolone (Oxandrin®)	5mg BID	PO	**Tablets**: 2.5 mg, 10 mg	• C-III controlled substance. • Testosterone derivative. • Contraindicated in breast or prostate cancer, or hypercalcemia.
Cannabinoids				
Dronabinol (Marinol®)	2.5mg BID	PO	**Capsules**: 2.5 mg, 5 mg, 10 mg	• C-III controlled substance. • May be less effective than megestrol. • May cause intolerable CNS side effects. • Expensive.

Continued

Generic Name (Trade Name)	Adult Starting Dose	Routes	Common Strengths and Formulations	Comments
Other				
Cyproheptadine (Periactin®)	4mg TID	PO	**Tablets:** 4 mg **Oral solution:** 2 mg/5 mL	• Limited data on effectiveness. • Associated with sedation and depression.

See Drug Dosing for Liver and Renal Disease for additional drug information.

References

1. Muscaritoli M, Anker S, Argiles J, Aversa Z, et al. Consensus definition of sarcopenia, cachexia and pre-cachexia: joint document elaborated by special interest groups (SIG) "cachexia-anorexia in chronic wasting diseases" and "nutrition in geriatrics." *Clin Nutr.* 2010;29:154-159.
2. Fearon K, Strasser F, Anker SD, et al. Definition and classification of cancer cachexia: an international consensus. *Lancet Oncol.* 2011;12:489-495.
3. Solano J, Gomes B, Higginson I. Comparison of symptom prevalence in far advanced cancer, AIDS, heart disease, chronic obstructive pulmonary disease, and renal disease. *J Pain Symptom Manage.* 2006;31(1):58-69.
4. Salacz M. Megestrol Acetate for Cancer Anorexia/Cachexia. Fast Facts and Concepts. October 2003; 100. Available at: https://www.capc.org/fast-facts/100-megestrol-acetate-cancer-anorexiacachexia/
5. Maccio A, Madeddu C, Mantovani G. Current pharmacotherapy options for cancer anorexia and cachexia. *Expert Opin Pharmacother.* 2012;13(17):2453-2472.
6. Ross DD, Alexander CS. Management of Common Symptoms in Terminally Ill Patients: Part I. Fatigue, Anorexia, Cachexia, Nausea and Vomiting. *Am Fam Physician.* 2001;64:807-814
7. Giacosa A, Frascio F, Sukkar S, Roncella S. Food intake and body composition in cancer cachexia. *Nutrition.* 1996;12:S20-S23
8. Suzuki H, Asakawa A, Amitani H, Nakamura N, Inui A. Cancer cachexia: pathophysiology and management. *J Gastroenterol.* 2013;48:574-594.
9. Campanelli C, American Geriatrics Society 2012 Beers Criteria Update Expert Panel. American Geriatrics Society Updated Beers Criteria for potentially inappropriate medication use in older adults. J Am Geriatr Soc 2012;60(4):616-631.
10. Ruiz Garcia V, López-Briz E, Carbonell Sanchis R, et al. Megestrol Acetate for Treatment of Anorexia-Cachexia Syndrome. *Cochrane Database Syst Rev.* 2013, Issue 3.1-193.
11. Shih A, Jackson KC III. Role of Corticosteroids in Palliative Care. *J Pain Palliat Care Pharmacother.* 2007; 21(4): 69-76.
12. Riechelmann RP, Burman D, Tannock IF, Rodin G, Zimmermann C. Phase II trial of mirtazapine for cancer-related cachexia and anorexia. *Am J Hosp Palliat Med.* 2010;27:106-110.
13. Prommer EE. Palliative Oncology: Thalidomide. *Am J Hosp Palliat Med.* 2010; 27(3):198-204.

Treatment Algorithm for Anorexia

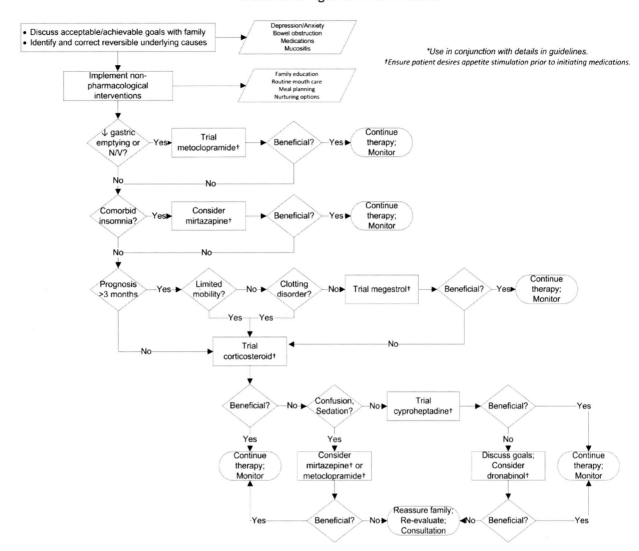

*Use in conjunction with details in guidelines.
†Ensure patient desires appetite stimulation prior to initiating medications.

Anxiety

Introduction and Background[1]
- Anxiety is characterized by apprehensive anticipation of future danger or misfortune accompanied by psychological symptoms such as worrying, vigilance and rumination as well as by physical feelings such as tension, jitters, palpitations, dyspnea, chest discomfort, or abdominal distress.
- Anxiety is a mood state associated with preparation for possible, upcoming negative events.
- Transient feelings of anxiety guide us to avoid situations that might lead to risk or harm and are adaptive and healthy ("fight or flight").
- Much like pain, patients experience significant distress and suffering when anxiety loses this adaptive or "signal" function, persists despite the absence of an anxiety-provoking stimulus, or becomes excessive.
- Anxiety is closely related to fear, but fear has an identified cause or source of worry (e.g., fear of death). The patient may not be able to attribute to his or her anxiety to a specific fearful stimulus.

Prevalence[2,3]
- The prevalence of clinically significant anxiety in patients receiving palliative care is not well studied, but has been reported to be 21-23%. Patient and family stress and anxiety tends to increase as patients approach the dying process.
- Anxiety disorders are the most prevalent class of mental disorders (6%) overall; anxiety is a common cause of distress at life's end.

Causes[3,4]
- Many medical conditions can precipitate anxiety (Table 1).
- Review patient medical history for alcohol and other substance abuse disorders. Adverse effects of medications may also mimic anxiety or contribute to anxiety symptoms such as akathisia, tachycardia, tremor, dizziness.
- Post-traumatic stress disorder (PTSD) may re-emerge as death approaches, even after decades of latency, with anxiety, avoidance behaviors, increased arousal, and vivid re-experiencing of traumatic events (as intrusive thoughts, daydreams, or nightmares).

Table 1. Potential Causes of Anxiety

Category	Conditions
Exacerbation of medical conditions	adjustment disorders, panic disorder, generalized anxiety disorder, obsessive compulsive disorder, PTSD, phobias
Changes in life situation	Loss of control, loss of self-esteem, loss of independence, alterations in environment (i.e., moving to facility for increased care needs)
Direct or indirect effects of terminal illness	Lack of knowledge concerning illness, uncontrolled symptoms (e.g., pain, dyspnea, nausea and vomiting), delirium, depression, hypoxemia, sepsis, impending cardiac or respiratory failure, spiritual, or existential concerns
Drug withdrawal	Drug withdrawal states (e.g., alcohol and sedative-hypnotic drugs)

Table 2. Medications That May Exacerbate Anxiety

Class	Medications
Anti-emetics	Metoclopramide, prochlorperazine, promethazine
Antipsychotics	Aripiprazole, chlorpromazine, haloperidol, olanzapine, quetiapine, risperidone
CNS Stimulants	Amphetamines, armodafinil, caffeine, methylphenidate, modafinil
COPD/Pulmonary	Albuterol, arformoterol, formoterol, indacaterol, levalbuterol, salmeterol, theophylline, vilanterol
Corticosteroids	Dexamethasone, methylprednisolone, prednisolone, predisone
Decongestants	Phenylephrine, pseudoephedrine
Thyroid agents	Levothyroxine, liothyronine, liotrix

Clinical Characteristics

- Behaviors or actions that indicate anxiety:
  - o Intense worry or dread
  - o Irritability
  - o Inability to concentrate
  - o Poor coping skills
  - o Maladaptive behaviors (e.g., treatment non-adherence, social withdrawal, or avoidance)
  - o Limited participation in palliative care treatment goals
- Symptoms and physical presentation of anxiety:
  - o Anorexia
  - o Hyperventilation
  - o Insomnia
  - o Nausea
  - o Palpitations
  - o Sweating
- Anxiety can worsen if other conditions are already present (e.g., insomnia, depression, fatigue, gastrointestinal upset, dyspnea, or dysphagia).
- Pathological anxiety has the following characteristics:
  - o Takes on a "life of its own."
  - o May be of an intensity that exceeds the patient's capacity to bear.
  - o Lasts longer than expected in a given situation.
  - o Produces anxiety behaviors and physical symptoms.
- Reassess the patient for anxiety with any change in behavior or any change in the underlying medical condition using the following steps:
  - o Search for causes of anxiety or fear – ask the patient!
  - o Assess for formal anxiety disorders.
  - o Assess for other problems that might lead to the emergence of anxiety.
  - o Ask about anxiety that predated the hospice diagnosis and any history of effective treatments.

Non-Pharmacological Treatment[2-4]

- Vigilance: regularly assess patients for anxiety; maintain a high level of suspicion for anxiety in terminal illness.
- Offer emotional support and reassurance when appropriate.
- Err on the side of treatment - be willing to palliate anxiety.
- Assess treatment response and side effects frequently.
- Incorporate social workers, spiritual care counselors, and psychologists into the patient's plan of care. Understand that the limited stamina and attention span of seriously ill patients may make counseling impractical in the hospice setting.
- Cognitive and behavioral therapies can be beneficial, including simple relaxation exercises or distraction strategies (i.e., focusing on something pleasurable or at least emotionally neutral).
  - o Guided imagery can reduce anxiety and lessen the need for anxiolytic medications.
- When an underlying cause of anxiety can be identified, treatment is initially aimed at managing the precipitating problem. Monitor to see if anxiety improves or resolves as the underlying cause is addressed.

Pharmacotherapy[6-11]

- Benzodiazepines are considered the drugs of choice for the management of anxiety in end-of-life care. For the relative potencies of benzodiazepines, refer to the *Benzodiazepine Equivalency Table* in the Appendix.
- If patients have a life expectancy greater than 2-3 months, selective serotonin receptor inhibitors (SSRIs) and serotonin norepinephrine reuptake inhibitors (SNRIs) may be appropriate to treat anxiety. An SSRI or an SNRI can also provide relief of comorbid depression.
- Antipsychotics and anticonvulsants have been used as monotherapy or in combination with antidepressants for the management of generalized anxiety disorder.

Clinical Pearls

- The primary goal of therapy for anxiety is patient comfort. Aim to prevent anxiety, and reduce stressors if possible. A combination of non-pharmacological approaches and pharmacotherapy may be required to adequately control symptoms.
- Most anxiolytics cause some sedation, initiate medications at the lower end of the dose range and titrate to effect. Depending on patient medical history, higher anxiolytic doses may be required.
- Psychostimulants such as methylphenidate while effective for depression, may make anxiety worse.

Pharmacological Management of Anxiety

Generic Name (Trade Name)	Adult Starting Dose	Routes	Common Strengths and Formulations	Comments
Benzodiazepines				
Alprazolam (Xanax®)	0.25 mg every 4 to 8 hours PRN or ATC	PO SL PR	**Tablets:** 0.25 mg, 0.5 mg, 1 mg, 2 mg **Oral solution:** 1 mg/mL	• C-IV controlled substance. • Beneficial for panic attacks. • Short-acting; may produce "rebound" anxiety between doses as tolerance develops. • Risk for withdrawal if tolerant patient abruptly stops medication.
Clonazepam (Klonopin®)	0.5 mg – 1 mg every 8 to 12 hours PRN or ATC	PO SL PR	**Tablets:** 0.5 mg, 1 mg, 2 mg **Oral disintegrating tablets:** 0.125 mg, 0.25 mg, 0.5 mg, 1 mg, 2 mg	• C-IV controlled substance. • Active metabolites may accumulate and contribute to sedation. • Most useful in presence of seizures and myoclonus.
Diazepam (Valium®)	2 mg-5 mg every 6-12 hours PRN or ATC	PO SL PR IV IM	**Tablets:** 2 mg, 5 mg, 10 mg **Oral solution:** 5 mg/mL, 1 mg/mL **Injection:** 5 mg/mL	• C-IV controlled substance. • Diazepam rectal gel expensive; tablets well absorbed PO, SL, or PR. • Due to prolonged duration and active metabolites, dose no more frequently than every 6-8 hours (adult) or 12-24 hours (geriatric). • Active metabolites may accumulate and contribute to sedation.
Lorazepam (Ativan®)	0.25 mg-0.5 mg every 4 to 12 hours PRN or ATC	PO SL PR SC IV IM	**Tablets:** 0.5 mg, 1 mg, 2 mg **Oral solution:** 2 mg/mL **Injection:** 2 mg/mL, 4 mg/mL	• C-IV controlled substance. • May use tablets sublingually or rectally instead of oral concentrate. • Short-acting; no active metabolites.
Antidepressants: *Selective Serotonin Reuptake Inhibitors (SSRIs)*				
Citalopram (Celexa®)	20 mg Daily	PO	**Tablets:** 10 mg, 20 mg, 40 mg **Oral solution:** 10 mg/5 mL	• Onset of effect in 1 week; full response may take 8-12 weeks after initiation of treatment. • Monitor anxiety in first few days therapy; consider addition of a benzodiazepine PRN. • Risk of QT prolongation at doses greater than 20mg in elderly. • Increased risk of GI bleeding when used with aspirin, NSAIDs, and other anticoagulants.

Continued

Generic Name (Trade Name)	Adult Starting Dose	Routes	Common Strengths and Formulations	Comments
Antidepressants: *Selective Serotonin Reuptake Inhibitors (SSRIs), continued*				
Escitalopram (Lexapro®)	5-10 mg Daily	PO	**Tablets:** 5 mg, 10 mg, 20 mg **Oral solution:** 1 mg/mL	• Onset of effect in 1 week; full response may take 8-12 weeks after initiation of treatment. • Monitor anxiety in first few days to a week of therapy; consider addition of a benzodiazepine PRN. • Increased risk of GI bleeding when used with aspirin, NSAIDs, and other anticoagulants.
Fluozetine (Prozac®)	10-20 mg Daily	PO	**Tablets:** 10 mg, 20 mg, 60 mg **Capsules:** 10 mg, 20 mg, 40 mg **Oral solution:** 20 mg/5mL	• Onset of effect in 1-2 weeks; full response may take 8-12 weeks after initiation of treatment. • Monitor anxiety in first few days to a week of therapy; consider addition of a benzodiazepine PRN. • Increased risk of GI bleeding when used with aspirin, NSAIDs, and other anticoagulants. • Long half-life allows abrupt discontinuation with no withdrawal symptoms.
Paroxetine (Paxil®)	10 mg Daily	PO	**Tablets:** 10 mg, 20 mg, 30 mg, 40 mg **Suspension:** 10 mg/5mL **CR tablets:** 12.5 mg, 25 mg, 37.5 mg	• Continue as existing therapy, but not recommended as initial therapy due to short half-life and discontinuation syndrome. • SSRI with highest incidence of anticholinergic side effects. • Withdrawal symptoms can occur with missed doses.
Sertraline (Zoloft®)	25-50 mg Daily	PO	**Tablets:** 25 mg, 50 mg, 100 mg **Oral solution:** 20 mg/mL	• Onset of effect in 1 week; full response may not be seen until 8-12 weeks after initiation of treatment. • May worsen anxiety in first few days to a week of therapy; consider addition of a benzodiazepine PRN. • Increased risk of GI bleeding when used with aspirin, NSAIDs, and other anticoagulants. • First line therapy for depression and generalized anxiety in elderly patients.

Continued

Generic Name (Trade Name)	Adult Starting Dose	Routes	Common Strengths and Formulations	Comments
Antidepressants: *Serotonin / Norepinephrine Reuptake Inhibitors*				
Duloxetine (Cymbalta®)	20-30 mg Daily	PO	**Capsules:** 20 mg, 30 mg, 60 mg	• Second line to SSRIs. • Do not discontinue abruptly. • Monitor blood pressure periodically. • Capsule contents may be sprinkled on applesauce for easier swallowing. Do not give with chocolate pudding. • Also FDA-indicated for neuropathic and chronic pain.
Venlafaxine (Effexor®)	25 mg Daily or BID	PO	**Tablets:** 25 mg, 37.5 mg, 50 mg, 75 mg, 100 mg **ER tablets:** 37.5 mg, 75 mg, 150 mg, 225 mg **ER capsules:** 37.5 mg, 75 mg, 150 mg	• Second line to SSRIs. • Do not discontinue abruptly. • Do not crush extended release (ER) tablets. • IR tabs require BID dosing. • Also off-label use for neuropathic pain.
Antipsychotics: *Conventional*				
Chlorpromazine (Thorazine®)	10-25 mg Q8h PRN or ATC	PO SL PR IM	**Tablets:** 10 mg, 25 mg, 50 mg, 100 mg, 200 mg **Injection:** 25 mg/mL	• More sedating than haloperidol. • Use with caution in ambulatory patients due to risk of orthostatic hypotension. • Concentrated oral solution (100 mg/mL) may be compounded for sublingual administration. • Associated with QT prolongation. • Avoid use in patients with Lewy Body Dementia, Parkinson's disease.
Haloperidol (Haldol®)	0.5-1 mg BID PRN or ATC	PO SL PR SC IV IM	**Tablets:** 0.5 mg, 1 mg, 2 mg, 5 mg, 10 mg, 20 mg **Oral solution:** 2 mg/mL **Injection:** 5 mg/mL	• Oral solution and tablets can be given PO, SL, or PR. • Low doses have few side effects, but monitor for EPS, including akathisia (which can mimic anxiety) or other abnormal movements. • Associated with QT prolongation. • Avoid use in patients with Lewy Body Dementia, Parkinson's disease.
Antipsychotics: *Atypical*				
Olanzapine (Zyprexa®)	2.5-5 mg Daily	PO	**Tablets:** 2.5 mg, 5 mg, 7.5 mg, 10 mg, 15 mg, 20 mg **Oral disintegrating tablets:** 5 mg, 10 mg, 15 mg, 20 mg	• Generally, no benefit over haloperidol or chlorpromazine. • Associated with hyperglycemia and metabolic syndrome. • Useful if anxious patient unable to tolerate benzodiazepines *and* conventional antipsychotics. • Monitor for EPS, including akathisia, or other abnormal movements.

Continued

Generic Name (Trade Name)	Adult Starting Dose	Routes	Common Strengths and Formulations	Comments
Antipsychotics: *Atypical*				
Quetiapine (Seroquel®)	25 mg BID	PO	**Tablets:** 25 mg, 50 mg, 100 mg, 200 mg, 300 mg, 400 mg **ER tablets:** 50 mg, 150 mg, 200 mg, 300 mg, 400 mg	• ER tablets are expensive. • Antipsychotic of choice in patients with Parkinson's disease or Lewy Body Dementia. • May increase blood glucose levels. • Most sedating of the atypical antipsychotics.
Risperidone (Risperdal®)	0.25mg-0.5 mg BID	PO	**Tablets:** 0.25 mg, 0.5 mg, 1 mg, 2 mg, 3 mg, 4 mg **Oral solution:** 1 mg/mL **Oral disintegrating tablets:** 0.25 mg, 0.5 mg, 1 mg, 2 mg, 3 mg, 4 mg	• Generally, no benefit over haloperidol or chlorpromazine. • Can increase blood glucose levels. • Orally disintegrating tablets more expensive than conventional tablets. • Oral solution may be mixed with coffee, milk, orange juice, water; incompatible with tea or cola.
Anticonvulsants				
Gabapentin (Neurontin®)	300 mg QHS	PO	**Capsules:** 100 mg, 300 mg, 400 mg **Tablets:** 600 mg, 800 mg **Oral solution:** 250 mg/5mL **ER tablets:** 300 mg, 600 mg	• Start at low dose and increase according to response. • ER tablets should be taken with evening meal. Do not crush or chew. • For GFR <15mL/min: administer 300mg on alternate days or 100mg at night initially, increase according to tolerability.
Pregabalin (Lyrica®)	50 mg at QHS	PO	**Capsules:** 25 mg, 50 mg, 75 mg, 100 mg, 150 mg, 200 mg, 225 mg, 300 mg **Oral solution:** 20 mg/mL	• C-V controlled substance. • May have faster onset of benefit compared to gabapentin. • Most evidence for anticonvulsants for the treatment of anxiety. • Studies suggest most benefit for anxiety when titrated to 200 mg/day.

See Drug Dosing for Liver and Renal Disease for additional drug information.

References

1. American Psychiatric Association: Diagnostic and Statistical Manual of Mental Disorders, Fifth Edition. Arlington, VA, American Psychiatric Association, 2013. http://dsm.psychiatryonline.org.
2. Payne DK, Massie, MJ. Anxiety in palliative care. In: Chochinov HM, Breitbart W, eds. *Handbook of Psychiatry in Palliative Medicine*. New York, NY: Oxford University Press; 2000:63-74.
3. Hinshaw D, Carnahan J, Johnson D. Depression, anxiety and asthenia in advanced illness. *J Am Coll Surg* 2002;195(2):271-278.
4. Cooper K, Stollings S. Guided imagery for anxiety. *Fast Facts and Concepts*. January 2009;211. Available at https://www.capc.org/fast-facts/211-guided-imagery-anxiety/
5. Kinzbrunner B et al. Delirium, depression and anxiety. In: Kinzbrunner B, Policzer J, eds. *End-of-Life-Care: A Practical Guide*, 2nd ed: New York, NY: McGraw-Hill Professional; 2011: 276-279.

6. Henderson, M, MacGregor, E, Sykes, N, Hotopf, M. The use of benzodiazepines in palliative care. *Palliat Med.* 2006;20(4): 407-412.
7. Buoli M, Caldiroli A, Caletti E, Paoli RA, Altamura AC. New approaches to the pharmacological management of generalized anxiety disorder. *Expert Opin. Pharmacother.* 2013;14(2):175-184.
8. Calabrese JR. Efficacy of typical and atypical antipsychotics for primary and comorbid anxiety symptoms or disorders: a review. *J of Clin Psychiatry* 2006; 67(9):1327-1340.
9. Vulink NC, Figee M, Denys D. Review of atypical antipsychotics in anxiety. *Eur Neuropsychopharmacol.* 2011;21(6): 429-49.
10. Allgulander, C. Antipsychotics in anxiety disorders. *Eur Psychiatry* 2009;24(Suppl 1):S119.
11. Mula M, Pini S, Cassano GB. The role of anticonvulsant drugs in anxiety disorders: a critical review of the evidence. *J Clin Psychopharmacol* 2007;27:263-72.
12. Baldwin D, Anderson I, Nutt D, Allgulander C, et al. Evidence-based pharmacological treatment of anxiety disorders, post-traumatic stress disorder and obsessive-compulsive disorder: a revision of the 2005 guidelines from the British Association for Psychopharmacology. *J Psychopharm* 2014;28(5):403-439.

Treatment Algorithm for Anxiety

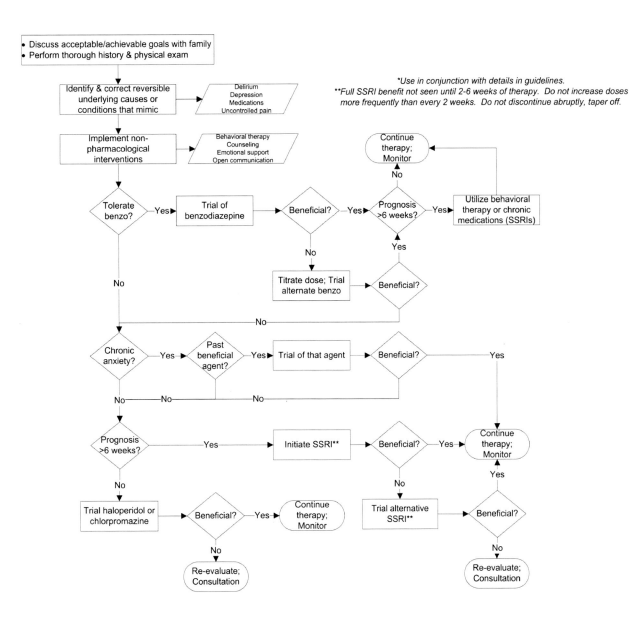

*Use in conjunction with details in guidelines.
**Full SSRI benefit not seen until 2-6 weeks of therapy. Do not increase doses more frequently than every 2 weeks. Do not discontinue abruptly, taper off.*

Ascites and Edema

Introduction and Background[1]
- Edema occurs as a result of an imbalance of the forces which control fluid exchange. Edema may be localized to one part of the body, or generalized throughout the body.
- Ascites is accumulation of fluid in the peritoneal space, between the lining of the abdomen and the organs in the abdominal cavity.
- Anasarca is severe, generalized edema with widespread fluid accumulation throughout the body's extracellular space.
- In various advanced illnesses, edema is a common symptom, and underlying causes are not always identifiable or reversible.
- Edema at end of life may result from malignancy, cardiac or liver failure, or medications.

Prevalence[2-4]
- Studies suggest that more than 50% of patients with end stage heart disease experience edema.
- Following mastectomy and axillary lymph node dissection for breast cancer, up to 49% of patients report arm lymphedema, with increasing occurrence in the years following surgery.
- Ascites can be a presenting feature in about 50% of malignancies.

Causes[1,3-9]
- Edema is usually caused by venous obstruction, increased capillary permeability, and increased plasma volume secondary to sodium and water retention.
- Dependent edema is often caused by limited mobility and usually affects the lower extremities.
- Pitting edema is caused by fibrotic changes from edema being present for an extended period of time. When the edematous area is pressed with a finger, the indentation remains.
- Cerebral edema occurs with brain trauma, cerebral infarction, tumor, infection, or hemorrhage.
- Heart failure results in cardiogenic pulmonary edema and peripheral edema secondary to insufficient pumping by the heart (left ventricular dysfunction) and poor circulation.
- Hypoalbuminemia leads to reduced oncotic pressure, decreased intravascular volume, and accumulation of interstitial fluid. Secretion of anti-diuretic hormone, increased water retention, and decreased urine output can then occur.
- Lymphedema occurs as the result of insufficiency in the lymphatic system and inefficient lymph transport, leading to swelling of a limb. Arm lymphedema is associated with surgical removal or damage to lymph nodes especially in patients with breast cancer.
- Ascites often occurs with liver disease as well as ovarian, uterine, or gastrointestinal cancers due to changes in portal and oncotic pressure and microvascular permeability.
- Medications can increase the risk of peripheral edema. Review medication profiles for potential contributing medications. Discontinue use of the medication, if possible. See Table 1 for medications associated with edema.

Table 1. Medications Associated with Edema

Acyclovir	Gabapentin	Naproxen
Amlodipine	Hydralazine	Pioglitazone
Carvedilol	Hydrocortisone (oral)	Prednisolone
Celecoxib	Ibuprofen	Prednisone
Clonidine	Megestrol	Rosiglitazone
Estrogen	Metoprolol	Verapamil

Clinical Characteristics[1,3-9]
- Peripheral edema is the accumulation of fluid in the feet, ankles, and legs, often the result of heart, kidney, or liver failure.
- Ascites is usually due to liver failure or malignancy and often accompanied by abdominal pain, nausea, anorexia, or vomiting.

- Malignant ascites indicates malignant cells in the peritoneal cavity (peritoneal carcinomatosis) and is associated with abdominal cancers (ovarian, colorectal, pancreatic, uterine) as well as extra-abdominal cancers (lymphoma, lung, breast).
- Lymphedema is the swelling of tissue resulting from failure of the lymphatic system. Accumulation of protein-rich fluid causes proliferation of fatty tissue, inflammation, and progressive fibrosis.
- Pulmonary edema is the diffuse extravascular accumulation of fluid in pulmonary tissues and surrounding air spaces
- Cerebral edema is the accumulation of excessive water in the extra- or intra-cellular spaces of the brain, usually the result of a tumor, hemorrhage, ischemia, or hypoxia.
- Numerical scales for grading peripheral edema (0 – 4+ pitting) are used. In addition to the scale, specific location, presence of pitting, and extent of the edema. For consistency in documentation, measure pitting in millimeters with a measuring tape.

Grade	Depth of Pitting
1+	2 mm
2+	4 mm
3+	6 mm
4+	8 mm

Non-Pharmacological Treatment[1,3,4,9-12]

- If possible, elevate affected extremities using pillows, footstools, reclining chairs.
- Initiate fluid and salt restricted diets only if such restriction is not overly burdensome to the patient.
- Paracentesis for symptomatic ascites
  - Fluid removal from paracentesis is temporary but may quickly relieve symptoms such as dyspnea in up to 90% of patients
  - Permanent drains or peritoneovenous shunts may be considered when ascites is uncontrolled despite repeated paracenteses or fluid rapidly reaccumulates after large volume paracentesis. Such interventions are typically reserved for patients with longer term survival prognosis.
  - Large volume paracenteses (3-5 liters) may cause hypotension, protein loss, intravascular volume depletion, and dehydration. Patients generally tolerate smaller volume (1-2 liters) fluid removal, though more frequent paracentesis may be needed.
- Lymphatic massage
  - Massage therapists or physical therapists trained in lymphedema management including manual lymph drainage (MLD) or complete decongestive therapy (CDT) can assist with range of motion and massage techniques for patient and caregivers. Frequency of massage should depend on severity of symptoms and patient tolerance.
  - Massaging should begin centrally in the neck or trunk area; this will help clear out the main lymphatic pathways, aiding in drainage from the limb.
- Tissue compression with wraps or garments (e.g., compression stockings or sleeves) will promote fluid reabsorption, reducing edema in limbs.
- Level of compression for garments varies from 8mmHg to 50 mmHg; patient should be assessed to determine appropriate level of compression to manage symptoms. Highest levels of compression (40-50 mmHg) should only be used when prescribed by a physician.

Pharmacotherapy[1,7-10]

- In patients receiving diuretics, monitor weights daily. Frequent weight measurement may not be feasible for patients who are chair- or bedbound and those too weak to transfer or stand.
- Weight loss should be limited to 0.5 kg per day if no peripheral edema is present. If peripheral edema is also present, limit weight loss to 1 kg lost per day.
- Patients on chronic diuretic therapy to control edema are at risk of hypokalemia, orthostatic hypotension, and dehydration. Monitor for signs and symptoms with each visit. Depending on the patient's goals of care, periodic lab work to assess electrolyte balance may be helpful.
- Thiazides and loop diuretics (except ethacrynic acid) contain a sulfa moiety, so there is a slight risk for cross-reaction in patients with sulfa allergies. Most patients with sulfa antibiotic allergies tolerate diuretics. Avoid use if the patient has a known history of severe reaction to sulfa drugs.

- Prednisone has more mineralocorticoid activity than dexamethasone, increasing sodium and water retention. For patients with edema, use dexamethasone as the corticosteroid of choice.
- When converting from one loop diuretic to another, approximate equivalent *oral* doses are: furosemide 40 mg = bumetanide 1 mg = torsemide 20 mg = ethacrynic acid 50 mg.
- Oral bioavailability of furosemide is 50%; sublingual administration provides bioavailability near 60%.
- Using spironolactone and furosemide to manage ascites may only be minimally effective if ascites is due to malignancy.

Clinical Pearls[1,7-13]

- Presence of malignant ascites is an indicator of advanced disease and is generally associated with a poor prognosis. Focus treatment on palliation of symptoms.
- Evaluate upper body skin turgor to determine hydration status of patient. Poor upper body skin turgor may indicate volume depletion and dehydration, despite the presence of ascites or peripheral edema.
- Unilateral, new-onset edema may indicate presence of deep vein thrombosis (DVT).
- If possible, avoid giving late-day doses of diuretics to reduce nocturia and sleep disruption.

Pharmacological Management of Ascites & Edema

Generic Name (Trade Name)	Adult Starting Dose	Routes	Common Strengths and Formulations	Comments
Loop Diuretics				
Furosemide (Lasix®)	20 mg Daily	PO SL PR SC IM IV	**Tablets:** 20 mg, 40 mg, 80 mg **Oral solution:** 10 mg/mL, 8 mg/mL **Injection:** 10 mg/mL	• Drug of choice for pulmonary congestion and edema • Oral bioavailability about 50% • IV dose is ½ of equivalent PO dose, 40 mg PO = 20 mg IV
Bumetanide (Bumex®)	0.5 mg Daily	PO IV IM	**Tablets:** 0.5 mg, 1 mg, 2 mg **Injection:** 0.25 mg/mL	• Oral bioavailability about 100% • PO and IV doses are same • May work if resistant to furosemide
Torsemide (Demadex®)	10 mg Daily	PO IV	**Tablets:** 5 mg, 10 mg, 25 mg, 100 mg **Injection:** 10 mg/mL	• Oral bioavailability about 100% • PO and IV doses are same • May work if resistant to furosemide
Carbonic Anhydrase Inhibitor				
Acetazolamide (Diamox®)	250 mg Daily	PO	**Capsules ER:** 500 mg **Tablets:** 125 mg, 250 mg	• Primarily used to decrease intracranial pressure (ICP) in cerebral edema. • May crush tablets if needed.
Thiazide-Type Diuretics				
Metolazone (Zaroxolyn®)	2.5 mg Daily	PO	**Tablets:** 2.5 mg, 5 mg, 10 mg	• Works synergistically with loop diuretics; use only if loop diuretic is ineffective alone. • When using as needed, give 30-60 minutes before loop diuretic for optimal effect. Dose timing not necessary with chronic use.
Hydrochlorothiazide (Microzide®)	25 mg Daily	PO	**Capsules:** 12.5 mg **Tablets:** 12.5 mg, 25 mg, 50 mg	• Ineffective in CrCl < 30 mL/min unless used with a loop diuretic. • Can cause hyperuricemia, use cautiously if history of gout. • Thiazide diuretics can decrease renal calcium excretion, avoid use in patients with hypercalcemia.

Continued

Generic Name (Trade Name)	Adult Starting Dose	Routes	Common Strengths and Formulations	Comments
Thiazide-Type Diuretics, *continued*				
Chlorothiazide (Diuril®)	250 mg Daily	PO IV	**Tablets:** 250 mg, 500 mg **Oral suspension:** 250 mg/5mL **Injection:** 500 mg	• Ineffective in CrCl < 30 mL/min unless used with a loop diuretic. • Can cause hyperuricemia, use cautiously if history of gout. • Thiazide diuretics can decrease renal calcium excretion, avoid use in patients with hypercalcemia.
Chlorthalidone (Thalitone®)	50 mg Daily	PO	**Tablets:** 25 mg, 50 mg, 100 mg	• Ineffective in CrCl < 30 mL/min unless used with a loop diuretic. • Can cause hyperuricemia, use cautiously if history of gout. • Thiazide diuretics can decrease renal calcium excretion, avoid use in patients with hypercalcemia.
Potassium-Sparing Diuretics				
Spironolactone (Aldactone®)	25 mg Daily	PO	**Tablets:** 25 mg, 50 mg, 100 mg	• Drug of choice for ascites in 100 mg:40 mg ratio with furosemide. • Aldosterone antagonist. • Avoid use if CrCl <10 mL/min • Gynecomastia possible, especially at higher doses
Eplerenone (Inspra®)	25 mg Daily	PO	**Tablets:** 25 mg, 50 mg	• Aldosterone antagonist. • Avoid use if CrCl < 50 mL/min. • High potential for drug interactions and hyperkalemia.
Triamterene (Dyrenium®)	50 mg Daily	PO	**Tablets:** 50 mg, 100 mg	• No aldosterone effects. • Avoid use if CrCl < 50 mL/min. • Can cause hyperuricemia, use cautiously if history of gout.

See Drug Dosing for Liver and Renal Disease for additional drug information.

References

1. O'Brien JG, Chennabhotla SA, Chennubhotla RV. Treatment of edema. *Am Fam Physician.* 2005;71(11):2111-2117.
2. McMillan SC, Dunbar SB, Zhang W. The prevalence of symptoms in hospice patients with end-stage heart disease. *J Hosp Palliat Nurs.* 2007;9(3):124-131.
3. Petrek JA, Senie RT, Peters M, et al. Lymphedema in a cohort of breast carcinoma survivors 20 years after diagnosis. *Cancer.* 2001;91(6):1368-1377.
4. Chung M, Kozuch P. Treatment of malignant ascites. *Curr Treat Options Oncol.* 2008;9(25):215-233.
5. Phelps KR. Edema, chapter 29. In: *Clinical Methods: The History, Physical, and Laboratory Examinations.* 3rd ed. Boston, MA: Butterworth Publishers; 1990. Available at http://www.ncbi.nlm.nih.gov/books/NBK348/.
6. Kempski O. Cerebral edema. *Semin Nephrol.* 2001;21(3):303-307.
7. Sangisetty S, Miner T. Malignant ascites: a review of prognostic factors, pathophysiology and therapeutic measures. *World J Gastrointest Surg* 2012;4(4):87-95
8. Lexi-Comp Online. Lexi-Drugs Online. Lexi-Comp, Inc: Hudson, Ohio. Accessed December 27, 2013.
9. Trayes K, Studdiford J, Edema: diagnosis and management. *Am Fam Physician.* 2013;88(2):102-110.
10. Generali J, Cada D. Furosemide: sublingual administration. *Hospital Pharm* 2008;43(4):297-298

11. Hunt SA, Abraham WT, Chin MH, et al. 2009 ACCF/AHA heart failure guidelines. *Circulation*. 2009;119:3391-e479.

12. Martin ML, Hernandez MA, Avendano C. Manual lymphatic drainage therapy in patients with breast cancer related lympoedema. *BMC Cancer*. 2011;11(94). Available at http://www.biomedcentral.com/1471-2407/11/94.

13. Niederhuber JE, Armitage JO, Doroshow JH, et al. Malignant effusions, chapter 54. In: *Abeloff's Clinical Oncology*. 5th ed. London, England: Churchill Livingstone, an imprint of Elsevier Inc; 2013;794-805.

14. Runyon B. Management of adult patients with ascites due to cirrhosis: update 2012. In American Association for the Study of Liver Diseases (AASLD), 2013. Available at http://www.aasld.org/practiceguidelines/Pages/guidelinelisting.aspx.

15. Runyon D. Care of patients with ascites. *N Engl J Med* 1994;330(5):337-342.

Treatment Algorithm for Ascites & Edema

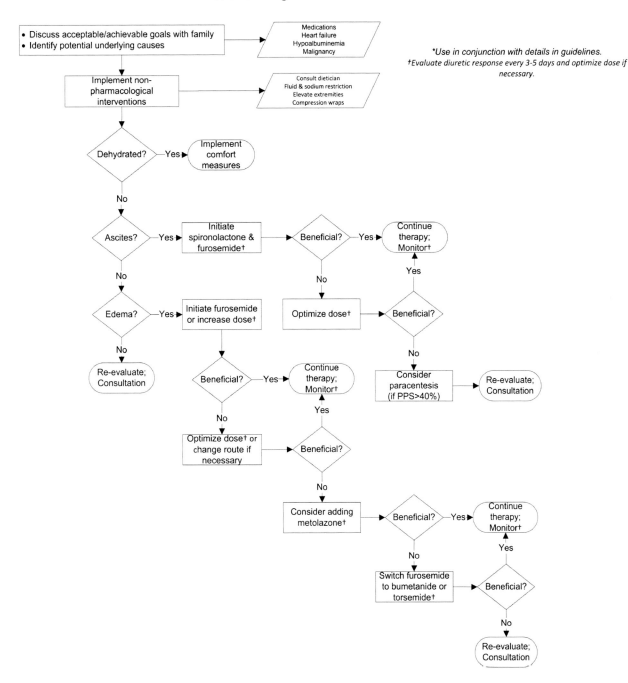

Bowel Obstruction

Introduction and Background [1-3]
- The most common cancers associated with bowel obstruction are colorectal, gastric, uterine and ovarian, but obstruction can occur in any advanced malignancy.
- Patients who have had abdominal surgery or abdominal radiation appear to be at higher risk of developing a bowel obstruction.

Prevalence [2-5]
- Up to 28% of colorectal cancer patients, and up to 51% of ovarian cancer patients will develop a malignant bowel obstruction.
- The most common location for obstructions related to colorectal cancer is the sigmoid colon.
- Bowel obstruction is most common during the advanced stages of terminal disease, and in elderly patients with significant comorbidities.
- In up to 76% of patients with ovarian cancer, the bowel obstruction is multifocal.

Causes [1,2,6]
- Compression from outside the intestinal tract, as well as narrowing or occlusion of the intestinal lumen (e.g., inflammation, fibrosis, trauma, tumor, adhesions, and hernias) delays the propulsion of the intestinal contents, causing bowel distension.
- Bowel distension leads to further accumulation of intestinal fluid, which stretches the bowel wall.
- When intestinal contents do not move through the bowel, but peristaltic activity continues, colicky pain may result. Additionally, a hypertensive state may develop in the intestinal lumen, producing an inflammatory response, damaging the intestinal epithelium.
- Venous drainage from the obstructed segment is impeded, leading to intestinal gangrene or perforation.
- Fluid and electrolytes accumulate in the gut wall, which can lead to hypotension and multi-organ failure.

Clinical Characteristics [1,2]
- Common general symptoms include: abdominal pain (colicky and/or continuous), abdominal distension, nausea and vomiting, and the absence of bowel movements.
- Obstructions higher in the GI tract, such as the pylorus or duodenum, may be associated with less pain and distention, but often produce severe emesis.
- Obstruction in the lower segments of the small intestine typically present with more colicky pain, moderate distention, and hyperactive bowel sounds.
- Large intestine obstruction presents commonly with lower abdominal pain, may be associated with severe abdominal distention, and can have emesis which is more delayed.
- Large intestine obstructions can lead to paradoxical diarrhea, which results from a leak of fluid stool around the fecal impaction.

Non-Pharmacological Treatment [2-5]
- Surgical approaches are considered the primary treatment for mechanical obstructions in patients without a malignancy causing their obstruction.
- For patients with a malignant bowel obstruction, there is no evidence of an improved outcome or survival following surgical correction.
- The short-term use of naso-gastric (NG) tubes is often useful, but invasive, and may be more of a burden than a benefit for the patient.
  - NG tubes can cause nose and throat pain, erosion of nasal cartilage, abscess formation, and social isolation.
  - Consider discontinuing the NG tube when NG output is less than 100 mL/day.
- Use of percutaneous endoscopic gastrostomy (PEG) and jejunostomy (J) tubes may be effective; intermittent venting allows the patient to continue oral intake and maintain an active lifestyle.
- The endoscopic placement of a metal stent at the site of the obstruction can be used for palliative purposes. Additionally, the placement of an intestinal stoma may bypass the blockage. However, these approaches may not be appropriate for patients with a short life expectancy, or those with multiple sites of obstruction.

Pharmacotherapy [1,2,5-8]

- Pharmacotherapy is the cornerstone of treatment for bowel obstruction for patients with poor functional status and short life expectancy.
- The goal of non-surgical management for patients with an intestinal obstruction is to decrease pain, nausea, and secretions into the bowel.
- Avoid oral (PO) medication administration due to unpredictable absorption.
- Consider rectal and sublingual routes of medication delivery, if appropriate. Subcutaneous or intravenous medications should also be considered.
- For irreversible and complete bowel obstruction, a trial of an anticholinergic antispasmodic (hyoscyamine or glycopyrrolate) may decrease bowel contractions and provide pain relief.
- Parenteral opioids and anti-emetics should also be considered to relieve pain and nausea, respectively.
- Anticholinergic medications can cause or worsen delirium; titrate doses carefully. Glycopyrrolate, a quaternary amine compound, does not cross the blood brain barrier and has a very low risk of delirium or other CNS effects.
- For a partial, functional bowel obstruction, a prokinetic agent such as metoclopramide may relieve nausea. Avoid use of metoclopramide in the presence of a complete bowel obstruction.
- Corticosteroids may provide benefit in complete or partial bowel obstruction by reducing inflammation and edema around the obstruction. Dexamethasone is the preferred corticosteroid for managing symptoms of bowel obstruction.
- Corticosteroids may also exhibit an antiemetic effect.
- Combination pharmacotherapy is often necessary for symptom relief, decreasing the need for larger doses of anticholinergic medications.
- Octreotide (Sandostatin®) has shown benefit for patients refractory to other therapies.
- Octreotide may be ineffective as a sole pharmacotherapy agent, and may have improved efficacy in combination with an anticholinergic medication and/or corticosteroids.
- There is conflicting data regarding the use of parenteral hydration:
  - Parenteral hydration may lead to exacerbation of symptoms due to fluid retention, and may increase gastrointestinal secretions.
  - Parenteral hydration can relieve symptoms of delirium, myoclonus, and hallucinations due to dehydration, as well as reverse a build-up of opioid metabolites that can lead to delirium.
  - Hydration should be avoided if it prolongs the dying process, and the care plan should be individualized in collaboration with the patient, family, and palliative care team.

Clinical Pearls [1,2,4,5,7]

- Aggressively treat nausea and reduce vomiting. Provide effective pain relief as needed with opioids.
- Discuss NPO (*nil per os*, nothing by mouth) status with patient and/or family. Caution patients that emesis may occur with eating or drinking.
- Assess for delirium with anticholinergic medication use.
- Consider adding an additional medication class if the patient has a partial response but maintains symptoms after 2-3 doses of the previous agent.
- Review the patient's medication profile to ensure that no other medications are complicating the patient's GI motility.

Pharmacological Management of Bowel Obstruction

Generic Name (Trade Name)	Adult Starting Dose	Routes	Common Strengths and Formulations	Comments
Anti-Emetics				
Haloperidol (Haldol®)	0.5-1 mg BID PRN or ATC	SL PR SC IV IM	**Tablets:** 0.5 mg, 1 mg, 2 mg, 5 mg, 10 mg, 20 mg **Oral solution:** 2 mg/mL **Injection:** 5 mg/mL	• Drug of choice as anti-emetic due to versatility of dosing. • Tablets and oral solution may be given SL or PR. • Avoid use in Parkinson's disease or Lewy Body Dementia.

Continued

Generic Name (Trade Name)	Adult Starting Dose	Routes	Common Strengths and Formulations	Comments
Anti-Emetics, *continued*				
Metoclopramide (Reglan®)	10 mg Q6H PRN	SL PR SC IV IM	**Tablets:** 5 mg, 10 mg **Oral disintegrating tablets:** 5 mg, 10 mg **Oral solution:** 5 mg/5 mL **Injection:** 5 mg/mL	• Avoid use if complete obstruction. • ODT formulation is expensive. • Monitor for confusion and EPS especially in elderly patients. • Higher doses increase EPS risk.
Prochlorperazine (Compazine®)	25 mg Q12H PRN	PR IM	**Tablets:** 5 mg, 10 mg **Suppository:** 25 mg **Injection:** 5 mg/mL	• For patients unable to tolerate haloperidol. • Suppositories are expensive.
Promethazine (Promethazine®)	25 mg Q6H PRN	PR IM	**Tablets:** 12.5 mg, 25 mg, 50 mg **Oral solution:** 6.25 mg/5 mL **Suppository:** 12.5 mg, 25 mg, 50 mg **Injection:** 25 mg/mL, 50 mg/mL	• For patients unable to tolerate haloperidol. • Suppositories are expensive • Sedating • Avoid direct IV administration due to risk of tissue damage and necrosis.
Corticosteroids				
Dexamethasone (Decadron®)	4 mg Daily	SC IV IM	**Injection:** 4 mg/mL, 10 mg/mL	• Most commonly recommended corticosteroid for bowel obstruction. • Administer IV over 5-10 minutes, rapid bolus associated with perianal pain. • Other corticosteroids may be used, see corticosteroid equivalency table in appendix.
Anticholinergics				
Glycopyrrolate (Robinul®)	0.2 mg Q8H PRN	SC IV	**Injection:** 0.2 mg/mL	• Drug of choice for reducing secretions in GI tract. • Does not cross blood-brain barrier minimizing CNS side effects.
Hyoscyamine (Levsin®)	0.125 mg Q6H PRN	SL SC IV	**Tablets:** 0.125 mg **Injection:** 0.5 mg/mL	• Tablets may leave chalky residue when given SL. • Preferred alternative to parenteral glycopyrrolate.
Scopolamine (Transderm Scop®)	1.5 mg Q72H	TD	**Patch:** 1.5 mg	• Do not cut or alter patches. • Patches may take 6-8 hours for onset of action. • Patches are expensive. • Injection removed from market in 2015.
Somatostatin Analog				
Octreotide (Sandostatin®)	0.1 mg Q8H PRN	SC IV	**Injection:** 0.05 mg/mL, 0.1 mg/mL, 0.2 mg/mL, 0.5 mg/mL, 1 mg/mL	• Expensive • Drug of choice for VIPomas and metastatic carcinoid tumors • Usually requires addition of anticholinergic and corticosteroid for bowel obstruction symptom management.

See Drug Dosing for Liver and Renal Disease for additional drug information.

References

1. Ripamonti C, Mercadante S. How to use octreotide for malignant bowel obstruction. *J Support Oncol.* 2004;2(4):357-364.
2. Mercadante S. Assessment and management of mechanical bowel obstruction. In Portenoy RK, Bruera E. eds. *Topics in Palliative Care*, Vol 1. New York, NY: Oxford University Press, 1997:113-130.
3. Jatoi A, Podratz KC, Gill P, Hartmann LC. Pathophysiology and palliation of inoperable bowel obstruction in patients with ovarian cancer. *J Support Oncol.* 2004;2(4):323–337.
4. Frago R, Ramirez E, Millan M, Kreisler E, Del Valle E, Biondo S. Current management of acute malignant large bowel obstruction: a systematic review. *Am J Surg.* 2014;207(1):127-138
5. Dolan E. Malignant bowel obstruction: a review of current treatment strategies. *Am J Hosp Palliat Med.* 2011;28(8):576-582.
6. Ripamonti C, Easson A, Gerdes H. Management of malignant bowel obstruction. *Eur J Cancer.* 2008;44(8):1105-1115.
7. von Gunten C, Muir JC. Fast Facts and Concepts #45. Medical Management of Bowel Obstructions, 2nd Edition. *J Palliat Med.* 2009;12(12):1151-1152.
8. Feuer DJ, Broadley KE. Systematic review and meta-analysis of corticosteroids for the resolution of malignant bowel obstruction in advanced gynaecological and gastrointestinal cancers. Systematic Review Steering Committee. *Ann Oncol.* 1999;10:1035-1041.

Treatment Algorithm for Bowel Obstruction

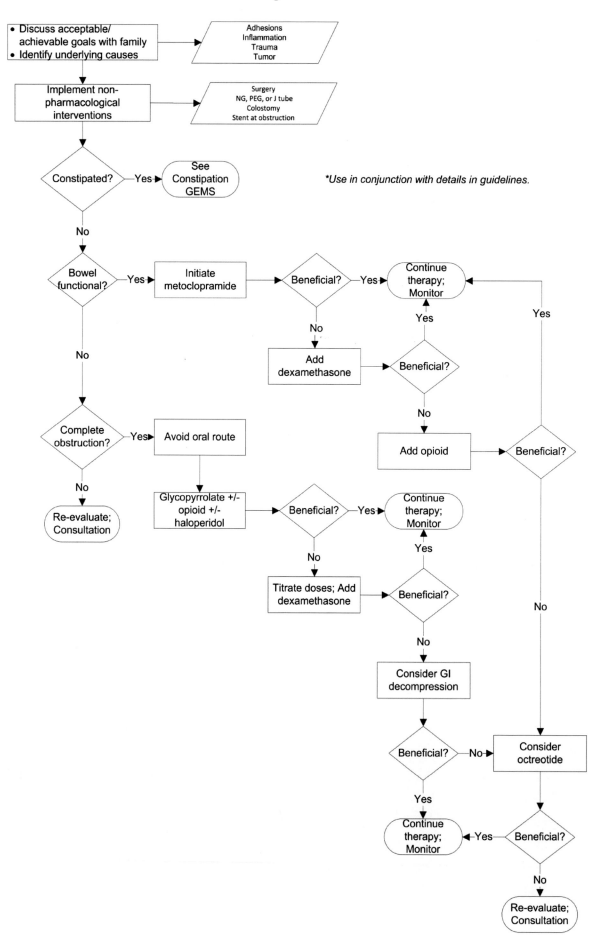

Constipation

Introduction and Background [1,2]

- Constipation is caused by the slow movement of fecal matter through the large intestine allowing excess fluid and electrolyte absorption from the colon while delaying elimination. This slowed process results in the painful passage of dry, hard stools.
- Constipation remains a substantial issue for patients with a limited life expectancy, especially as a result of opioid analgesic use.
- Normal bowel frequency is patient-specific but usually less than 3 bowel movements per week may indicate constipation. However, simply monitoring bowel frequency may lead to undertreatment of associated symptoms.

Prevalence [3-5]

- Constipation is a common complaint in healthcare settings, occurring in up to 20% of the general population.
- Rates of constipation in patients treated with maintenance opioids approach 90%.
- Recent literature suggests approximately 50% of hospice patients experience constipation even without opioid pharmacotherapy.

Causes [1-8]

- Understanding the underlying causes of constipation will help direct prevention and treatment. Three major factors are decreased fluid and food intake, reduced mobility, and medications (primarily opioids).
- Table 1 lists common causes, some of which may be correctable. Table 2 lists medications known to contribute to constipation.
- Hemorrhoids or anal fissures can be a cause and a painful complication of constipation. Fear of painful bowel movements may limit the patient's willingness to take laxatives or to use suppositories.
- Constipation is often multifactorial and a combination of both pharmacological and non-pharmacological approaches may be necessary to successfully treat constipation.

Table 1. Common Causes of Constipation

Lifestyle	
Decreased food intake	Inadequate fiber intake
Decreased mobility	Inadequate fluid intake
Disease States and Syndromes	
Amyotrophic lateral sclerosis (ALS)	Hypokalemia
Colitis	Hypothyroidism
Depression	Irritable bowel syndrome (IBS)
Diabetes	Multiple sclerosis
Diverticular disease	Parkinson's disease
End organ failure	Post-stroke muscle control deficits
Hemorrhoids, anal fissure	Spinal cord compression
Hypercalcemia	Tumor in gastrointestinal tract
Environmental/Cultural Factors	
Lack of comfort or privacy	Lack of assistance with toileting
Cultural sensitivities regarding defecation	Inability to reach toilet

Table 2. Medications Causing Constipation

Medication Class	Examples
Antacids	Calcium carbonate, aluminum hydroxide, bismuth subsalicylate
Anticholinergics	Hyoscyamine, oxybutynin, tolterodine, scopolamine, glycopyrrolate, benztropine
Antidepressants	Amitriptyline, doxepin, paroxetine, mirtazapine
Antiemetics	Ondansetron, granisetron, promethazine, prochlorperazine
Antiepileptics	Carbamazepine, lamoTRIgine, oxcarbazepine, phenobarbital, phenytoin, pregabalin, primidone
Antihistamines	Diphenhydramine, dimenhydrinate, meclizine, hydroxyzine
Antihypertensives	Verapamil, diltiazem, nifedipine, clonidine
Antiparkinson agents	Carbidopa-levodopa, amantadine, pramipexole, ropinirole, rotigotine
Antipsychotic drugs	Lithium, haloperidol, chlorpromazine
Bile acid sequestrants	Cholestyramine, colestipol
Chemotherapy	Vincristine, vinblastine, bleomycin, cytosine
Diuretics	Furosemide, hydrochlorothiazide, torsemide, bumetanide, chlorthalidone
Iron supplements	Ferrous sulfate, ferrous gluconate
NSAIDs	Ibuprofen, naproxen, meloxicam, diclofenac
Opioid analgesics	Codeine, morphine, hydrocodone, methadone, fentanyl, hydromorphone, tramadol, tapentadol, oxymorphone, oxycodone, buprenorphine, meperidine

Clinical Characteristics [1,2,5,6]

- Symptoms associated with constipation include abdominal pain, bloating, flatulence, and feeling of incomplete evacuation.
    - Leakage of fluid feces around in impacted mass may mimic diarrhea.
- Bristol Stool Chart describes seven types of feces and is a tool for assessing intestinal transit time [8]

Stool Type	Stool Description
1	Separate hard lumps, like nuts.*
2	Sausage-shaped but lumpy.*
3	Like a sausage or snake but with cracks on its surface.
4	Like a sausage or snake, smooth and soft.
5	Soft blobs with clear-cut edges.
6	Fluffy pieces with ragged edges, a mushy stool.
7	Watery, no solid pieces.
* Type 1 and 2 may indicate constipation	

- Complications of constipation can include agitation, anorexia, confusion, nausea, vomiting, pain, and urinary dysfunction.
- Proper assessment and physical examination are essential in providing good bowel regimens for patients with a terminal diagnosis.
    - Establish patients' normal bowel pattern and habits, including prior and current use of laxatives.
    - Note any changes in dietary intake (including fluids) and/or physical activity.
    - Continually assess bowel pattern since causal factors are likely long-standing.
    - Note any changes in medications, especially those listed in Table 2.

Non-Pharmacological Treatment [1,2,5,7]

Fluid

- Increase fluid intake within patient limits.
    - Prevention of constipation requires as much as 2 liters of fluid per day.
- Foods with high water content
    - Soups, fruits, gelatin desserts, yogurt, mousse, sauces, and milky desserts.
- Senna tea

- o Add 3-4 ounces of senna tea leaves to 2.5 cups boiling water and let steep for 5 minutes. Strain and remove tea leaves.

Fiber [7,10,11]

- Fiber alone is insufficient for treatment of opioid-induced constipation.
  - o May increase risk of obstruction or impaction in patients with decreased intestinal motility or opioid-induced constipation.
- Accompany increased fiber intake with increased fluid intake to prevent worsening of constipation.
  - o At least 1.5 liters of fluid are required for safe use of fiber supplements.
  - o May cause impaction without adequate water intake.
- High-fiber intake is contraindicated in patients with an increased risk of bowel obstruction (including patients with a past history of a bowel obstruction or status-post colostomy).
- Use caution with high-fiber intake in patients with limited mobility, decreased fluid intake, or on opioid analgesics.
- Dried plums (prunes) were found to be more effective than psyllium fiber use in patients with chronic constipation.
- High fiber recipes:
  - o Power pudding: Blend together 1 cup prune juice, 1 cup bran cereal, and 1 cup applesauce. Take 2 tablespoons (one ounce) daily. Refrigerate up to 1 week.
  - o Yakima paste: Boil 1 lb prunes, 1 lb raisins, 1 lb figs, and 16 oz brewed senna tea for 5 minutes; add 1 cup brown sugar and 1 cup lemon juice and mix to form paste; freeze and serve 1-3 teaspoons daily and titrate as needed.

Environmental/Optimized Toileting

- Provide patients with appropriate privacy, bedside commodes, and other assistive devices if possible.
- Avoid bedpans if possible as they inhibit privacy and correct positioning.
- A footstool may aid in optimal positioning by raising intra-abdominal pressure and facilitating the opening of bowels.
- Encourage patient to attempt a bowel movement 20-30 minutes after breakfast since the most powerful gastro-colic reflex occurs in the morning.

Complementary therapy [12]

- Abdominal massage may help prevent and/or relieve constipation by increasing peristalsis.
  - o Health-care professional or self-administered massage may stimulate defecation through activation of stretch receptors and stimulation of somato-autonomic reflexes and parasympathetic nervous system.
  - o Good option in patients with chronic constipation due to effectiveness, lack of side effects, and low cost.
  - o Various techniques have been used including light-pressure effleurage for 7 minutes, kneading and vibration for 15-20 minutes, and propulsive massage for 10 minutes.
    - ▪ Massage may have to be preformed repeatedly of for extended periods of time to see benefit.
  - o Contraindications include abdominal obstruction, abdominal mass, intestinal bleeding, abdominal radiation therapy, strangulated hernia, and < 6 weeks post-abdominal surgery.

Pharmacotherapy [2,3,6]

- The goal of pharmacotherapy is preventing constipation where possible and re-establishing comfortable bowel habits in patients who are constipated.
- Determine nature of stools and cause of constipation to select appropriate laxative; use oral laxatives if possible.
- Patients with dysphagia, fecal impaction, or disrupted innervations to lower bowel may require a rectal suppository or enema.
- Patients using opioids to treat pain or dyspnea.
  - o Initiate a stimulant laxative, with or without a stool softener, for all patients being initiated on an opioid regimen.

- o   Alternatives include osmotic laxatives such as polyethylene glycol, lactulose, or sorbitol.
- Patients not using opioids
  - o   Stool softeners such as docusate (Colace®) may be preferred.
  - o   Alternatives include osmotic laxatives (polyethylene glycol, lactulose, sorbitol).
- Patients with rectum containing hard feces
  - o   Glycerin suppositories or oil-based enema to clear rectum by softening the fecal mass and stimulating defecation. If no results or incomplete results, perform manual disimpaction.
  - o   Add a stool softener to current bowel regimen if not already present.
  - o   If a stool softener is part of current bowel regimen, evaluate fluid intake and increase within patient limits if possible. Increase dose of stool softener if appropriate.
  - o   Consider addition of daily polyethylene glycol.
- Patients with a full rectum containing soft feces
  - o   Bisacodyl suppository or sodium phosphate enema to clear rectum.
  - o   Treat with an oral stimulant laxative (e.g. senna or bisacodyl) to promote bowel motility.
  - o   Add a stimulant laxative to the preventative regimen.
- Palatability considerations
  - o   Crushed Senna-S tablets are unpalatable and not recommended.
  - o   Docusate liquid has an unpleasant, bitter taste, and a combination liquid of senna and docusate is not available. If a liquid formulation is needed, monotherapy with senna liquid is preferred.

Clinical Pearls [4,13-15]

- Avoid mineral oil liquid, particularly in bedbound patients, due to high risk of aspiration.
- For high impactions, give 3-6 Vaseline balls (white petrolatum) orally instead of liquid mineral oil. [13]
  - o   Vaseline balls: Pea size frozen balls of white petrolatum rolled in powdered sugar.
  - o   Discontinue use of docusate before initiation of Vaseline balls.
- Linaclotide has not been sufficiently studied in elderly patients, and the studies conducted excluded patients receiving anticholinergic or opioid medications. [14]
- Methadone may decrease the therapeutic effect of lubiprostone.
- The safety of methylnaltrexone (Relistor) has not been fully evaluated. Reserve methylnaltrexone for opioid-induced constipation where conventional laxatives have failed. [4]
- Patients, especially those with chronic non-cancer pain, tend to underreport constipation from opioids and may attempt to self-treat with several over-the-counter laxatives for a longer period of time. [15]
- In September 2014 an oral peripheral opioid antagonist, naloxegol (Movantik), was approved by the FDA for opioid-induced constipation. Market availability is expected in early 2015. Naloxegol is marketed as an oral alternative to the injection-only product Methylnaltrexone (Relistor).

Pharmacological Management of Constipation

Generic Name (Trade Name)	Adult Starting Dose	Routes	Common Strengths and Formulations	Comments
Stool Softeners				
Docusate (Colace®)	100 mg BID	PO PR	**Capsules:** 50 mg, 100 mg, 240 mg, 250 mg **Tablets:** 100 mg **Oral solution:** 50 mg/5 mL, 20 mg/5 mL **Enema:** 100 mg/5 mL 283 mg/5 mL	• Ineffective without adequate fluid intake. • Crushing tablets or capsules is not recommended; not palatable. • Oral solution may cause mouth and throat irritation. • Not sufficient for OIC without stimulant (senna or bisacodyl). • Onset of action, 12-72 hours.

Continued

Generic Name (Trade Name)	Adult Starting Dose	Routes	Common Strengths and Formulations	Comments
Stimulant Laxatives				
Bisacodyl (Dulcolax®)	5 mg PO Daily 10 mg PR Daily PRN	PO PR	**Tablets:** 5 mg **Suppositories:** 10 mg	• May combine with oral stool softener. • Suppositories may not be effective if rectum full of stool. • Onset of action, 6-12 hours (oral).
Senna (Senokot®, Ex-Lax®)	2 tabs Daily	PO	**Tablets:** 8.6 mg, 15 mg **Oral solution:** 8.8 mg/5 mL	• May be used with stool softener. • Comes in combination product with docusate. • Onset of action, 6-12 hours.
Docusate + Senna (Senna-S®)	2 tabs Daily	PO	**Tablets:** Docusate 50 mg + Senna 187 mg	• Senna + docusate may be no more effective than senna alone for OIC. • Onset of action, 6-12 hours.
Osmotic Laxatives				
Glycerin	1 PR Daily PRN	PR	**Suppositories:** 1 g, 2 g	• For as needed use if hard, dry stool in rectum.
Milk of magnesia	30 mL Daily	PO	**Tablets:** 400 mg **Oral solution:** 400 mg/5 mL	• Saline laxative. • Associated with increased cramping and electrolyte disturbances • Onset of action, 30 minutes to 3 hours.
Sorbitol 70%	30 mL Daily	PO	**Oral solution:** 70%	• More costly than stimulants with no improved efficacy. • Associated with increased cramping and flatulence. • Onset of action, 12-96 hours.
Lactulose (Chronulac®)	30 mL Daily PRN	PO	**Oral solution:** 10 g/15 mL	• More costly than stimulants with no improved efficacy. • Associated with increased cramping and flatulence. • Onset of action, 12-96 hours.
Polyethylene Glycol 3350 (Miralax®)	17 g Daily	PO	**Powder:** 17 g/packet, 238 g	• May mix in water, juice, soda, coffee, or tea. • Onset of action, 12-96 hours.
Opioid Antagonist, Peripherally-Acting				
Methylnaltrexone (Relistor®)	Patients 38-62 kg: 8 mg Daily PRN Patients 62-114 kg: 12 mg Daily PRN	SC	**Injection:** 8 mg/0.4 mL, 12 mg/0.6 mL	• Indicated for second-line treatment of OIC, after oral stimulant laxatives and suppositories have failed. • Weight-based dosing 0.15mg/kg • Onset of action, 30-60 minutes.
Naloxegol (Movantik®)	25 mg QAM on empty stomach	PO	**Tablets:** 12.5 mg, 25 mg	• Indicated for treatment of OIC in patients with chronic noncancer pain. • Take naloxegol on empty stomach at least 1 hour before or 2 hours after, the first meal of the day. • Do not crush or chew tablets. • Avoid grapefruit, grapefruit juice.

Continued

Generic Name (Trade Name)	Adult Starting Dose	Routes	Common Strengths and Formulations	Comments
Enemas				
Castile Soap Enema	1 enema Daily PRN	PR	**Enema kit:** includes soap packet for large volume enema	• Also known as "soap suds" enema. • Soap facilitates penetration of water into fecal matter. • Onset of action, 15-30 minutes.
Mineral Oil Enema (Fleet Oil Enema®)	1 enema Daily PRN	PR	**Enema:** 133 mL	• Oral mineral oil not recommended due to aspiration risk. • Onset of action, 30-60 minutes.
Sodium Phosphates Enema (Fleet Enema®)	1 enema Daily PRN	PR	**Enema:** 66 mL, 133 mL, 230 mL	• Saline laxative. • Onset of action, 15-30 minutes. • Associated with increased cramping and electrolyte disturbances. • FDA black box warning for acute phosphate nephropathy.
Other				
Linaclotide (Linzess®)	145 mcg Daily	PO	**Capsules:** 145 mcg, 290 mcg	• Expensive. • Take with food to decrease nausea. • Indicated only for constipation-predominant IBS or chronic idiopathic constipation. • Do not open or chew capsules.
Lubiprostone (Amitiza®)	24 mcg BID	PO	**Capsules:** 8 mcg, 24 mcg	• Expensive. • Take with food to decrease nausea. • Do not open or chew capsules. • Concurrent use with methadone may diminish effectiveness of lubiprostone.

See Drug Dosing for Liver and Renal Disease for additional drug information.

References
1. Fallon M, O'Neill B. ABC's of palliative care: constipation and diarrhea. *BMJ* 1997;315: 1293-1296.
2. Librach SL, Bouvette M, De Angelis C, et al. Consensus recommendations for the management of constipation in patients with advanced, progressive illness. *J Pain Symptom Manage* 2010; 40(5):761-73.
3. Miles CL, Fellowes D, Goodman ML, Wilkinson S. Laxatives for the management of constipation in palliative care patients. *Cochrane Database Syst Rev* 2006;4:CD003448.
4. Candy B, Jones L, Goodman ML, et al. Laxatives or methylnaltrexone for the management of constipation in palliative care patients. *Cochrane Database Syst Rev* 2011;1:CD003448.
5. Sykes N. Constipation and diarrhea. In: Walsh DT, Caraceni AT, Fainsinger R, et al, editors. *Palliative Medicine*. Philadelphia, PA: Elsevier; 2009. http://www.expertconsultbook.com/. Accessed October 30, 2013.
6. Mancini I, Bruera E: Constipation in advanced cancer patients. *Support Care Cancer.* 1998; 6(4):356-364.
7. Larkin PJ, Sykes NP, Centeno C, et al. The management of constipation in palliative care: clinical practice recommendations. *Palliat Med* 2008; 22:796-807.
8. Deepak P, Ehrenpreis E. Constipation. *Dis Month* 2011;57(9):511-517
9. Lewis SJ, Heaton KW. Stool form scale as a useful guide to intestinal transit time. *Scand J Gastroenterol* 1997; 32:920-4.
10. Herndon CM, Jackson KC, Hallin PA. Management of opioid-induced gastrointestinal effects in patients receiving palliative care. *Pharmacotherapy* 2002; 22(2):240-50.

11. Attaluri A, Donahoe R, Valestin J, Brown K, Rao S. Randomised clinical trial: dried plums (prunes) vs psyllium for constipation. *Aliment Pharmacol Ther* 2011;33:822-828.

12. Sinclair M. Use of abdominal massage to treat chronic constipation. *J Body Mov Ther* 2011;15(4):436-445.

13. Tavares CN, Kimbrel JM, Protus BM, Grauer PA. Petroleum jelly (Vaseline® balls) for the treatment of constipation: a survey of hospice and palliative care practitioners. *Am J Hosp Palliat Care* 2014;31(8):797-803.

14. Lembo AJ, Schneier HA, Shiff SJ, et al. Two randomized trials of linaclotide for chronic constipation. *N Engl J Med* 2011; 365:527-36.

15. Knezevic N, Chiweshe J, Khare V, Candido K. Is the constipation problem adequately addressed in patients using opioids and non-opioids for chronic non-cancer pain? Poster no.111 presented at: American Academy of Pain Medicine (AAPM) 2014 Annual Meeting, March 6-9, 2014; Phoenix, AZ.

Treatment Algorithm for Constipation

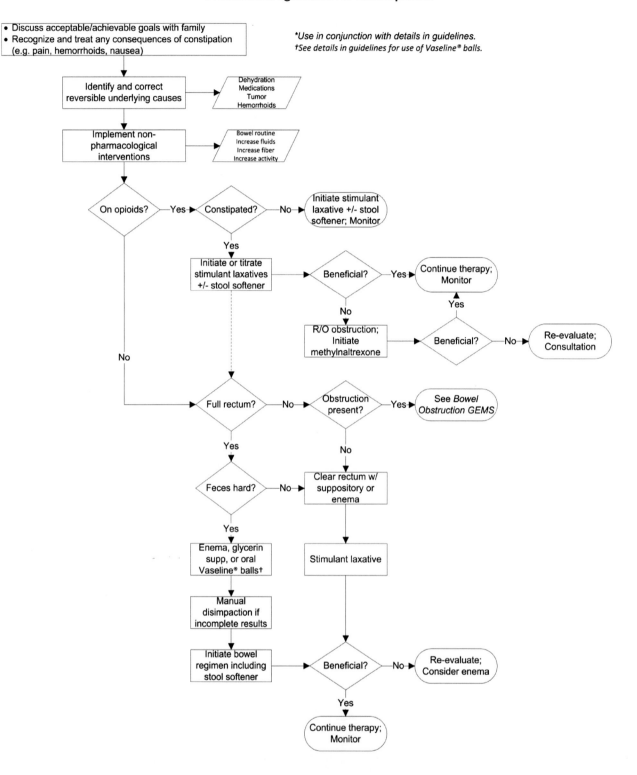

- Discuss acceptable/achievable goals with family
- Recognize and treat any consequences of constipation (e.g. pain, hemorrhoids, nausea)

*Use in conjunction with details in guidelines.
†See details in guidelines for use of Vaseline® balls.

Identify and correct reversible underlying causes → Dehydration / Medications / Tumor / Hemorrhoids

Implement non-pharmacological interventions → Bowel routine / Increase fluids / Increase fiber / Increase activity

On opioids? —Yes→ Constipated? —No→ Initiate stimulant laxative +/- stool softener; Monitor

Constipated? —Yes→ Initiate or titrate stimulant laxatives +/- stool softener → Beneficial? —Yes→ Continue therapy; Monitor

Beneficial? —No→ R/O obstruction; Initiate methylnaltrexone → Beneficial? —Yes→ Continue therapy; Monitor

Beneficial? —No→ Re-evaluate; Consultation

On opioids? —No→ Full rectum? —No→ Obstruction present? —Yes→ See *Bowel Obstruction GEMS*

Obstruction present? —No→ Clear rectum w/ suppository or enema

Full rectum? —Yes→ Feces hard? —No→ Clear rectum w/ suppository or enema

Clear rectum w/ suppository or enema → Stimulant laxative

Feces hard? —Yes→ Enema, glycerin supp, or oral Vaseline® balls† → Manual disimpaction if incomplete results → Initiate bowel regimen including stool softener → Beneficial? —No→ Re-evaluate; Consider enema

Stimulant laxative → Beneficial? —No→ Re-evaluate; Consider enema

Beneficial? —Yes→ Continue therapy; Monitor

Cough

Introduction and Background[1-5]

- Cough is described as a violent expulsion of air from the lungs associated with a characteristic sound.
- Although cough is an airway defense process that helps to clear the lower airways of debris, persistent or chronic cough can result in significant suffering on the part of the patient and family and can negatively impact quality of life.
- Treatment goals for cough at end of life include improving patient comfort, reducing cough frequency and intensity, and enhancing cough effectiveness.

Prevalence[6-8]

- Cough is a commonly experienced symptom in patients at end of life.
- The prevalence of cough at end of life can vary widely with ranges of 10% to more than 80% reported depending on the patient population in question.
- In lung cancer, cough is a very common symptom, occurring with a frequency of 40% to over 80%.

Causes[9-10]

- A thorough history and physical examination can determine possible reversible causes of cough.
- Identify and treat reversible causes of cough if doing so meets patient/family goals of care.
- Assessment should include timing of onset of symptoms as well as cough/sputum characteristics and a detailed description of any additional cough-related symptoms (pain, dyspnea, nausea, etc).

Table 1. Potential Causes of Cough

Cause	Examples
Allergens	Cigarette or wood smoke, pet dander, plants, dust, cockroaches, feather pillows, mold, mildew
Cardiac	Heart failure
Infection	Viral or bacterial, bronchiolitis, bronchitis, pneumonia, tuberculosis
Malignancy	Tumor, lung cancer, mesothelioma
Medications	Angiotensin converting enzyme (ACE) inhibitors, angiotensin receptor antagonists (ARB), antibiotics (amphotericin, erythromycin, aminoglycosides, sulfonamides), inhaled steroids
Pulmonary	Asthma, bronchospasm, chronic obstructive pulmonary disease (COPD), pleural effusion, bronchiectasis, interstitial lung disease, upper airway cough syndrome (postnasal drip)
Psychological	Psychogenic cough (habit cough syndrome), Tourette syndrome
Other	Radiation therapy, aspiration (including foreign body), gastroesophageal reflux (GERD), respiratory tract secretions, seizures, rheumatic disease

Clinical Characteristics[9-13]

- Acute cough lasts less than 3 weeks, subacute cough ranges from 3 to 8 weeks. Cough is considered chronic if lasting longer than 8 weeks.
- Persistent cough can have a significant negative impact on quality of life, causing physical and psychosocial complications.
- Persistent coughing can cause or contribute to anorexia, exhaustion, sleep deprivation, depression, gastroesophageal reflux events, urinary incontinence, rib fractures, syncope, or dizziness.
- Potential complications of cough emphasize the importance of effectively treating cough. Treat any underlying causes when feasible and within the patient's goals of care.
- Avoid minimizing any complaints of cough.
- Most persistent cough can be the result of more than one condition; assess for multiple factors could be contributing to the cough.

Non-Pharmacological Treatment[14]

- Avoid smoking, second-hand smoke, or other respiratory irritants.
- Humidified air may help to soothe irritated airways.
- Help patients maintain an upright posture or elevate of head of bed if GERD is a contributing factor.
- Candies, lozenges, honey, and non-medicated syrups soothe throat irritation and decrease coughing.

- Use thickened liquids or pureed foods if cough is triggered by aspiration. However, consider the impact of the altered diet on the patient's quality of life.
- Discuss worsening or refractory cough as a sign of disease progression (lung cancer, COPD, heart failure) with patients and family members.

Pharmacotherapy[9-10]

- Direct therapy at suspected causes of cough whenever possible (Table 2).
- Determine if cough is productive (wet, mucus-clearing) or non-productive (dry, hacking)
    - Productive cough – expectorants are preferred over suppressants to help loosen
    - Non-productive cough – suppressants are preferred
- Empiric therapy with a cough suppressant or expectorant may be necessary during the assessment and treatment of underlying causes, when a cause cannot be identified, or when addressing the underlying cause is not appropriate or feasible based on the patient's prognosis and patient/family goals of care.
- The goals of cough treatment should also be established:
    - Is the goal to enhance effectiveness of cough?
    - Is the goal to reduce severity/frequency of cough?

Table 2. Treatment Based on Cause of Cough

Cause	Treatment
Bacterial respiratory infection	Antibiotics
COPD or Asthma	Inhaled bronchodilators, corticosteroids
Gastroesophageal reflux disease (GERD)	H2 receptor antagonists, proton pump inhibitors
Common cold (viral)	Nasal decongestants, antihistamines
Upper airway cough syndrome	Nasal decongestants, antihistamines
Allergens	Antihistamines
Medications	Discontinue causative medications (ACE inhibitors, ARBs, inhaled steroids)
Respiratory tract secretions	Anticholinergics (glycopyrrolate, hyoscyamine, atropine, scopolamine)
Pleural effusions	Thoracentesis

Clinical Pearls[12,15-18]

- All opioids have antitussive activity. There is no evidence to support the addition of a second opioid (codeine or hydrocodone) for cough in patients already using opioids for other symptom control. For patients already on opioids for other symptoms (e.g. pain, dyspnea), dosage increases may be necessary to control cough symptoms.
- Adequate treatment of cough may require scheduled doses of medications (in addition to PRN doses) to proactively manage cough symptoms.
- Non-medicated syrups (e.g. simple syrup, corn syrup, cherry syrup) or honey may be options for patients with refractory cough.
- Effectiveness of guaifenesin for cough is controversial. Patients report subjective improvement, but therapeutic benefit has not been demonstrated in clinical trials.
- Nebulized ipratropium may reduce cough frequency and severity in patients with chronic bronchitis or upper respiratory tract infection.

Pharmacological Management of PRODUCTIVE Cough

Generic Name (Trade name)	Adult Starting Dose	Routes	Common Strengths and Formulations	Comments
Expectorants				
Guaifenesin (Robitussin®, Mucinex®)	400 mg Q4H PRN **ER:** 600 mg BID	PO	**Oral solution:** 100 mg/5 mL **Tablets:** 200 mg, 400 mg **ER Tablets:** 600 mg, 1200 mg	• If patient has no swallowing difficulties, using ER tablets may increase adherence. • Encourage adequate hydration when possible. • Do not crush or chew tablet.
Mucolytics				
Nebulized saline	Inhale 3 mL via nebulizer Q4H PRN	INH	**Nebulizer solution:** 3 mL, 5 mL, 15 mL	• May help to loosen and thin secretions and aid in expectoration.

Pharmacological Management of NONPRODUCTIVE Cough

Generic Name (Trade name)	Adult Starting Dose	Routes	Common Strengths and Formulations	Comments
Expectorant + Suppressant				
Guaifenesin + Dextromethorphan (Robitussin DM®, Mucinex DM®)	10 mL Q4H PRN 1 tab BID	PO	**Oral solution:** 10-100 mg/5 mL **ER Tablets:** 600-30 mg, 1200-60 mg	• Do not crush, chew, or break tablet. Take with a full glass of water without regard to meals. • Use of the extended release product may increase adherence if product is effective and needed around the clock.
Guaifenesin + Codeine Liquid (Robitussin AC®)	10 mL Q4H PRN	PO	**Oral solution:** 10-100 mg/5 mL	• C-V controlled substance. • Due to opioid content, initiate laxative to prevent constipation.
Suppressant				
Dextromethorphan (Robitussin CoughGels®, Delsym®)	15 mg Q4H PRN **ER suspension:** 60mg BID	PO	**Oral solution:** 20 mg/15 mL, 7.5 mg/5 mL, 10 mg/5 mL, 15 mg/5 mL **Capsule:** 15 mg **ER suspension:** 30 mg/5 mL	• Fewer GI and CNS effects than opioid therapy. • ER suspension contains Polistirex™, an ion-exchange resin to provide sustained release of drug over 8-12 hours.
Hydrocodone + Homatropine (Hycodan®, Tussigon®)	5 mg Q4H PRN	PO	**Oral solution:** 5-1.5 mg/5 mL **Tablets:** 5-1.5 mg	• C-II controlled substance. • Homatropine dose is subtherapeutic to discourage deliberate overuse. • Due to opioid content, initiate a laxative to prevent constipation.
Anesthetic Suppressant				
Benzonatate (Tessalon Perles®)	100 mg TID PRN	PO	**Capsules:** 100 mg, 150 mg, 200 mg	• Do not crush or chew capsules. • Avoid use if tetracaine allergy.
Lidocaine (Xylocaine®)	Inhale 5 mL (1%) via nebulizer Q4H PRN	INH	**Injection:** 1% (10 mg/mL) 2% (20 mg/mL) 4% (40 mg/mL)	• Avoid eating or drinking for 30 to 60 min after treatment to reduce risk of aspiration. • Use preservative free lidocaine to reduce risk of bronchospasm. • May dilute with normal saline if needed for nebulizer function.

Continued

Generic Name (Trade name)	Adult Starting Dose	Routes	Common Strengths and Formulations	Comments
Suppressant + Antihistamine				
Hydrocodone +Chlorpheniramine (Tussionex® Pennkinetic, TussiCaps®)	5 mL Q6H PRN **ER suspension:** 5 mL BID	PO	**Oral solution:** 5-4 mg/5 mL **ER suspension:** 10-8 mg/5 mL **ER capsules:** 5-4 mg, 10-8 mg	• C-II controlled substance. • Due to opioid content, initiate laxative to prevent constipation. • Monitor for anticholinergic side effects including dry mouth, constipation and confusion. • Do not use ER suspension or capsules more frequently than every 12 hours.

See Drug Dosing for Liver and Renal Disease for additional drug information.

References

1. Fontana GA. Before we get started: What is a cough? *Lung.* 2008;186(1)(suppl 1):S3-S6.
2. Brignall K, Jayaraman B, Birring SS. Quality of life and psychosocial aspects of cough. *Lung.* 2008;186(1)(suppl 1):S55-S58.
3. Wee B, Browning J, Adams A, et al. Management of chronic cough in patients receiving palliative care: a review of evidence and recommendations by a task group of the Association of Palliative Medicine of Great Britain and Ireland. *Palliat Med.* 2012;26(6):780-787.
4. Chan KS, Sham MMK, Tse DMW, Thorsen AB. Palliative medicine in malignant respiratory diseases. In: Doyle D, Hanks G, Cherny N, Calman K, eds. *Oxford Textbook of Palliative Medicine.* 3rd ed. Oxford: Oxford University Press;2003:608-610.
5. Leach RM. Palliative medicine and non-malignant end-stage respiratory disease. In: Doyle D, Hanks G, Cherny N, Calman K, eds. *Oxford Textbook of Palliative Medicine.* 3rd ed. Oxford: Oxford University Press;2003:899-901.
6. Watanabe S, Tarumi Y, Amigo P. Cough, hemoptysis, and bronchorrhea. In: Walsh TD, Caraceni AT, Fainsinger R, Foley KM, Glare P, Goh, C, Lloyd-Williams M, Nunez Olarte J, Radbruch L. *Palliative Medicine.* 1st ed. Philadelphia, PA: Elsevier; 2009. http://www.expertconsultbook.com.
7. Rodriguez KL, Hanlon JT, Perera S, et al. A cross-sectional analysis of the prevalence of undertreatment of nonpain symptoms and factors associated with undertreatment in older nursing home hospice/palliative care patients. *Am J Geriatr Pharmacother.* 2010;8(3):225-232.
8. Estfan B, LeGrand S. Management of cough in advanced cancer. *J Support Oncol.* 2004;2:523-527.
9. Irwin RS, Madison JM. The diagnosis and treatment of cough. *N Engl J Med.* 2000;343(23):1715-1721.
10. Irwin RS, Baumann MH, Bolser DC, et al. Diagnosis and management of cough executive summary: ACCP evidence-based clinical practice guidelines. *Chest.* 2006;129(1)(suppl 1):1S-23S.
11. Irwin RS. Complications of cough: ACCP evidence-based clinical practice guidelines. *Chest.* 2006;129(1)(suppl 1):55S-58S.
12. Homsi J, Walsh D, Nelson KA. Important drugs for cough in advanced cancer. *Support Care Cancer.* 2001;9(8):565-574.
13. Irwin RS, Madison JM. The persistently troublesome cough. *Am J Respir Crit Care Med.* 2002;165(11):1469-1474.
14. Jacobs LG. Managing respiratory symptoms at the end of life. *Clin Geriatr Med.* 2003;19(1):225-239.
15. Homsi J, Walsh D, Nelson KA, et al. A phase II study of hydrocodone for cough in advanced cancer. *Am J Hosp Palliat Care.* 2002;19(1):49-56.
16. Lingerfelt BM, Swainey CW, Smith TJ, Coyne PJ. Nebulized lidocaine for intractable cough near the end of life. *J Support Oncol.* 2007;5(7):301-302.
17. Yancy W, McCrory D, Coeytaux R, Schmidt K, et al. Efficacy and tolerability of treatments for chronic cough: a systematic review and meta-analysis. *Chest.* 2013;144(6):1827-1838.
18. Bolser D. Cough suppressant and pharmacologic protussive therapy. ACCP evidence-based clinical practice guidelines. *Chest.* 2006;129(1)(suppl 1):238S-249S.

Treatment Algorithm for Cough

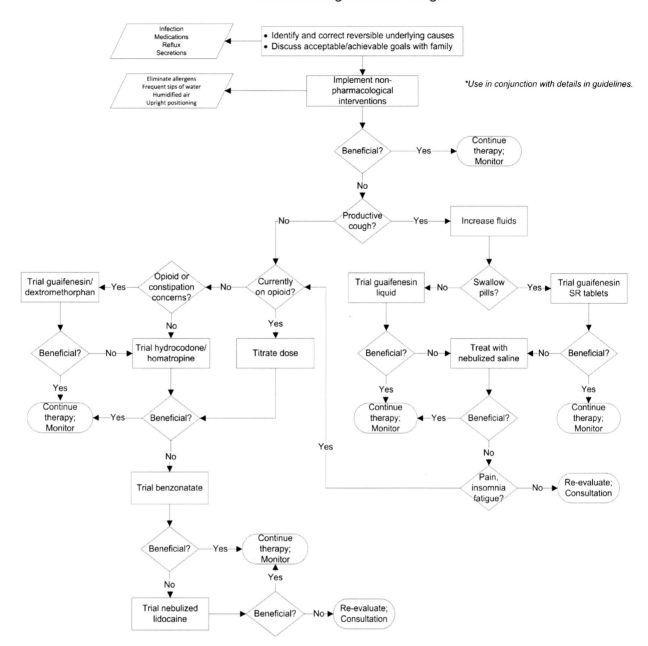

Use in conjunction with details in guidelines.

Depression

Introduction and Background[1-3]
- Depression is a medical condition in which a person experiences feelings of sadness, hopelessness, loss of interest and despair that affecting daily life.
- Depressive disorders (e.g., Major Depressive Disorder, Dysthymia) tend to be recurrent or chronic.
- Periods of discouragement, sadness, or distress are understandable as patients adapt or adjust to the diagnosis of a life-limiting illness. Elisabeth Kübler-Ross referred to this as the "depression" stage of grief and adaptation to loss.
- Clinical depression is not a normal phase of adaptation; it is a complication of life-limiting illness.
- Adaptation and clinical depression can be easily confused, depression is common in hospice patients and often goes unrecognized and untreated.
- Depression is commonly associated with requests for assisted or hastened death.
- Effective treatment of depression will reduce the burden of suffering and enhance quality of life.

Prevalence[4]
- Clinical depression in the hospice setting has been estimated at between 20% and 50%.
- More women experience clinical depression than men.
- Depression is most commonly experienced by patients with late stage cancer.

Causes[1]
- Undertreated symptoms such as pain, agitation/restlessness, anxiety or nausea.
- Spiritual concerns such as perceived loss of control, interpersonal problems, fear, grief or discouragement.
- Experiencing a sudden loss or receiving bad news.

Clinical Characteristics[1,3-6]
- The clinical features of a depressive episode as defined by DSM-V include depressed mood and the following symptoms, which can be remembered by using the acronym SIG-E-CAPS:
  - **S**leep disturbance
  - **I**nterest/pleasure reduction
  - **G**uilty feeling or thoughts of worthlessness
  - **E**nergy change/fatigue
  - **C**oncentration impairment
  - **A**ppetite/weight change
  - **P**sychomotor retardation or agitation
  - **S**uicidal thoughts
- A major depressive episode is characterized by the presence of depressed mood or loss of interest plus 4 or more of the remaining SIG-E-CAPS criteria for at least two weeks.
- At end-of-life, however, some of these criteria could result from serious physical disease itself.
- General clinical approach to depression includes:
  - Assess for any history of previous depressive episodes, including family history of depression, and response to treatment.
  - Assess correlation of depression onset or severity to changes in medical condition, treatment.
  - Assess substance abuse history.
  - Assess for presence of formal depressive disorders.
  - Search for factors which may complicate depression in the medically ill patient.
  - Don't be taken in by the myth of "appropriate depression."
  - Address any underlying general medical causes or complicating factors.
- Diagnostic confidence is increased by the presence of one or more of the following:

o marked anhedonia	o pervasive guilt	o suicidal ideation
o hopelessness	o feeling of being punished; that illness itself is a punishment	o intense, moribund ruminations
o helplessness		o frequent tearfulness
o worthlessness		o self-loathing

- Hopelessness is a particularly important because of its strong association with suicidal ideation and suicide attempts.
- Always inquire about the presence of suicidal thoughts and suicidal intent in a patient with signs or symptoms of depression.
- Untreated depression not only causes prolonged suffering but places the patient at risk for a prolonged or chronic depressive episode.
- In hospice, a clinical depressive episode is unlikely to resolve spontaneously. Failure to recognize and treat depression means the patient will suffer with depression throughout his or her remaining days.
- Traditional formal assessment tools for depression such as Geriatric Depression Scale (GDS) or the Hamilton Rating Scale for Depression (HAM-D) can be used for hospice patients, however, simply asking the patient "Are you depressed?" may be sufficient for depression screening.

Non-Pharmacological Treatment[1,4]

- Overall goals for treatment of depression in hospice care are symptom reduction, social support, and the maintenance of morale.
- Treatment of depression preserves patient dignity, helps to maintain hope and meaning, and demonstrates a commitment to non-abandonment.
- Include the social worker, spiritual care counselor, or other team members and visitors as accepted by the patient, in development of the treatment plan.
- Concurrent management of co-morbid physical symptoms and preservation or repair of important relationships can help reduce the severity of depression.
- Initiate treatment when depressed or sad mood interferes with the patient's quality of life.
- Cognitive or interpersonal psychotherapy can be effective in the treatment of depression; limited stamina and attention span of patients with advanced illness may render such therapies impractical.

Pharmacotherapy[1,7-12]

- Mood should improve gradually with antidepressant treatment. Insomnia may respond early while fatigue and low energy often persists longer. Full resolution of depressive symptoms may take weeks.
- Efficacy of antidepressants in clinical trials ranges from 30-80% and response to medication varies from patient to patient. There are no studies demonstrating that any particular antidepressant works better or worse than any other.
- Choose initial antidepressant therapy based on several considerations:
  - Does the patient have a personal history of beneficial response to a particular drug?
    - May be the most reliable predictor of drug treatment response.
  - Does the patient have a family history of beneficial response to a particular drug?
    - May affect influence of family members on treatment and encouragement of patient.
  - What is the side effect profile of the drug and are any of the typical side effects potentially beneficial for the patient?
    - For example, use of mirtazapine in a patient with anorexia and weight loss or insomnia.
  - What is the patient's anticipated prognosis?
    - Some patients report early response in 1-2 weeks with antidepressants; full clinical response may not be seen for 6-8 weeks.
    - CNS stimulants may provide more rapid benefit especially for patients with a prognosis of less than 2-4 weeks.
  - What is the cost of this drug compared to comparable alternatives?
    - Because no individual antidepressant has been determined to be superior to any other, cost may be considered in choosing initial therapy.
- If a patient has a suboptimal treatment response, consider the following:
  - If below the recommended therapeutic dose range, consider a dose increase.
  - If within the recommended therapeutic dose range of a recently started antidepressant, if patient safety and prognosis allows, consider monitoring response over 6-8 weeks while maintaining the current dose.
  - Consider changing medications within the same antidepressant class or to a different class.
  - Consider obtaining psychiatric consultation for combination or augmentation therapies.

- The most common causes of antidepressant non-response are:
  - Inadequate dose
  - Insufficient duration of therapy
  - Non-adherence to treatment
  - Comorbid substance use
  - Misdiagnosis
  - Intolerable side-effects
- Maintenance treatment of depression lasts at least an additional 16-20 weeks after achievement of full resolution of depression before considering discontinuation of therapy. In hospice, maintenance treatment for a hospice patient generally continues to end of life.
- If a decision is made to discontinue long term antidepressant therapy, a gradual taper over a several days to a few weeks minimizes the risk of depressive relapse and reduces symptoms associated with discontinuation of the antidepressant.
- Antidepressant discontinuation syndrome includes flu-like symptoms, insomnia, paresthesias, hyperarousal, dizziness, and relapse of depression. Paroxetine and venlafaxine are commonly associated with withdrawal symptoms even with missed doses, however all antidepressant medications have been associated with discontinuation syndrome symptoms especially when abruptly discontinued.
- The FDA requires a boxed warning on labeling and in prescribing information for antidepressants regarding the increased risk of suicidal thinking and behavior in young adults during initial treatment (generally the first 4-8 weeks). Always monitor depressed patients for the emergence of suicidal ideation or intent.
- Ketamine (Ketalar) is a newly studied option for treatment of refractory depression. Small studies and case reports have demonstrated rapid resolution of depressive symptoms after oral or parenteral ketamine dosing. A case series in hospice patients included one-time oral doses of 0.5mg/kg with observation. The solution for injection is mixed with cola or juice for palatability.

Clinical Pearls[1,8-11]

- CNS stimulants may be chosen first line due to the rapid therapeutic onset when the estimated life expectancy of the patient is short, but there are exceptions. Situations where one might choose a traditional antidepressant over a CNS stimulant include:
  - Unable to tolerate CNS stimulants.
  - History of poor response to CNS stimulants.
  - History of good response to traditional antidepressants.
  - Additional therapeutic benefit with traditional antidepressants (e.g., neuropathic pain, anorexia, insomnia).
- When starting therapy with a CNS stimulant, assess the patient daily and increase the dose in the smallest increment available until depression resolves or the patient experiences adverse effects.
- In patients with bipolar disorder antidepressant use without concurrent mood stabilizer or antipsychotic may risk precipitating mania. Always ask about a personal or family history of mania or bipolar disorder before starting a new antidepressant.

Pharmacological Management of Depression

Generic Name (Trade Name)	Adult Starting Dose	Routes	Common Strengths and Formulations	Comments
CNS Stimulants				
Dextro-amphetamine (Dexedrine®)	5 mg QAM	PO	**Tablets:** 5 mg, 10 mg **Oral solution:** 5 mg/5 mL	• C-II controlled substance. • May counteract opiate-induced sedation. • May precipitate delirium. • May induce tolerance with prolonged use. • Use immediate release preparations.

Continued

Generic Name (Trade Name)	Adult Starting Dose	Routes	Common Strengths and Formulations	Comments
CNS Stimulants, *continued*				
Methylphenidate (Ritalin®)	5 mg QAM	PO	**Tablets:** 5 mg, 10 mg, 20 mg **Chewable tablets:** 2.5 mg, 5 mg, 10 mg **Oral solution:** 5 mg/5 mL 10 mg/5 mL	• C-II controlled substance. • May counteract opiate-induced sedation. • May precipitate delirium. • May induce tolerance with prolonged use. • Use immediate release preparations.
Selective Serotonin Reuptake Inhibitors (SSRI)				
Citalopram (Celexa®)	20 mg Daily	PO	**Tablets:** 10 mg, 20 mg, 40 mg **Oral solution:** 10 mg/5 mL	• Useful if expected survival exceeds a few weeks. • Review CYP450 system mediated drug interactions. • Not constipating; low risk for precipitating delirium.
Escitalopram (Lexapro®)	5 mg Daily	PO	**Tablets:** 5mg, 10 mg, 20 mg **Oral solution:** 5 mg/5 mL	• Reliability of reputed faster onset of action unclear. • Useful if expected survival exceeds a few weeks. • Review CYP450 system mediated drug interactions. • Not constipating; low risk for precipitating delirium.
Fluoxetine (Prozac®)	10 mg Daily	PO	**Tablets:** 10 mg, 20 mg, 60 mg **Capsules:** 10 mg, 20 mg, 40 mg **Oral solution:** 20 mg/5 mL	• SSRI with longest half-life. • Useful if expected survival exceeds a few weeks. • Review CYP450 system mediated drug interactions. • Not constipating; low risk for precipitating delirium.
Sertraline (Zoloft®)	25 mg Daily	PO	**Tablets:** 25 mg, 50 mg, 100 mg **Oral solution:** 20 mg/mL	• Useful if expected survival exceeds a few weeks. • Review CYP450 system mediated drug interactions. • Not constipating; low risk for precipitating delirium.
Paroxetine (Paxil®, Pexeva®, Brisdelle®)	10 mg Daily	PO	**Tablets:** 10 mg, 20 mg, 30 mg, 40 mg **Capsules:** 7.5 mg **Oral suspension:** 10 mg/5 mL **ER Tablets:** 12.5 mg, 25 mg, 37.5 mg	• SSRI with highest risk of anticholinergic side effects • SSRI with shortest half-life, withdrawal symptoms can occur with missed doses. • ER formulations are expensive. • Capsule formulation only indicated for vasomotor symptoms of menopause. • Review CYP450 system mediated drug interactions.

Continued

Generic Name (Trade Name)	Adult Starting Dose	Routes	Common Strengths and Formulations	Comments
Serotonin-Norepinephrine Reuptake Inhibitors (SNRI)				
Venlafaxine (Effexor®)	Immediate release: 37.5 mg BID Extended release: 75mg Daily	PO	**Tablets:** 25 mg, 37.5 mg, 50 mg, 75 mg, 100 mg **ER Capsules:** 37.5 mg, 75 mg, 150 mg	• Can cause hypertension. • IR product requires BID dosing. • May treat neuropathic pain. • Withdrawal symptoms can occur with missed doses. • Capsules maybe opened and sprinkled on applesauce and swallowed without chewing. • Do not crush or chew capsules.
Duloxetine (Cymbalta®)	20mg Daily	PO	**Capsules:** 20 mg, 30 mg, 60 mg	• FDA-approved for diabetic neuropathy, chronic musculoskeletal pain, and fibromyalgia in addition to antidepressant indications. • Capsules maybe opened and sprinkled on applesauce and swallowed without chewing. • Capsules contain enteric coated granules, do not crush or chew.
Other Antidepressants				
Mirtazapine (Remeron®)	15 mg QHS	PO	**Tablets:** 7.5 mg, 15 mg, 30 mg, 45 mg **Oral disintegrating tablets:** 15 mg, 30 mg, 45 mg	• Antidepressant with mixed neurotransmitter and receptor effects: serotonin, norepinephrine, histamine, alpha-adrenergic. • Doses ≤ 30mg tend to have more sedation. • Useful for comorbid insomnia or anorexia.
Bupropion (Wellbutrin®)	100 mg BID	PO	**Tablets:** 75 mg, 100 mg **12-hr tablets:** 100 mg, 150 mg, 200 mg **24-h tablets:** 150 mg, 300 mg, 450 mg	• Primary effects on dopamine and norepinephrine. • May be used to augment SSRI in refractory depression. • Select dosage forms are brand only and expensive.

See Drug Dosing for Liver and Renal Disease for additional drug information.

References

1. Practice guideline for the treatment of patients with major depressive disorder. 3rd ed. Arlington, VA. American Psychiatric Association; 2010. Available at http://psychiatryonline.org/guidelines.aspx. Accessed November 14, 2013.
2. Breitbart W, Bruera E, Chochinov H, Lynch M. Neuropsychiatric syndromes and psychological symptoms in patients with advanced cancer. *J Pain Symptom Manage.* 1995; 10; 131-141.
3. American Psychiatric Association. Major depressive disorder. In: Diagnostic and statistical manual of mental disorders, 5th ed. Arlington, VA: American Psychiatric Association; 2013. Available at dsm.psychiatryonline.org. Accessed November 14, 2013.
4. Chochinov HM, Wilson KG, Enns M, Lander S: "Are you depressed?" Screening for depression in the terminally ill. *Am J Psychiatry.* 1997; 154: 674-676.
5. Yesavage JA, Brink TL, Rose TL, et al. Development and validation of a geriatric depression screening scale: Preliminary Report. *J Psychiat Res.*1983; 17:37-49.
6. Hamilton M, A rating scale for depression. *J Neurol Neurosurg Psychiatry.* 1960; 23:56-62

7. Berman RM, Cappiello A, Oren DA, et al. Antidepressant effects of ketamine in depressed patients. *Biol Psychiatry.* 2000; 47:351-354.

8. Masand PS, Tesar GE: Use of stimulants in the medically ill. *Psychiatr Clin North Am.* 1996; 19:515-547.

9. Shuster JL, Breitbart W, Chochinov HM: Psychiatric aspects of excellent end-of-life care. *Psychosomatics,*1999; 40:1, 1-4.

10. Balt S. Assessing and enhancing the effectiveness of antidepressants. [Internet]. *Psychiatr Times* 2014;June 13, 2014. Available at http://www.psychiatrictimes.com/depression/assessing-and-enhancing-effectiveness-antidepressants. Accessed July 23, 2014.

11. Warner C, Bobo W, Warner C, Reid S, Rachal J. Antidepressant discontinuation syndrome. *Am Fam Physician.* 2006;74(3):449-456. Available at http://www.aafp.org/afp/2006/0801/p449.html. Accessed July 23, 2014.

12. U.S. Food and Drug Administration (FDA). Antidepressant use in children, adolescents, and adults. May 2, 2007. Available at http://www.fda.gov/Drugs/DrugSafety/InformationbyDrugClass/ucm096273.htm. Accessed July 23, 2014.

13. Irwin S, Iglewicz A. Oral ketamine for the rapid treatment of depression and anxiety in patients receiving hospice care. *J Palliat Med* 2010;13(7):903-908

Treatment Algorithm for Depression

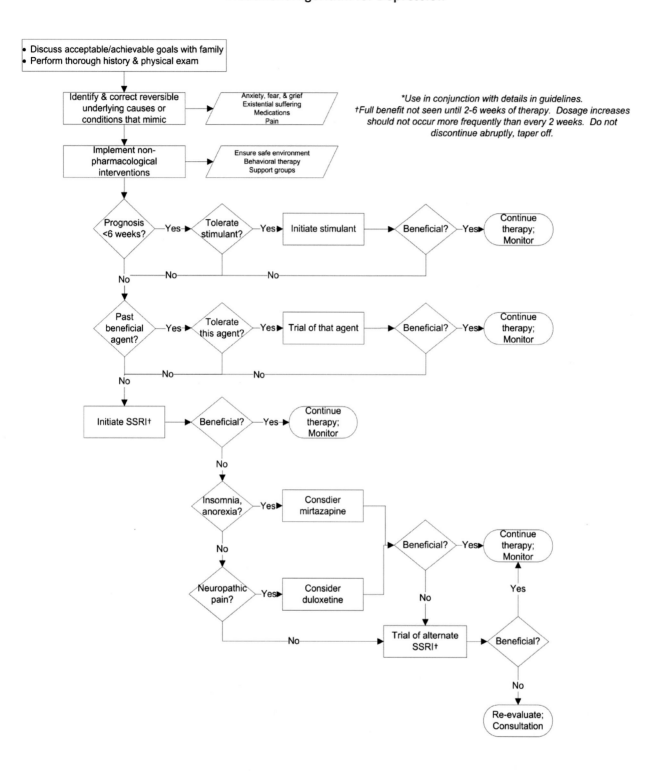

- Discuss acceptable/achievable goals with family
- Perform thorough history & physical exam

Identify & correct reversible underlying causes or conditions that mimic

Anxiety, fear, & grief
Existential suffering
Medications
Pain

*Use in conjunction with details in guidelines.
†Full benefit not seen until 2-6 weeks of therapy. Dosage increases should not occur more frequently than every 2 weeks. Do not discontinue abruptly, taper off.

Implement non-pharmacological interventions

Ensure safe environment
Behavioral therapy
Support groups

Prognosis <6 weeks? → Yes → Tolerate stimulant? → Yes → Initiate stimulant → Beneficial? → Yes → Continue therapy; Monitor

No / No / No

Past beneficial agent? → Yes → Tolerate this agent? → Yes → Trial of that agent → Beneficial? → Yes → Continue therapy; Monitor

No / No / No

Initiate SSRI† → Beneficial? → Yes → Continue therapy; Monitor

No

Insomnia, anorexia? → Yes → Consdier mirtazapine → Beneficial? → Yes → Continue therapy; Monitor

No / No

Neuropathic pain? → Yes → Consider duloxetine

No → Trial of alternate SSRI† → Beneficial? → Yes → Continue therapy; Monitor

No → Re-evaluate; Consultation

Diarrhea

Introduction and Background[1-2]

- Diarrhea is passage of liquid or unformed stools at an increased frequency; however, "frequency" is patient-specific. Diarrhea results from an imbalance of the absorption and secretion properties of the intestinal tract. The imbalance may be from decreased absorption or increased secretion.
- Diarrhea may be an acute (< 2 weeks), persistent (2-4 weeks), or chronic (> 4 weeks) problem.
- Treat the cause of the diarrhea rather than just the symptom, if possible. In most cases, diarrhea is self-limiting, but can lead to dehydration, electrolyte imbalance, fatigue, and skin breakdown, especially in patients with poor oral intake and reduced mobility.

Prevalence[2]

- Diarrhea will occur in most people, associated with an acute illness and lasting less than a week.
- Diarrhea affects approximately 7 to 10% of patients at the time of hospice admission. Up to 80% of patients who have recently received chemotherapy or those with gastrointestinal carcinoid tumors have persistent or chronic diarrhea.

Causes

- Overmedication with laxatives is a common cause of diarrhea in palliative medicine.
- Bacterial and/or viral gastroenteritis, also commonly known as food poisoning or stomach flu, should be considered as a potential cause of diarrhea across age groups and diagnoses (Table 1).

Table 1. Characteristics of Common Gastroenteritis Pathogens[1,3]

Pathogen Examples	Characteristics & Associated Symptoms
Campylobacter	Watery, then bloody
Cryptosporidium	Watery, mucoid
Escherichia coli (E. coli)	Watery, then bloody; associated with vomiting
Giardia	Chronic, greenish
Norwalk virus (norovirus)	Watery, yellow or greenish; associated with vomiting and fever; highly contagious
Salmonella	Sometimes bloody or greenish; associated with fever
Shigella	Bloody, mucoid; associated with fever

Table 2. Causes of Diarrhea[1,3]

Causes	Examples
Bone marrow transplant	Graft-vs-host disease (GVHD), total-body irradiation
Chemotherapy	Capecitabine, cisplatin, taxanes, methotrexate, VEGFR blockers
Comorbid conditions	Diabetes, hyperthyroidism, inflammatory bowel diseases
Diet	Lactose intolerance, fruit juices, high-fat foods, sorbitol-containing foods, spicy foods, gas-forming foods and beverages
Drug adverse effects	Broad spectrum antibiotics, magnesium-containing antacids, colchicine, digoxin, metoclopramide, laxatives
Fecal	Constipation leading to impaction and obstruction
Infection	*Clostridium difficile* – see Risk Factors (Table 3). See also Table 1 for other pathogens and *Infection GEMS.*
Malignancies	Carcinoid syndrome, colon cancer, lymphoma, pancreatic cancer
Psychological	Stress, anxiety, Munchausen syndrome
Radiation therapy	Irradiation to abdomen, lumbar, pelvic region
Surgery/Procedures	Celiac plexus block, cholecystectomy, intestinal resection

Clinical Characteristics & Assessment[1,4,5]

- Diarrhea may also be objectively defined as more than 200 mL of water in the stool (more than 90% water) and is often accompanied by gas, abdominal pain, an urgency to defecate, nausea, and vomiting.
- If diarrhea is accompanied by fever, occult blood, steatorrhea, appetite changes, weight loss, or tenesmus (painful, ineffective straining to defecate), these may be signs of a more serious underlying condition.
- Diarrhea may be classified into four general types, based on mechanism:
    - *Osmotic* diarrhea may be caused by a non-absorbed substance that draws fluid into the intestinal lumen. This may occur with disorders such as pancreatitis, bile duct obstruction, celiac disease, or Whipple's disease. Osmotic diarrhea may also occur with ingestion of certain sugar substitutes (sorbitol, mannitol, xylitol) or lactose intolerance.
    - *Secretory* diarrhea may be caused by bacterial toxins, viruses, and some drugs. 90% of acute diarrhea is caused by infection and is often accompanied by vomiting, fever, and abdominal pain. Other causes include chronic alcohol ingestion, carcinoid tumor, Addison's disease, bowel resection or fistula, and partial bowel obstruction or impaction.
    - *Exudative or Inflammatory* diarrhea may result from inflammation, causing plasma proteins, mucus, and blood to appear in stool. It is usually accompanied by fever, pain and other manifestations of inflammation.
    - *Motility* disorders, such as diabetic neuropathy, hyperthyroidism, or irritable bowel syndrome, may cause decreased absorption.
- For patients with limited mobility requiring opioids for pain or symptom management, watery diarrhea may be a sign of a fecal impaction.
- Ask patient/caregiver assessment questions to determine appropriate therapy. Choice of agent should be individualized according to the patient's history and the primary cause of the diarrhea, if possible.
    - When did the diarrhea begin?
    - How frequent are the episodes?
    - Are there any other symptoms that may be related to the diarrhea?
    - Have any anti-diarrheal medications been used?
    - Has the diet been altered?
    - Are there any other persons that have had diarrhea that have contact with the patient?
    - What medications is the patient taking?
    - Are there any related co-morbidities (e.g., irritable bowel syndrome)?

Table 3. Risk Factors Associated with *C. difficile* Diarrhea[6,7]

Advanced age > 64 years
Immunosuppression due to cancer chemotherapy or HIV/AIDS infection
Nursing facility residents
Recent hospitalization, especially longer hospital stays
Medications
• Antibiotics, especially cephalosporins, fluoroquinolones, and clindamycin
• Proton pump inhibitors, possibly due to suppression of protective effect of stomach acid

Non-Pharmacological Treatment[1-5,8]

- For mild cases of diarrhea, the BRAT (bananas, rice, apples, toast) diet may reduce stool frequency.
- Eat small, frequent meals containing foods that are low in fiber, contain minerals, and do not stimulate or irritate the gastrointestinal tract.
- Avoid offending foods, including lactose-containing food (milk and dairy products), spicy foods, alcohol, caffeine-containing foods and beverages, certain fruit juices, gas-forming foods and beverages, high-fiber foods, and high-fat foods.
- Rehydrate the patient and replace electrolytes. Increase clear liquid intake as tolerated to balance fluid loss from diarrhea (e.g., water, sports drinks, broth, weak decaffeinated teas, caffeine-free soft drinks, clear juices, and gelatin).
- For patients with fecal incontinence, apply barrier cream or ointment to perianal area to help prevent skin breakdown.

Pharmacotherapy

- Medication selection for diarrhea is based on the most likely etiology. Regardless of the cause, oral rehydration therapy is an important component of symptom management. Parenteral rehydration, including hypodermoclysis, may be offered in severe dehydration if in line with patient and family goals of care.
- Discontinue laxative use temporarily. If diarrhea resolves, laxative may be restarted at a lower dose.
- Assess patient for possible infection prior to initiating anti-diarrheal medications.
- Empiric treatment with metronidazole is indicated if watery, foul-smelling diarrhea is present along with any risk factors for *C. difficile* infection (see Table 3).

Clinical Pearls

- Nausea with diarrhea, or foul-smelling diarrhea, may indicate an infectious process or toxin ingestion.
- Due to lack of evidence, use of probiotics is not recommended by the Infectious Disease Society of America (ISDA) for primary prevention of *C. difficile* infection.
- Stool culture analysis testing of feces samples can help determine if there are cells, mucus, fat, blood, parasites, or bacterial toxins in the stool. Obtaining feces samples can be difficult or uncomfortable, especially for the patient and family caregivers; this process may be reserved for severe or refractory cases of diarrhea.

Pharmacological Management of Diarrhea

Generic Name (Trade Name)	Adult Starting Dose	Routes	Common Strengths and Formulations	Comments
Anti-Motility Agents				
Diphenoxylate with atropine (Lomotil®)	2 tablets, then 1 tablet after each loose stool (not to exceed 8 per 24 hrs)	PO	**Solution:** 2.5mg/5ml **Tablets:** 2.5mg	• Not recommended in patients with bacterial diarrhea
Loperamide (Immodium AD®, Kaopectate II, Maalox Antidiarrheal®, Pepto® Diarrhea Control)	2 tablets, then 1 tablet after each loose stool (not to exceed 8 per 24 hrs)	PO	**Tablets/Capsules:** 2mg **Solution:** 1mg/5ml	• Not recommended in patients with bacterial diarrhea
Paregoric	5-10 ml QD-QID	PO	**Solution:** 2mg/5ml	• Not recommended in patients with bacterial diarrhea
Codeine	10-60 mg BID-QID	PO IM SC	**Tablets:** 15, 30, 60 mg **Solution:** 15 mg/ml **Injection:** 15, 30 mg/ml	• Not recommended in patients with bacterial diarrhea • Acetaminophen with codeine may be used instead of pure codeine, for cost and ease of prescribing.
Absorbents and Adsorbents				
Bismuth subsalicylate (Pepto-Bismol®, Kaopectate®, Maalox® Total Stomach Relief)	2 tablets (or 30 ml) every 30 min to 1 hr, (max 8 doses per 24 hrs)	PO	**Tablets:** Bismuth subsalicylate 262mg **Suspension:** Bismuth subsalicylate 262 mg/15ml	• Caution with concomitant aspirin; impaction may occur in debilitated patients • May turn stool dark or black in color • Do not use in immuno-compromised patients due to risk of bismuth encephalopathy

Continued

Generic Name (Trade Name)	Adult Starting Dose	Routes	Common Strengths and Formulations	Comments
Bulking Agents for Bulking Loose/Watery Stool				
Psyllium (Metamucil®, Fiberall®)	1 dose up to TID	PO	**Tablets:** 4 tablets / dose, **Powder:** 1 tbsp powder/dose **Wafers:** 2 wafers/ dose	• Separate drug administration times with other medication due to decreased absorption • Take with 8oz water
Methylcellulose (Citrucel®, FiberEase®)	2-4 caplets or 5-10 tsp 1 to 3 times daily	PO	**Caplets:** 500mg **Powder**	• Not useful in dehydrated patients • Take with 8oz water
Calcium polycarbophil (FiberCon®, Equalactin®, Phillips' Fibercaps®)	2 tablets (1 g) QD-QID (max 6 g per 24 hrs)	PO	**Caplet/tablets:** calcium polycarbophil 625mg (equivalent to 500mg polycarbophil)	• Epigastric pain and bloating may occur with large doses • Take with 8oz water
Cholestyramine (Questran®)	1 packet (4g) QD	PO	**Powder**: 4g pkt for reconstitution	• Effective in controlling chologenic (bile salt) or radiation-induced diarrhea
Infection: Antibiotics				
Metronidazole (Flagyl®)	250-500mg TID-QID for 10 - 14 days	PO IV	**Tablets:** 250mg, 500mg **Suspension:** Can make extemporaneously	• Drug of choice for *C.difficile* & *Giardia* infection • May be used empirically if diarrhea follows course of antibiotics • Length of therapy determined by severity of infection
Vancomycin (Vancocin®)	125mg QID for 10 - 14 days	PO	**Capsules:** 125mg **Solution:** Can make extemporaneously	• PO only, IV ineffective • Consider oral vancomycin if metronidazole ineffective • Resistance occurs quickly to enterococcus • Length of therapy determined by severity of infection
Infection: Probiotics				
Lactobacillus spp (Bacid®, Culturelle®, Lactinex®)	1-2 doses QD	PO	Active probiotic species and content varies by manufacturer	• Dietary supplement, *no FDA-approved indications* • No oral absorption, works locally in the lower GI tract • Review product specific ingredient lists prior to use; may contain allergens: milk, soy, yeast
Saccharomyces boulardii (Florastor®)	250mg BID	PO	**Capsules:** 250mg **Powder:** 250mg/pkt	• Avoid in patients with yeast allergy; *S. boulardii* is a live yeast probiotic • Risk of fungemia; avoid use in immunocompromised patients

Continued

Generic Name (Trade Name)	Adult Starting Dose	Routes	Common Strengths and Formulations	Comments
Carcinoid Syndrome				
Cyproheptadine (Periactin®)	4mg TID	PO	**Tablets:** 4mg	• 12-48mg/day in divided doses
Octreotide (Sandostatin®)	50mcg BID-TID titrating up as needed (mean daily dosage is 300 mcg)	SC IV	**Ampules:** 50, 100, 500 mcg (as acetate) **Multidose Vials:** 200, 1000mcg/mL	• For severe intractable diarrhea from carcinoid tumors
Steatorrhea/Pancreatic Insufficiency				
Pancrelipase (Multiple brands)	30,000 IU pancreatic lipase with each meal	PO	**Tablets:** various strengths	• Fatty stool from pancreatic insufficiency • +/- H_2 blocker or PPI

See Drug Dosing for Liver and Renal Disease for additional drug information.

References

1. Camilleri M, Murray JA. Chapter 40. Diarrhea and Constipation. In: Longo DL, Fauci AS, Kasper DL, Hauser SL, Jameson JL, Loscalzo J, eds. *Harrison's Principles of Internal Medicine*. 18th ed. New York: McGraw-Hill; 2012. http://www.accessmedicine.com/content.aspx?aID=9112979. Accessed June 13, 2013.

2. National Cancer Institute: PDQ® Gastrointestinal Complications. Bethesda, MD: National Cancer Institute. Date last modified 07/18/2012. Available at: http://cancer.gov/cancertopics/pdq/supportivecare/gastrointestinalcomplications/HealthProfessional. Accessed 06/13/2013.

3. National Digestive Diseases Information Clearinghouse (NDDIC). Viral gastroenteritis. Bethesda, MD: National Institutes of Health. Date last modified 4/23/2013. Available at: http://digestive.niddk.nih.gov/ddiseases/pubs/viralgastroenteritis/

4. Sykes N. Chapter 154. Constipation and diarrhea. In: Walsh D, Caraceni A, Fainsinger R, Foley K, Glare P, Goh C, et al, eds. *Palliative Medicine*. Philadelphia, PA: Saunders-Elsevier; 2009:846-854.

5. Horne J, Swanson L. Diarrhea. *US Pharmacist* 1997;22(5):1-14. Available at: http://legacy.uspharmacist.com/. Accessed 6/13/2013.

6. Association for Professionals in Infection Control and Epidemiology, Inc. (APIC). Guide to preventing *Clostridium difficile* infections: APIC implementation guide. Washington, DC: APIC; 2013. Available at http://www.apic.org/Professional-Practice/Implementation-guides. Accessed May 13, 2014.

7. Cohen S, Gerding D, Johnson S, et al. Clinical practice guidelines for Clostridium difficile infection in adults: 2010 update by the Society for Healthcare Epidemiology of America (SHEA) and the Infectious Disease Society of America (ISDA). *Infect Control Hosp Epidemiol* 2010;31(5):431-455.

8. Schiller LR, Sellin JH. Chapter 15. Diarrhea. In: Feldman M, Friedman LS, Brandt LJ, eds. *Sleisenger & Fordtran's Gastrointestinal and Liver Disease*. 9th ed. Philadelphia, Pa: Saunders Elsevier; 2010.

Treatment Algorithm for Diarrhea

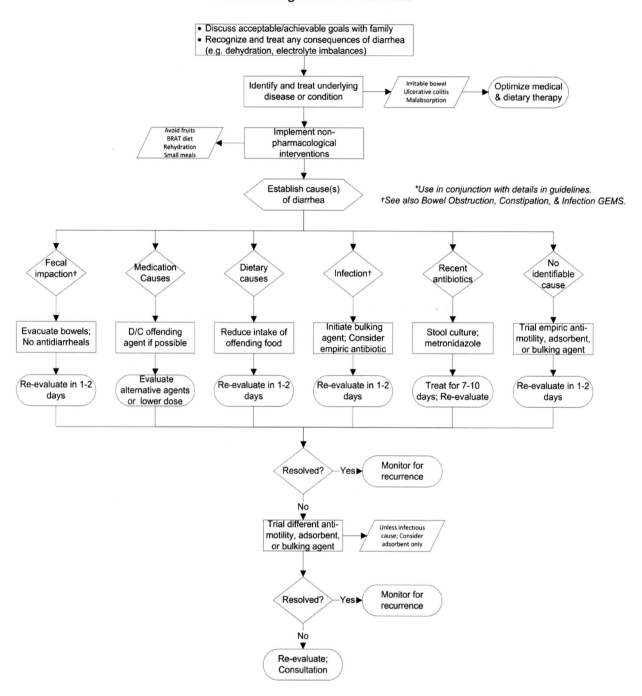

Dysphagia

Introduction and Background [1-4]
- Dysphagia is described as difficulty moving food from the mouth to the stomach.
- Normal swallowing is a coordinated process that involves a complex series of voluntary and involuntary neuromuscular contractions.
- Swallowing is typically divided into three distinct phases: oral, pharyngeal, and esophageal.
- Dysphagia can be caused by neurological, cognitive, muscular, or structural changes, as well as medications and weakness.
- In elderly patients with dysphagia, there is significant morbidity and mortality that result from choking, aspiration, dehydration, pneumonia, and malnutrition.
- Dysphagia can lead to physical discomfort while eating or drinking, as well as anxiety at mealtime or medication time.
- The inability to maintain nutrition through the oral route is a marker of the dying process. The presence of dysphagia may allow discussion of overall end of life goals.
- Management of dysphagia in palliative care consists of restoring safe and effective oral feeding according to the patient's goals of care.

Prevalence [1,2,5]
- Because of the multiple potential etiologies, the exact prevalence of dysphagia is unknown.
- Two of the more common situations associated with dysphagia include stroke (incidence range: 22-70%) and esophageal cancer (incidence 70%).
- Dysphagia is one of seven symptoms most commonly experienced during the last 48 hours of life.

Causes [1,2,4,6]
- Age-related changes in oropharyngeal and esophageal functioning
- Weakness and de-conditioning due to progression of underlying disease
- Medications:
  o CNS depressants cause impaired cognition which can affect swallowing
  o Anticholinergics cause xerostomia
  o Drugs that cause esophageal injury (e.g. NSAIDs, steroids, bisphosphonates, potassium chloride, tetracycline, iron preparations)
- Radiation therapy
- Esophageal strictures
- Reflux esophagitis, gastroesophageal reflux disease (GERD)
- Local tumor burden (e.g., head and neck, thyroid)
- Impaired motor function (e.g., stroke)
- Neurodegenerative disease (e.g., Parkinson's disease, stroke, multiple sclerosis, dementia, amyotrophic lateral sclerosis, myasthenia gravis)
- Localized infection (e.g., candidiasis, herpes)

Clinical Characteristics [1,2,4,6]
- Dysphagia is usually associated with coughing or choking on food or fluids; but it may also present as the inability to swallow medications, decreased oral intake, or weight loss.
- Patients may describe the sensation of food being stuck in the throat, vocal changes, pain while swallowing, shortness of breath following eating or drinking, or the appearance of drooling.
- Dysphagia may be classified as oropharyngeal or esophageal (Table 1).
- Oropharyngeal dysphagia refers to difficulty in passage of the food bolus from the mouth to the esophagus. Neurological disorders that affect skeletal muscles often lead to oropharyngeal dysphagia.
- In esophageal dysphagia, there is disordered passage of the food bolus through the esophagus.

Table 1. Signs and Symptoms of Dysphagia by Phases

Phase	Signs & Symptoms
Oral or pharyngeal	<ul><li>Coughing or choking while swallowing</li><li>Difficulty initiating swallowing</li><li>Inability to chew or propel food into pharynx</li><li>Sialorrhea (excessive production of saliva)</li><li>Unexplained weight loss</li><li>Change in dietary habits</li><li>Recurrent pneumonia</li><li>Change in voice or speech (wet voice)</li><li>Nasal regurgitation</li></ul>
Esophageal	<ul><li>Sensation of food sticking in the chest or throat</li><li>Chest pain</li><li>Late regurgitation hours after eating</li><li>Oral or pharyngeal regurgitation</li><li>Change in dietary habits</li><li>Recurrent pneumonia</li></ul>

Non-Pharmacological Treatment [1-3,5]

- Artificial nutrition and hydration have not been proven effective in prolonging life, preventing aspiration, or improving nutrition in patients with dementia.
- Patients with dysphagia may choose to continue oral intake. Provide patient and family information on the risks of dehydration, malnutrition, and aspiration.
- Depending on patient goals of care and estimated life expectancy, self-expanding metal stent insertion may be an option for palliation of dysphagia in patients with esophageal cancer.
- Prior to placing a feeding tube, establish goals of care and a plan for periodic re-evaluation of benefits.
- Dietary modification, including the use of soft or pureed foods, thickening agents, thorough chewing of food, and staying upright while eating, may allow for easier swallowing.
- Frequent, small meals may reduce fatigue while maintaining caloric intake.
- Removing environmental distractions during meal times may also be important in certain settings.
- Ice chips, sugarless candy, or artificial saliva may help with xerostomia or mucositis-induced dysphagia.
- Dental concerns, including oral ulcers and tooth disease or decay should be ruled out as causes of pain or refusal to eat.
- Some patients can learn to hold their breath before swallowing to allow for full laryngeal closure. Additionally, to prevent aspiration of pharyngeal and laryngeal residue, patients can cough and swallow after an initial swallow to clear the residue.
- The National Dysphagia Diet was established in 2002 by the American Dietetic Association to establish a standard terminology for dietary texture modification for patients with swallowing disorders (Table 2).

Table 2. National Dysphagia Diet (NDD) Texture Terminology[6-8]

Terminology	Description
Food	
Level 1: Pureed	Homogenous, very cohesive, pudding-like, requires very little chewing ability
Level 2: Mechanical Altered	Cohesive, moist, semi-solid foods, requiring some chewing
Level 3: Advanced	Soft foods that require more chewing ability
Regular	All foods allowed
Liquid	
Thin	Water, orange juice
Nectar-like	Tomato juice, fluid-type yogurt
Honey-like	Curd-type yogurt, cream soup, orange juice, thin soup with thickener
Spoon-thick	Pudding, mashed potatoes

Pharmacotherapy [1,9-11]

- Medication use in dysphagia follows two paths:
  - ○ Treating underlying causes
  - ○ Providing symptom relief
- Combine both treatment of underlying causes and symptomatic relief whenever possible (Table 3).

Table 3. Treatment Options for Dysphagia[1,9-11]

Cause of Dysphagia	Treatment Options
Candidiasis	Non-systemic antifungals such as nystatin suspension possibly combined with a local anesthetic (e.g., lidocaine) if localized pain is present. If ineffective or undesirable, consider oral fluconazole and a systemic opioid.
Esophageal spasm	Anticholinergic medications
GERD/Reflux	H_2 receptor antagonist (H2RA) or proton pump inhibitor (PPI)
Mucositis	Topical viscous lidocaine as a single ingredient or in combination with other agents to provide localized analgesia. Use caution with local anesthetics, as some patients may have worsening of their swallowing reflex.
Anatomical swelling	Steroids, such as dexamethasone, may be useful for temporary reduction. Steroids can cause GI ulceration and worsen dysphagia. Weigh risk vs. benefit of starting steroid therapy.
Tumor burden	Palliative chemotherapy or radiation therapy may be of some benefit for patients where tumor burden is the main concern.
Xerostomia	Review medication profile for potential causes and consider saliva substitutes, alcohol-free mouthwashes and rinses. *See Xerostomia GEMS.*

Clinical Pearls [9]

- Some food thickeners can adversely affect the taste of foods.
- Positioning patient as close to a 90-degree angle as possible makes swallowing easier and safer.
- When a patient is unable to consume a variety of foods, nutritional support in the form of supplements may offer means of assuring adequate nutrition.
- When offering nutritional support, allow patient to taste several different products to find the most palatable.
- Many supplements taste best when chilled, rather than at room temperature.
- Orally disintegrating tablets, transdermal, rectal, buccal delivery systems, as well as altered-thickness liquid medications may ease medication administration.

Pharmacological Management of Dysphagia

Generic Name (Trade Name)	Adult Starting Dose	Routes	Common Strengths and Formulations	Comments
Anticholinergics for Esophageal Spasm				
Glycopyrrolate (Robinul®)	PO: 1 mg BID PRN SC/IV: 0.1 mg BID	PO SC IV IM	**Injection:** 0.2 mg/mL **Tablets:** 1 mg, 2 mg **Oral solution:** 1 mg/5 mL	• Oral solution is expensive; oral absorption can be erratic. • Does not cross blood brain barrier minimizing CNS side effects (e.g., sedation, confusion).
Hyoscyamine (Levsin®)	PO/SL: 0.125 mg Q4H PRN	PO SL SC IM IV	**Tablets:** 0.125 mg **SL Tablets:** 0.125 mg **ER Tablets:** 0.375 mg **Oral solution:** 0.125 mg/5 mL	• Oral solution is expensive. • Available in sublingual formulation for administration in patients who cannot swallow.

Continued

Generic Name (Trade Name)	Adult Starting Dose	Routes	Common Strengths and Formulations	Comments
Anticholinergics for Esophageal Spasm, *continued*				
Scopolamine (Transderm Scop®)	1 patch every 3 days	TD	**Patch:** 1.5 mg	• Difficult to titrate due to single patch strength and delayed onset of effect. • Do not cut patches.
Antifungals for Candidiasis				
Nystatin (Mycostatin®)	Swish & swallow 5-10 mL QID for 14 days	PO	**Oral solution:** 2.5 mg/5 mL	• First-line therapy for oral thrush. • PRN use not recommended.
Fluconazole (Diflucan®)	200 mg PO x 1 day, then 100 mg Daily for 13 days	PO	**Tablets:** 50 mg, 100 mg, 150 mg, 200 mg **Suspension:** 40 mg/mL	• Reduce dose and frequency in patients with renal dysfunction. • Can be crushed. • Use when systemic therapy needed to treat esophageal candidiasis.
Corticosteroids for Inflammation/Swelling				
Dexamethasone (Decadron®)	8mg Daily	PO IV SC IM	**Tablets:** 0.5 mg, 0.75 mg, 1 mg, 1.5 mg, 2 mg, 4 mg, 6 mg **Oral solution:** 1 mg/mL **Injection:** 4 mg/mL	• May titrate to 32mg/day • Administer IV over 5-10 minutes, rapid bolus associated with perianal pain. • May give dose once daily or BID (morning and noon) to prevent insomnia.
H₂ Receptor Antagonists (H2RA) for GERD				
Famotidine (Pepcid®)	10-20 mg Daily	PO	**Tablets:** 10 mg, 20 mg, 40 mg **Suspension:** 40 mg/5 mL **Injection:** 10 mg/mL	• OTC products more cost effective than prescription. • Due to fewer side effects and drug interaction profile, famotidine is the preferred H2RA in geriatrics.
Ranitidine (Zantac®)	75-150 mg Daily	PO	**Tablets:** 75 mg, 150 mg, 300 mg **Syrup:** 15 mg/mL **Injection:** 25 mg/mL	• OTC products more cost effective than prescription. • Greater risk of confusion with higher doses, especially in geriatric patients or those with renal insufficiency.
Proton Pump Inhibitors (PPI) for GERD				
Lansoprazole (Prevacid®, Prevacid24HR®)	15-30 mg Daily	PO	**Capsules:** 15 mg, 30 mg **Oral disintegrating tablets:** 15 mg, 30 mg	• OTC products more cost effective than prescription. • All PPIs have similar effectiveness. • Evaluate the need to continue. Can step down to H2RA.

Continued

Generic Name (Trade Name)	Adult Starting Dose	Routes	Common Strengths and Formulations	Comments
Proton Pump Inhibitors (PPI) for GERD, *continued*				
Omeprazole (Prilosec®, Prilosec OTC®)	20-40 mg Daily	PO	**Capsules:** 10 mg, 20 mg, 40 mg **Tablets:** 20 mg	• Omeprazole OTC tends to be the most cost effective PPI. All PPIs have similar effectiveness. • Evaluate the need to continue. Can step down to H2RA. • Capsules may be opened and contents added to a bite of applesauce.
Pantoprazole (Protonix®)	40 mg Daily	PO	**Tablets:** 20 mg, 40 mg **Packets:** 40 mg	• Consider therapeutic interchange to an OTC PPI. All PPIs have similar effectiveness. • Evaluate the need to continue. Can step down to H2RA.
Topical Anesthetic for Mucositis				
Lidocaine viscous	Swish & spit 5-10 mL Q4H PRN	PO, topical	**Oral solution:** 2% viscous	• Lidocaine will numb the mouth and throat, advise patients to eat and drink cautiously after use. • Lidocaine is commonly included in "magic mouthwash" preparations.

See Drug Dosing for Liver and Renal Disease for additional drug information.

References

1. Pollens R, Hillenbrand K, Sharp, H. Dysphagia. In: Murphy K, Carroll C, Hetherington P, Bartz J, eds. *Palliative Medicine.* 1st ed. Philadelphia, PA: Saunders; 2009: 871-876.
2. Howden C. Management of acid-related disorders in patients with dysphagia. *Am J Med.* 2004;117 (5A)(suppl 1):44S-48S.
3. Weissman DE. Swallow studies, tube feedings, and the death spiral, 2nd edition. Fast Facts and Concepts. October 2007; 84. https://www.capc.org/fast-facts/84-swallow-studies-tube-feeding-and-death-spiral/.
4. Bramwell, B. Compliance to treatment in elderly dysphagic patients: potential benefits of alternate dosage forms. *Int J Pharm Compd.* 2009;13(6):498-505.
5. Sreedharan A, Harris K, Crellin A, et al. Interventions for dysphagia in oesophageal cancer. *Cochrane Database Syst Rev.* 2009(4):CD005048.
6. Understanding and implementing dysphagia diets. *Dietary Manager.* 2004:18-20.
7. American Dietetic Association. National Dysphagia Diet: Standardization for Optimal Care, 2002.
8. McCallum SL. The National Dysphagia Diet: Implementation at a regional rehabilitation center and hospital system. *J Am Diet Assoc.* 2003; 103(3):381-384.
9. Rosielle D. Oropharyngeal Candidiasis. Fast Facts and Concepts. December 2005;147. Available at: https://www.capc.org/fast-facts/147-oropharyngeal-candidiasis/.
10. Sheehan NJ. Dysphagia and other manifestations of oesophageal involvement in the musculoskeletal diseases. *Rheumatology.* 2008;47:746-752.
11. Goldstein N, Genden E, Morrison RS. Palliative care for patients with head and neck cancer. *JAMA.* 2008;299(15):1818-1825.

Treatment Algorithm for Dysphagia

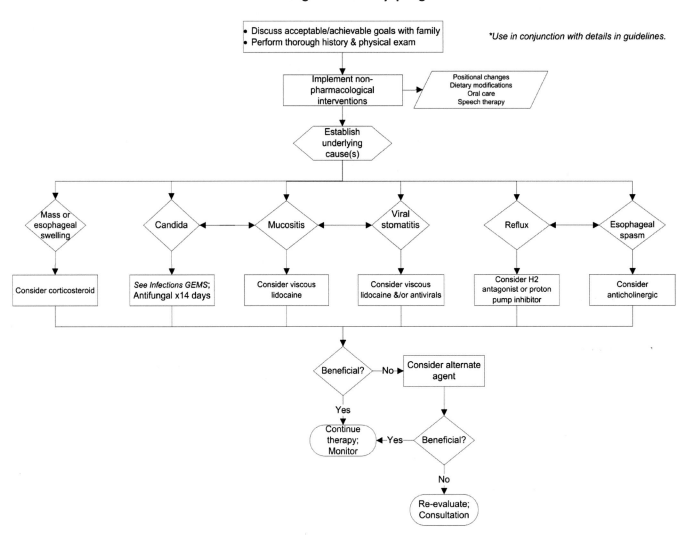

Dyspnea

Introduction and Background[1]
- Dyspnea is a distressing subjective breathing discomfort described as shortness of breath, air hunger, increased effort to breath, chest tightness, rapid breathing, incomplete exhalation, or feeling of suffocation.
- Dyspnea is subjective, multidimensional, and personal and may be affected by past experiences.
- The goal of therapy is to decrease the patient's perception of breathlessness.

Prevalence[2-3]
- Approximately 70% of palliative care patients experience dyspnea, particularly those with chronic obstructive pulmonary disease (90-95%), heart failure (HF; 60-88%), and cancer (10-70%).

Causes [1,4,5]
- Physical, psychosocial, and spiritual factors can all contribute to dyspnea.
- The causes of dyspnea can vary widely and patients often have multiple contributing factors (Table 1). Some underlying causes may be beneficially treated. Other causes cannot be reversed and treatment focuses on supportive care (Table 2).

Table 1. Factors Contributing to Dyspnea

Contributing Factors	Examples
Physical	Fluid, tumor, weakness, injury, obesity
Psychosocial	Fear of impaired function and inability to carry out normal tasks
Spiritual	Fear of imminent death, fear of suffocation

Table 2. Pathophysiological Mechanisms of Dyspnea

Mechanisms	Causes	Treatment Options
Non-Reversible Causes		
Airway obstruction	Tumor, congenital anomalies of the airway, obesity	Non-pharmacological, opioid +/- benzodiazepine
Cardiac	Heart failure, pulmonary hypertension	
Muscle weakness	Cachexia, neuromuscular degenerative conditions (Amyotrophic lateral sclerosis (ALS), muscular sclerosis, myasthenia gravis), deconditioning	
Parenchymal failure	Cystic fibrosis , pneumonia, interstitial disease(pulmonary fibrosis)	
Reversible Causes		
Anxiety	Fear of difficulty breathing, sensation of suffocation	Benzodiazepine
Blood disorders	Anemia, metabolic acidosis	Consider red blood cell transfusion
Bronchospasm	Asthma	Bronchodilator +/- corticosteroid
Cough	Secretions, Infection, tumor	Expectorant or nebulized saline
Fluid in respiratory tract	Secretions, Infection, inflammation (tracheitis), Edema,	Reduction of fluids; furosemide; corticosteroid
Abdominal pressure	ascites	paracentesis, loop diuretic + spironolactone
Pain	Rib pain (fracture, metastasis), inflammation (pleuritic pain)	Opioid +/- corticosteroid
Pulmonary embolism	Clotting disorder	Anticoagulants for prevention and treatment
Pneumothorax or effusion	Malignancy, interstitial lung disease	Consider therapeutic thoracentesis
Secretions	Dehydration, medications	Weak cough reflex: anticholinergic

See Anxiety, Pain, Cough, Secretion, and Infection GEMS

Clinical Characteristics[1,2,5]

- Respiratory rate, blood gas values, and pulmonary function testing poorly correlate with patients' perception of breathlessness.
- Breathing can be abnormal without being uncomfortable, as well as uncomfortable without abnormality.
- Respiratory effort and dyspnea are not the same. For example, patients may experience relief of dyspnea from opioids without change in respiratory rate.
- Since dyspnea is a subjective sensation, self-report is the only reliable indicator.
- The impact of dyspnea on function is an important clinical manifestation. Decrease in activities such as walking, eating, talking as a result of dyspnea is distressing both to the patient and the family.
- Anxiety frequently accompanies dyspnea and often exacerbates the perception of shortness of breath, leading to a downward spiraling cycle of anxiety and dyspnea.

Non-Pharmacological Treatment[1-2,4-7]

- Deep, slow breathing; breathing into a paper bag.
- Improve air circulation and quality:
    - Provide a draft, using fans or open windows
        - Stimulates trigeminal nerve with central inhibitory effects on dyspnea
        - Attach ribbons to fan to visualize air movement
    - Adjust temperature and humidity with air conditioner or humidifier
- Reposition to comfort, usually to a more upright position (30-90 degree incline).
- Self-hypnosis, hypnosis directed by a professional skilled in hypnotherapy, or guided imagery.
- Encourage relaxation.
    - Calm, quiet environment
    - Reduce the need for exertion
    - Massage or therapeutic touch
    - Pet, water, or music therapy
- Minimize dyspnea triggers.
    - Avoid strong odors, perfumes, and smoke
- Provide companionship (isolation and spiritual issues can worsen symptoms).
- Enlist support of the entire interdisciplinary team (spiritual care, social workers, and counselors) to facilitate ongoing discussions surrounding symptoms and medication use to alleviate fears and myths.
- Anticipate and proactively prepare the patient and family for worsening symptoms.

Pharmacotherapy[1-3,6-15]

- Pharmacological treatment is aimed at decreasing the perception of dyspnea with opioids and benzodiazepines; avoid using medications simply to decrease the respiratory rate.
- Opioids suppress respiratory awareness, decrease response to hypoxia and hypercapnia, and have sedative properties. Opioids provide vasodilation in the lungs, therefore improving the ventilation/perfusion ratio in the lungs.
- Appropriately titrated, opioids have been shown to be safe and effective in the treatment of dyspnea. Doses should be titrated to minimal effective dose, often much lower than conventional pain doses.
- In patients also receiving opioids for pain, total daily dose can be converted to an extended-release opioid with a short-acting opioid available for dyspnea or pain episodes.
- Benzodiazepines have a role if anxiety is significant, providing additional and sustained anxiolytic properties.
- Oxygen therapy is a well-tolerated, relatively non-threatening intervention that can reverse hypoxemia and provide relief from dyspnea in some situations. However, oxygen is rarely beneficial in the active phase of dying.
- Noninvasive positive pressure ventilation can be useful to assist fatigued muscles and allow patients to take a deeper breath, which may help overcome the feeling of dyspnea; however do not initiate at end of life. In some patients, oxygen masks may heighten anxiety due to a smothering effect. Masks may also limit communication and eating.
- In some cases, an underlying pathology can be established; treatment should focus on reversing the cause of dyspnea. Opioids may be used temporarily while these therapies take effect.

Clinical Pearls [1,8,10-18]

- When using opioids, anticipate side effects and prevent constipation upon initiation of opioid.
- Do not use methadone for treating dyspnea. Methadone is not beneficial for treating dyspnea.
- Use of nebulized opioids for the treatment of dyspnea is controversial. Study results have been inconsistent.
    - Nonrandomized studies, case reports, and chart reviews describe anecdotal improvement in dyspnea using nebulized opioids.
    - Studies using nebulized opioids have provided inconclusive or negative results.
- Disadvantages of nebulized opioids compared to oral or other dosage forms include increased costs and a more complicated method of delivery. In patients with impaired alveolar surface or thick secretions (e.g. metastatic lung disease, cystic fibrosis), absorption will be limited, decreasing effectiveness.
- Nebulized opioids may be advantageous in patients that are not able or willing to take an oral agent or cannot tolerate adverse effects.
    - Fentanyl is more lipophilic than morphine or hydromorphone which may contribute to higher systemic bioavailability and therefore more patient-reported benefit for dyspnea.
    - Studies have not shown benefit with nebulized morphine or nebulized hydromorphone versus nebulized saline.
- Nebulized furosemide appears effective for dyspnea refractory to other conventional therapies however the effectiveness is controversial.
    - Hypothesized mechanism of action of nebulized furosemide is its ability to enhance pulmonary stretch receptor activity, inhibition of chloride movement through the membrane of the epithelial cell, and its ability to increase the synthesis of bronchodilating prostaglandins.
- For patients intolerant to benzodiazepines, promethazine or chlorpromazine may be effective for dyspnea as an adjuvant to opioid use. Although promethazine and chlorpromazine are both phenothiazines, a third phenothiazine, prochlorperazine, showed no benefit for dyspnea and more adverse effects than promethazine. Prochlorperazine is not recommended for dyspnea management.

Pharmacological Management of Dyspnea

Generic Name (Trade Name)	Adult Starting Dose	Routes	Common Strengths and Formulations	Comments
Opioids				
Hydromorphone (Dilaudid®)	2 mg Q4H PRN	PO SL PR SC IV	**Tablets:** 2 mg, 4 mg, 8 mg **Oral solution:** 1 mg/mL **Injection:** 1 mg/mL, 2 mg/mL, 4 mg/mL, 10 mg/mL	• C-II controlled substance. • Opioid dosing for dyspnea may start at ¼ to ½ the analgesic dose. • Nebulized hydromorphone has not been shown effective.[10] • Monitor for signs of neurotoxicity with higher doses (myoclonus, hyperalgesia, allodynia).
Morphine (Roxanol®)	2.5 mg Q4H PRN	PO SL PR SC IV	**Oral solution:** 10 mg/5 mL; 20 mg/5 mL; 20 mg/mL **Tablets:** 15, 30 mg **Injection:** 1, 2, 4, 5, 8, 10, 15, 25, 50 mg/mL	• C-II controlled substance. • Opioid dosing for dyspnea may start at ¼ to ½ the analgesic dose. • Nebulized morphine has not been shown effective.[10] • Caution in renal impairment. • Monitor for signs of neurotoxicity with higher doses (myoclonus, hyperalgesia, allodynia).
Oxycodone (Oxyfast®, Roxicodone®)	5 mg Q4H PRN	PO SL PR	**Oral solution:** 5 mg/5 mL, 20 mg/mL **Tablets:** 5mg, 10mg, 15mg, 20mg, 30 mg	• C-II controlled substance. • Opioid dosing for dyspnea may start at ¼ to ½ the analgesic dose. • May be preferred in patients with renal failure.

Continued

Generic Name (Trade Name)	Adult Starting Dose	Routes	Common Strengths and Formulations	Comments
Benzodiazepines				
Alprazolam (Xanax®)	0.25mg TID PRN	PO SL PR	**IR tablets:** 0.25 mg, 0.5 mg, 1 mg, 2 mg **Oral solution:** 1 mg/mL	• C-IV controlled substance. • IR tablets may be crushed for SL administration or given PR. • Short-acting, may produce rebound anxiety between doses. • Highest risk for withdrawal if patient abruptly stops medication.
Clonazepam (Klonopin®)	0.25mg BID PRN	PO SL PR	**Tablets:** 0.5 mg, 1 mg, 2 mg **Oral disintegrating tablets:** 0.125 mg, 0.25 mg, 0.5 mg, 1 mg, 2 mg	• C-IV controlled substance. • Tablets may be crushed for SL administration or given PR. • Long-acting, may provide sustained baseline control of anxiety.
Diazepam (Valium®)	2mg TID PRN	PO SL PR IM IV	**Tablets:** 2 mg, 5 mg, 10 mg **Oral solution:** 5 mg/mL, 1 mg/mL **Injection:** 5 mg/mL	• C-IV controlled substance. • Tablets may be crushed for SL administration or given PR. • Active metabolite can accumulate in patients with renal insufficiency.
Lorazepam (Ativan®)	0.5mg Q6H PRN	PO SL PR SC IV	**Tablets:** 0.5 mg, 1 mg, 2 mg **Oral solution:** 2 mg/mL **Injection:** 2 mg/mL, 4 mg/mL	• C-IV controlled substance. • Tablets may be crushed for SL administration or given PR.
Nebulized Agents				
Albuterol (AccuNeb®)	2.5mg Q4H PRN (3mL of 0.083% solution) **MDI:** 2 puffs Q4H PRN	Inh	**Solution, nebulization:** 0.083% [2.5 mg/3 mL]; 0.042% [1.25 mg/3 mL]; 0.5% [2.5 mg/0.5 mL] **Metered dose inhaler:** 90mcg/ACT	• Preferred for dyspnea associated with wheezing and bronchoconstriction. • Discontinue if paradoxical bronchospasm. • Avoid caffeine due to increased side effects of albuterol. • Use MDI only if patient can effectively use an inhaler.
Fentanyl (Sublimaze®)	25mcg Q2H PRN	Inh	**Injection:** 0.05 mg/mL preservative free	• C-II controlled substance. • Nebulized fentanyl produces less bronchospasm than nebulized morphine.[10-12] • Bioavailability of inhaled fentanyl varies by inhalation device.[17] • Dilute fentanyl injection solution with 2 mL 0.9% NS & administer via nebulizer.
Furosemide (Lasix®)	20mg QID	Inh	**Injection:** 10 mg/mL preservative free	• Minimal systemic absorption, little or no diuretic effect reported.[14,16] • If edema or lung congestion is contributing to dyspnea, treat with an oral or injectable furosemide. • Dilute furosemide injection solution with 2 mL 0.9% NS & administer via nebulizer.

Continued

Generic Name (Trade Name)	Adult Starting Dose	Routes	Common Strengths and Formulations	Comments
Nebulized Agents				
Levalbuterol (Xopenex®)	0.63mg Q6H PRN **MDI:** 2 puffs Q6H PRN	Inh	**Solution, nebulization:** 0.63 mg/3 mL, 1.25 mg/ 3mL **Metered dose inhaler:** 45mcg/ACT	• Reserve for patients with bronchospasm or excessive side effects with albuterol. • Dose no more frequently than q6-8 hours. Overuse of levalbuterol will cause tachycardia, tremor, anxiety. • Use MDI only if patient can effectively use an inhaler. • Expensive.
Sodium chloride 0.9% (saline nebulization solution)	3mL Q4H PRN	Inh	**Solution, nebulization:** 0.9%	• Thins secretions, moisturizes airways. • Use in between bronchodilator doses to reduce overuse of inhaled medications.
Corticosteroids				
Dexamethasone (Decadron®)	4mg Daily	PO PR IM IV	**Tablets:** 1 mg, 2 mg, 4 mg, 6 mg **Oral solution:** 1 mg/mL **Injection:** 4 mg/mL, 10 mg/mL	• Give with food or milk to decrease GI disturbances. • Avoid administering later in the day due to insomnia. • Minimal mineralocorticoid activity. • Withdraw gradually after long-term therapy.
Prednisone (Deltasone®)	20mg Daily	PO	**Tablets:** 1, 2.5, 5, 10, 20, 50 mg **Oral solution:** 1 mg/mL, 5 mg/mL	• Give with food or milk to decrease GI disturbances. • Avoid administering later in the day due to insomnia. • Associated with more fluid retention and edema than dexamethasone.

See Drug Dosing for Liver and Renal Disease for additional drug information.

References

1. Shadd J, Dudgeon D. Chap 159, Dyspnea In: Expert Consult: Walsh TD, Caraceni AT, Fainsinger R. *Palliative Medicine.*. http://www.expertconsultbook.com; Accessed June 8, 2014
2. Cuervo pinna MA, Mota vargas R, Redondo moralo MJ, Sánchez correas MA, Pera blanco G. Dyspnea--a bad prognosis symptom at the end of life. *Am J Hosp Palliat Care*. 2009;26(2):89-97.
3. Gomutbutra P, O'riordan DL, Pantilat SZ. Management of moderate-to-severe dyspnea in hospitalized patients receiving palliative care. *J Pain Symptom Manage*. 2013;45(5):885-91.
4. Hayen A, Herigstad M, Pattinson KT. Understanding dyspnea as a complex individual experience. *Maturitas*. 2013;76(1):45-50.
5. Von Gunten C, Thomas J. Management of dyspnea. *J Support Oncol* 2003;1(1):23-34.
6. Karnal AH, Maguire JM, Wheeler JL, et al. Dyspnea review for the palliative care professional: treatment goals and therapeutic options. *J Palliat Med* 2012;15(1):106-114.
7. Currow DC, Ward AM, Abernethy AP. Advances in the pharmacological management of breathlessness. *Curr Opin Support Palliat Care* 2009;3:103-106.
8. Viola R, Kiteley C, Lloyd N S, Mackay J A, Wilson J, Wong R K. The management of dyspnea in cancer patients: a systematic review. *Support Care Cancer*. 2008;16(4): 329-37.

9. Navigante AH, Castro MA, Cerchietti LC. Morphine Versus Midazolam as Upfront Therapy to Control Dyspnea Perception in Cancer Patients While Its Underlying Cause Is Sought or Treated. *J Pain Symptom Manage* 2010;39 (5):820-830, May 2010

10. Gomutbutra P, O'Riordan D, Kerr K, Pantilat S. Benzodiazepines and the Management of Dyspnea in Palliative Care Patients *(411-A)*. *J Pain Symptom Manage* 2012;43(2):374.

11. Ferraresi V. Inhaled opioids for the treatment of dyspnea. *Am J Health-Syst Pharm* 2005;62:319-320.

12. Graff G, Stark J, Grueber R. Case report: nebulized fentanyl for palliation of dyspnea in a cystic fibrosis patient. *Respiration* 2004;71(6):646–649.

13. Coyne PJ, Viswanathan R, Smith TJ. Nebulized fentanyl citrate improves patients' perception of breathing, respiratory rate, and oxygen saturation in dyspnea. *J Pain Symptom Manage* 2002;23(2):157–160.

14. Charles MA, Reymond L, Israel F. Relief of incident dyspnea in palliative cancer patients: a pilot, randomized controlled trial comparing nebulized hydromorphone, systemic hydromorphone and nebulized saline. *J Pain Symptom Manage* 2008;36(1):29-38.

15. Newton PJ, Davidson PM, Macdonald P, et al. Nebulized furosemide for the management of dyspnea: Does the evidence support its use? *J Pain Symptom Manage* 2008;36(4):424-441.

16. McIver B, Walsh D, Nelson K. Use of chlorpromazine for symptom control in dying cancer patients. *J Pain Symptom Manage* 1994;9(5):341-345.

17. Boyden J, Connor S, Otolorin L, Nathan S, Fine P, Davis M, Muir J. Nebulized medications for the treatment of dyspnea: a literature review. *J Aerosol Med Pulm Drug Deliv* 2014 June 10. [epub ahead of print]. DOI 10.1089/jamp.2014.1136.

18. MacLeod D, Habib A, Ikeda K, Spyker D, Cassella J, et al. Inhaled fentanyl aerosol in healthy volunteers: pharmacokinetics and pharmacodynamics. *Anesth Analg* 2012;115(5):1071-1077.

19. Lexi-Comp Online, Lexi-Drugs Online, Hudson, Ohio: Lexi-Comp, Inc.; June 15, 2014.

Treatment Algorithm for Dyspnea

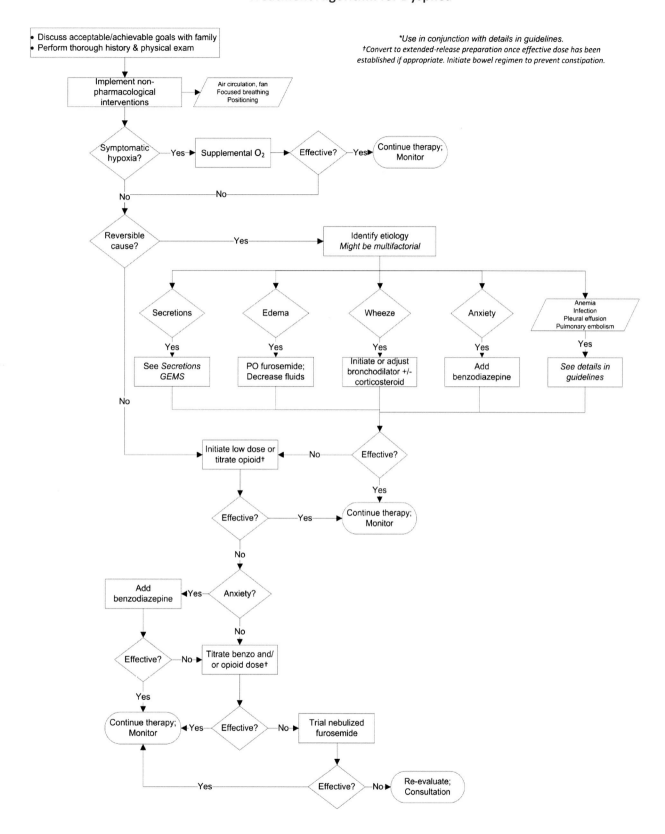

Fatigue

Introduction and Background[1-5,7]
- Fatigue is a prevalent, subjectively reported symptom that often accompanies depression, insomnia, and pain in patients with a terminal diagnosis.
- About 30% of the healthy population reports episodic fatigue, but this symptom is more severe in patients with chronic illnesses. For patients receiving hospice care, fatigue is often multi-factorial and generally not relieved with rest.

Prevalence[1, 4-5, 7]
- Fatigue is the most common symptom reported by patients with chronic, debilitating illnesses.
- Up to 90% of patients with cancer report significant fatigue.
- Sometime within the first year after a stroke, at least half of patients report fatigue.

Causes[1-2, 7]
- Causes of fatigue at end of life are often multifactorial (Figure 1), including physical, psychosocial, and sleep disturbance factors.
- Depending on goals of care and proximity to end of life, sedating medications, such as opioids, should be reviewed for efficacy versus sedation effects. If opioids are tapered, pain should be monitored to ensure it does not become intolerable.
- Daytime oversedation or "hangover sedation" is common when a sedative/hypnotic is given for insomnia, especially if the medication is dosed late at night.

Table 1. Causes of Fatigue at End of Life

Disease and disease progression	Cancer, cerebrovascular accident (CVA), chronic obstructive pulmonary disease (COPD), heart failure, multiple sclerosis (MS), human immunodeficiency virus (HIV), amyotrophic lateral sclerosis (ALS), systemic infections
Medications	Opioids, anxiolytics, hypnotics, anticonvulsants, antihistamines, beta-blockers, chemotherapy, radiation, antidepressants, muscle relaxants, anticholinergics
Unrelieved symptoms	Anemia, metabolic disorders, insomnia, pain, muscle deconditioning, depression
Psychosocial	Spiritual concerns, boredom, chronic stress

Clinical Characteristics[1-2,6]
- Fatigue is comprised of physical, emotional, and cognitive components.
- In addition to a generalized feeling of tiredness, patients often report feeling weak, having difficulty concentrating, and not feeling motivated.
- Though difficult to differentiate from depression, fatigue is not thought to induce feelings of worthlessness or recurrent thoughts of death.
- Patients are more likely to report physical characteristics of fatigue than mental attributes.

Non-Pharmacological Treatment[1,9-10]
- Prioritize energy expenditure. Communicate limitations with friends, family, and other visitors.
- Improve sleep hygiene with relaxing bedtime routine (warm bath, relaxing music, aromatherapy).
- Establish daytime routines with mental stimulation and physical exercise, if possible.
- Consider modestly increased physical activity, tailored to a patient's tolerance and ability.
- Increase psychosocial and spiritual support as accepted by patient.
- Evaluate and correct any potentially reversible causes of fatigue, if possible.
  - Dehydration may be addressed by encouraging oral fluid intake. Consider parenteral fluid replacement with hypodermoclysis if within patient's goals of care.

Pharmacotherapy[1,5,8,11-21]
- Neither donepezil nor amantadine is effective to manage fatigue.
- Corticosteroids have been shown to improve energy levels, but effectiveness wanes over time.

- Methylphenidate can be used on a PRN basis to provide bursts of energy lasting for a few hours. This may be beneficial allow a patient to participate in prioritized activities.
- If fatigue is related to anemia, erythropoiesis-stimulating agents (ESAs) may be effective to improve symptoms, but it can take up to 12 weeks for hemoglobin to reach 12 g/dL. ESAs (epoetin alfa, darbepoetin alfa) and other colony-stimulating factors are not recommended for patients with anemia related to malignancy unless the patient is currently undergoing chemotherapy.
- Selective serotonin reuptake inhibitors (SSRIs) are usually not effective to improve fatigue symptoms independent of depression. Buproprion may improve symptoms of fatigue independent of depression after routine doses for 2-4 weeks.

Clinical Pearls[1,8,11,20]

- At the very end of life, fatigue may be a protective response against suffering. Avoid treatment if physical or existential discomfort worsens.
- If sedation is due to opioid use, adjuvant agents or opioid-sparing analgesics may be used to decrease opioid requirements and decrease sedative effects.
- Once pain is adequately controlled, patient may experience "catch up" sleep for a day or two that is not medication induced sedation.

Pharmacological Management of Fatigue

Generic Name (Trade Name)	Adult Starting Dose	Routes	Common Strengths and Formulations	Comments
Corticosteroids				
Dexamethasone (Decadron®)	4mg Daily	PO PR IM IV	**Tablets**: 1 mg, 2 mg, 4 mg, 6 mg **Oral solution:** 1 mg/mL **Injection**: 4 mg/mL, 10 mg/mL	• Give with food or milk to decrease GI disturbances. • Avoid administering later in the day due to insomnia. • Minimal mineralocorticoid activity. • Taper long-term therapy gradually.
Prednisone (Deltasone®)	20mg Daily	PO	**Tablets**: 1 mg, 2.5 mg, 5 mg, 10 mg, 20 mg, 50 mg **Oral solution:** 1 mg/mL, 5 mg/mL	• Give with food or milk to decrease GI disturbances. • Avoid administering later in the day due to insomnia. • Associated with more fluid retention and edema than dexamethasone.
CNS Stimulants				
Dextro-amphetamine (Dexedrine®)	5 mg QAM	PO	**Tablets:** 5 mg, 10 mg **Oral solution:** 5 mg/5 mL	• C-II controlled substance. • May counteract opiate-induced sedation. • May precipitate delirium. • May induce tolerance with prolonged use. • Use immediate release preparations.
Methylphenidate (Ritalin®)	5 mg QAM	PO	**Tablets**: 5 mg, 10 mg, 20 mg **Chewable tablets:** 2.5 mg, 5 mg, 10 mg **Oral solution:** 5 mg/5 mL 10 mg/5 mL	• C-II controlled substance. • May counteract opiate-induced sedation. • May precipitate delirium. • May induce tolerance with prolonged use. • Use immediate release preparations.

See Drug Dosing for Liver and Renal Disease for additional drug information.

References

1. Radbruch L, Strasser F, Elsner F, Goncalces JF, et al. Fatigue in palliative care patients – an EAPC approach. *Palliat Med* 2008;22:13-22.
2. Donovan KA and Jacobsen PB. Fatigue, depression, and insomnia: evidence of a symptom cluster in cancer. *Semin Oncol Nurs* 2007;23(2):127-135.
3. Lou JS, Weiss MD, and Carter GT. Assessment and management of fatigue in neuromuscular disease. *Am J Hosp Palliat Med* 2010;27(2):145-157.
4. National Institutes of Health State-of-the-Science Panel. National Institutes of Health State-of-the-Science Conference Statement: Symptom management in cancer: pain, depression, and fatigue, July 15-17, 2002. *J Natl Cancer Inst Monogr* 2004;32:9-16.
5. Harris, JD. Fatigue in chronically ill patients. *Curr Opin Supp Palliat Care.* 2008;2:180-186.
6. Hardy SE and Studenski SA. Qualities of fatigue and associated chronic conditions among older adults. *J Pain Symptom Manage* 2010;39(6):1033-1042.
7. Lerdal A, Bakken LN, Kouwenhoven SE, Pedersen G, et al. Poststroke fatigue – a review. *J Pain Symptom Manage* 2009;38(6):928-949.
8. Calabrich A and Katz A. Management of anemia in cancer patients. *Future Oncol* 2011;7(4):507-517.
9. Oldervall LM, Loge JH, Paltiel H, Asp MB, et al. The effect of a physical exercise program in palliative care: a phase II study. *J Pain Symptom Manage* 2006;31(5):421-430.
10. Maddocks M, Mockett S, and Wilcock A. Re: the effect of a physical exercise program in palliative care: a phase II study. *J Pain Symptom Manage* 2006;32(6):513-515.
11. Bruera E, Roca E, Cedaro L, Carraro S, et al. Action of oral methylprednisolone in terminal cancer patients: a prospective randomized double-blind study. *Cancer Treat Rep* 1985;69(7-8):751-754.
12. Pucci E, Tato PB, D'Amico R, Giuliani G, et al. Amantadine for fatigue in multiple sclerosis. *Cochrane Database Syst Rev* 2007;1:CD002818.
13. Bruera E, El Osta B, Valero V, Driver LC, et al. Donepezil for cancer fatigue: a double-blind, randomized, placebo-controlled trial. *J Clin Oncol* 2007;25(23):3475-3481.
14. Minton O, Richardson A, Sharpe M, Hotopf M, et al. Drug therapy for the management of cancer-related fatigue. *Cochrane Database Syst Rev* 2010;7:CD006704.
15. Roscoe JA, Morrow GR, Hickok JT, Mustian KM, et al. Effect of paroxetine hydrochloride (Paxil) on fatigue and depression in breast cancer patients receiving chemotherapy. *Breast Cancer Res Treat* 2005;89:243-249.
16. Sheng P, Hou L, Wang X, Wang X, et al. Efficacy of modafinil on fatigue and excessive daytime sleepiness associated with neurological disorders: a systematic review and meta-analysis. *PLoS ONE* 2013;8(12):e81802.
17. Cruciana RA, Zhang JJ, Manola J, Cella D, et al.L-Carnitine supplementation for the management of fatigue in patients with cancer: an eastern cooperative oncology group phase III, randomized, double-blind, placebo-controlled trial. *J Clin Oncol* 2012;30(31):3864-3869.
18. Bruera E, Valero V, Driver L, Shen L, et al. Patient-controlled methylphenidate for cancer fatigue: a double-blind, randomized, placebo-controlled trial. *J Clin Oncol* 2006;24(13):2073-2078.
19. Carroll JK, Kohli S, Mustian KM, Roscoe JA, et al. Pharmacologic treatment of cancer-related fatigue. *Oncologist* 2007;12(suppl 1):43-51.
20. Yennurajalingam S, Frisbee-Hume S, Palmer JL, Delgado-Guay MO, et al. Reduction of cancer-related fatigue with dexamethasone: a double-blind, randomized, placebo-controlled trial in patients with advanced cancer. *J Clin Oncol* 2013;31(25):3076-3082.
21. Minton O, Richardson A, Sharpe M, Hotopf M, et al. A systematic review and meta-analysis of the pharmacological treatment of cancer-related fatigue. *J Natl Cancer Inst* 2008;100:1155-1166.
22. Cullum JL, Wojciechowski AE, Pelletier G, and Simpson JSA. Bupropion sustained release treatment reduced fatigue in cancer patients. *Can J Psychiatry* 2004;49:139-144.

Treatment Algorithm for Fatigue

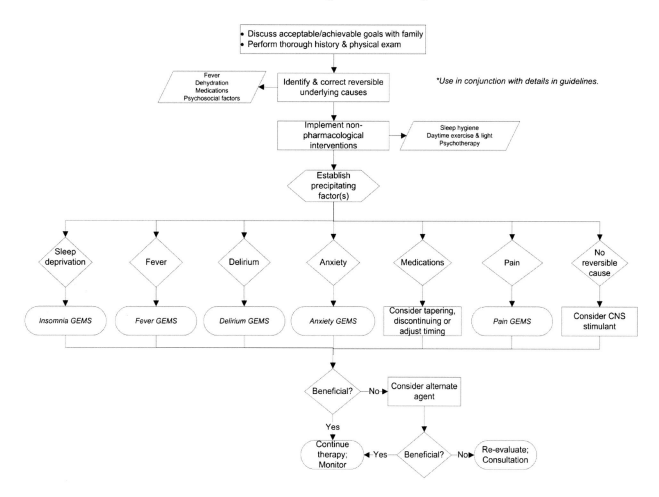

Fever

Introduction and Background[1,2]

- Normal body temperature is considered to be 37° C or 98.6° F. Human body temperature normally follows a circadian rhythm, or 24 hour cycle. Body temperature is lowest in the predawn hours and rises as the day progresses.
- The anterior hypothalamus contains heat-sensitive receptors controlling the body's thermoregulation and the core body temperature. This control mechanism can be reset, like a home thermostat, to a higher temperature in response to a fever-producing substance (pyrogen).
- Fever is defined as an elevation of body temperature that exceeds the normal daily variation and occurs in conjunction with an increase in the hypothalamic set point for body temperature.
- Fever (pyrexia) is often accompanied by other symptoms which include sweating and shivering (spontaneous rapid muscle spasms that generate additional heat) or rigors (exaggerated shivering).
- Temperature regulation in the body is dependent on maintaining a balance between heat production and heat loss.
- Fever of unknown origin (FUO) is "an illness lasting at least 3 weeks with a fever higher than 38° C on more than one occasion and which lacks a definitive diagnosis after 1 week of evaluation in a hospital".[2]
- Elevated temperature may be secondary to hyperthermia (characterized by fever > 41.5°C or 106.7° F) resulting from heat stroke, hyperthyroidism, or medications that affect thermoregulation. Malignant hyperthermia is a rare genetic disorder causing elevated temperature following administration of anesthetic agents (e.g., succinylcholine, halothane).
- Neuroleptic malignant syndrome is a life-threatening adverse reaction to dopamine-blocking medications, such as conventional and atypical antipsychotics. Symptoms include high fever, unstable blood pressure, muscular rigidity and autonomic dysfunction.

Prevalence[1,3-6]

- Most hospice patients will develop fever at some point in their illness.
- Though its prevalence has not been well studied in the hospice population, fever is a frequent symptom in patients when death is imminent.

Causes[1-7]

- Assess for reversible causes of fever (Table 1).
- Infection in hospice patients may be attributed to many circumstances including alteration in physical defense mechanisms (e.g., mucositis), decreased immune response (neutropenia), presence of foreign objects (urinary or venous catheters) and aspiration.

Table 1. Causes of Fever

Categories	Etiologies
Drugs	
• Antibiotics	Penicillins, cephalosporins, sulfonamides, nitrofurantoin, amphotericin B, vancomycin
• Cytotoxic agents	Bleomycin, interferon, interleukin, radiation
• Immune therapy agents	Biological response modifiers, growth factors
• CNS agents	Selective serotonin reuptake inhibitors (SSRIs), tricyclic antidepressants (TCAs), opioids, benzodiazepines, antiepileptic drugs (AEDs), antipsychotics
• Miscellaneous	Allopurinol, hydralAZINE
Infection	Viral or bacterial, febrile neutropenia, human immunodeficiency virus (HIV)
Inflammatory	Graft-versus-host disease (GVHD), rheumatoid arthritis, systemic lupus erythematosus, Kawasaki disease
Miscellaneous	Blood transfusion, gastrointestinal hemorrhage, cardiovascular accident (CVA)
Neurologic	Dysregulation of autonomic balance, status epilepticus, sympathetic storming
Neoplasm	Tumor fever, Hodgkin's disease, lymphoma, leukemia, neuroblastoma, renal cell carcinoma, osteogenic sarcoma

- Tumor fever, also known as paraneoplastic fever, can occur with several types of cancers. The most common cancers associated with fever are:
  - Hodgkin's disease
  - Lymphoma
  - Leukemia
  - Renal cell carcinoma
  - Myxoma
  - Osteogenic sarcoma
- Antipsychotics (e.g., aripiprazole, clozapine, olanzapine, quetiapine, or haloperidol) may rarely cause high fever and diaphoresis, signs of neuroleptic malignant syndrome.
- When used in excess or with multiple serotonergic medications, Selective serotonin reuptake inhibitors (SSRIs), tricyclic antidepressants, monoamine oxidase inhibitors (MAOI) can cause serotonin syndrome, characterized by elevated temperature, tremor, myoclonus and diarrhea.
- Blood product transfusion sometimes causes a febrile reaction during the transfusion. Premedication with acetaminophen and diphenhydramine may reduce the incidence and severity of fever.

Clinical Characteristics[1,2,8]

- Clinically significant fever is a body temperature greater than 38° C (100.4° F). Very young or very old patients may have abnormal temperature elevations that do not meet this definition of fever, but still may cause symptoms and discomfort requiring treatment.
- Fever is almost always accompanied by headache, myalgia and malaise.
- Fever occurs in three phases:
  - Phase 1 (chill phase): pyrogen is introduced; cutaneous vasoconstriction and increased muscle activity cause heat production, manifested by chills and shivering.
  - Phase 2 (fever phase): heat production balances heat loss at the elevated temperature and shivering stops.
  - Phase 3 (flush phase): cutaneous vasodilatation occurs as a response to elevated body temperature and sweating promotes heat loss to the environment. The skin may appear pink/red or "flushed."
- Sweating, along with a decrease in the quantity of pyrogen or the administration of an antipyretic agent, will reset the core temperature to a lower or normal level.
- In the elderly population, thermoregulatory mechanisms are often diminished. Consequently, hyperthermia may result in arrhythmias, ischemia, mental status changes or heart failure due to the associated increase in metabolic demands.
- Persons with epilepsy may experience seizures triggered by fever. Additionally, fever has been reported as an adverse effect of some anticonvulsant medications related to AED hypersensitivity syndrome. See also *Seizures GEMS*.

Non-Pharmacological Treatment[1-3,9]

- Maintain patient in a dry, moderate temperature environment; avoid drafts or temperature fluctuation.
- In hot and humid environments, sponging the patient with tepid water will promote physical cooling.
- Do not use cold water or alcohol as these may lead to shivering with resulting temperature elevation and increased patient discomfort.
- Encourage fluid replacement and adequate nutrition. Fever is associated with dehydration and increased metabolic demands.
- If appropriate, discontinue medications that could cause fever.
- Non-pharmacological cooling techniques in combination with anti-pyretic medications may provide the best symptomatic relief for the patient.

Pharmacotherapy[1-7,9-11]

- Two classes of medications lower body temperature:
  - *Pure antipyretics*: medications with no effect in the absence of a pyrogen and with no effect on normal body temperature (e.g., acetaminophen, NSAIDs)
  - *Drugs that may cause hypothermia*: medications with direct effect on thermoregulatory functions resulting from serotonergic activity, or dopamine or alpha-2 adrenergic receptor

blockade (e.g., ethanol, chlorpromazine, thioridazine, haloperidol, risperidone, clozapine, olanzapine, quetiapine).
   o Hypothermia related to medication use may be dose related. Chlorpromazine is antipyretic in low doses and causes hypothermia in high doses.
- Dantrolene, a skeletal muscle relaxant, is used for treatment of malignant hyperthermia. Emergency management is typically reserved for intra-operative reactions to anesthetics and neuromuscular blocking agents (e.g., succinylcholine). Dantrolene is used in conjunction with surface cooling, intravenous and rectal cooling solutions to bring body temperature below 38° C.
- A single IV, IM, or SC dose of meperidine 25mg may be used to treat fever-related rigors or shivering. Avoid use of meperidine with serotonergic agents due to an increased risk of serotonin syndrome.

Clinical Pearls[1-7]
- While frequently recommended in pediatrics, alternating acetaminophen with an NSAID has not been studied in adults. This practice may be beneficial when either agent alone does not reduce fever.
- In neutropenic patients, determine the infectious cause of fever and treat accordingly; treat empirically if pathogen is not known. Discuss goals of therapy with patient prior to initiating antibiotics.
- Although an antibiotic may decrease symptoms, the benefits and burdens of the intervention must be weighed. Antibiotics may be considered in patients who are near death if the patient is requesting them or if the patient is experiencing symptoms causing suffering (e.g., seizures or pronounced mental status changes) as a result of a high fever (>40° C or 104°F).
- Avoid aspirin in children because of the risk of developing Reye's syndrome with resulting liver failure.
- Premedication with acetaminophen, NSAIDs, or corticosteroids when administering drugs associated with hyperthermia or blood products may reduce the incidence and severity of fever.
- Avoid routinely treating fever with antipyretic agents in the presence of infection. Reducing the fever may mask antimicrobial treatment failure.

Pharmacological Management of Fever

Generic Name (Trade Name)	Adult Starting Dose	Routes	Common Strengths and Formulations	Comments
Antipyretic				
Acetaminophen (Tylenol®, Feverall®)	650mg Q6H PRN	PO PR IV	**Tablets:** 325 mg, 500 mg, 650 mg **Capsules:** 500 mg **Suppositories:** 120 mg, 325 mg, 650 mg **Oral solution:** 160 mg/5 mL **Injection:** 10 mg/mL	• Maximum daily dose: 4000 mg. • Weigh risk vs benefit in patients with severe liver dysfunction. • FDA now recommends 325mg or less per dosage unit. • Injection (Ofirmev®) is expensive; hospital use only. • Chewable tablets available.
Non-Steroidal Anti-Inflammatory Drugs (NSAIDs)				
Aspirin	300mg Q6H PRN	PO PR	**Tablets:** 325 mg, 500 mg **Suppositories:** 300 mg, 600 mg	• Maximum daily dose: 4000 mg. • Avoid use in patients with severe liver disease or with bleeding risk. • More cost effective than indomethacin suppositories.
Ibuprofen (Motrin®, Advil®)	400mg Q6H PRN	PO IV	**Tablets:** 200 mg, 400 mg, 600 mg, 800 mg **Capsules:** 200 mg **Oral suspension:** 100 mg/5 mL **Injection:** 100 mg/mL	• Maximum daily dose: 3200mg. • Weigh vs risk benefit in patients with renal insufficiency. • Chewable tablets available. • Patients must be well hydrated prior to IV ibuprofen use.

Continued

Generic Name (Trade Name)	Adult Starting Dose	Routes	Common Strengths and Formulations	Comments
Non-Steroidal Anti-Inflammatory Drugs (NSAIDs), *continued*				
Naproxen (Naprosyn®, Aleve®)	250 mg Q8H PRN	PO	**Tablets:** 220 mg, 250 mg, 375 mg, 500 mg **ER tablets:** 375 mg, 500 mg, 750 mg **Capsules:** 220 mg **Oral suspension:** 125 mg/5 mL	• Maximum daily dose: 1250 mg (naproxen base). • Naproxen sodium (OTC) 220mg = naproxen base 200mg + 20mg sodium. • Weigh risk vs benefit in patients with renal insufficiency. • *Preferred agent for tumor fever.*
Indomethacin (Indocin®)	25mg Q8H PRN	PO PR	**Capsules:** 25 mg, 50 mg **Suspension:** 25 mg/5 mL **Suppositories:** 50 mg	• Maximum daily dose: 200 mg. • Associated with more GI distress than other NSAIDs. • Weigh risk vs benefit in patients with renal insufficiency. • Suppositories are expensive.
Malignant Hyperthermia				
Dantrolene (Dantrium®)	*Crisis:* 2.5mg/kg IV up to 4 doses (total 10mg/kg) *Post-crisis:* 1mg/kg Q4-6H for at least 24 hours	PO IV	**Capsules:** 25 mg, 50 mg, 100 mg **Injection:** 20 mg/vial	• For fever > 41.5°C or 106.7° F unresponsive to NSAIDs or acetaminophen. • Additional information at www.MHAUS.org or via the MH emergency hotline: 800-644-9737 • Also used PO as a skeletal muscle relaxant for patients with spasticity.

See Drug Dosing for Liver and Renal Disease for additional drug information.

Reference
1. Strickland M, Stovsky E. Fever near the end of life. *Fast Facts and Concepts.* August 2012;256. Available at https://www.capc.org/fast-facts/256-fever-near-end-life/.
2. Dalal S, Zhukovsky D. Pathophysiology and management of fever. *J Support Oncol* 2006;4:9-16.
3. Nagy-Agren S, Haley H. Management of infections in palliative care patients with advanced cancer. *J Pain Symptom Manage* 2002;24(1):64-70.
4. Chen L, Chou Y, Hsu P, Tsai S, et al. Antibiotic prescription for fever episodes in hospice patients. *Support Care Cancer* 2002;10:538-541.
5. Phipps M, Desai R, Wira C, Bravata D. Epidemiology and outcomes of fever burden among patients with acute ischemic stroke. *Stroke* 2011;42(12):3357-62.
6. Pinderhughes S, Morrison R. Evidence-based approach to management of fever in patients with end-stage dementia. *J Palliat Med* 2003;6(3):351-354.
7. Zell J, Chang J. Neoplastic fever: a neglected paraneoplastic syndrome. *Support Care Cancer* 2005;13:870-877.
8. Balamurugan E, Aggarwal M, Lamba A, Dang N, Tripathi M. Perceived trigger factors of seizures in persons with epilepsy. *Seizure.* 2013;22(9):743-747.
9. Hammond N, Boyle M. Pharmacological versus non-pharmacological antipyretic treatments in febrile critically ill adult patient: a systematic review and meta-analysis. *Aust Crit Care.* 2011;24(1):4-17.
10. Van Marum R, Wegewijs M, Loonen A, Beers E. Hypothermia following antipsychotic drug use. *Eur J Clin Pharmacol.* 2007;63(6):627-631.
11. Malignant hyperthermia. Lexi-Drugs Online. Hudson, Ohio:Lexi-Comp, Inc. Accessed August 18, 2014.

Treatment Algorithm for Fever

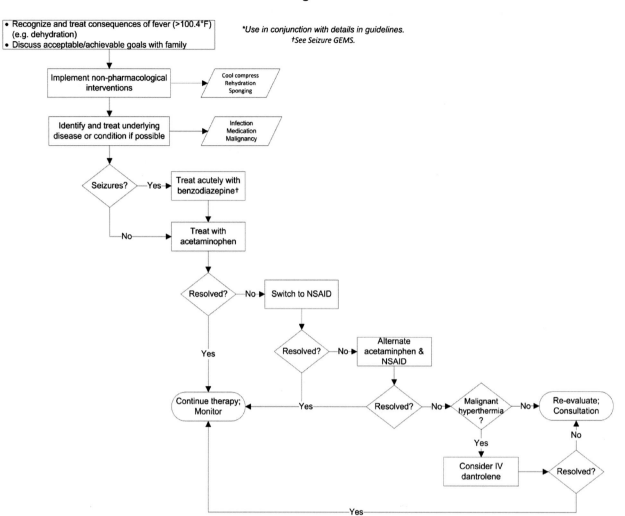

Hiccups

Introduction and Background [1-3]
- Hiccups (singultus, hiccoughs) are involuntary, synchronous contractions of the diaphragm and intercostal muscles. Spasms typically occur after peak inspiration and terminate by an abrupt closure of the glottis, producing the characteristic "hic" sound.
- Hiccups can interfere with oral intake, communication ability, and exacerbation of pain. They can also contribute to embarrassment, weight loss, fatigue, and insomnia.

Prevalence [2-3,6]
- Approximately 4,000 hospital admissions each year are due to severe, intractable hiccups.
- The incidence of hiccups in advanced cancer patients or those at the end of life has not been thoroughly studied, but may occur in up to 9%.
- Hiccups are more frequent in men than women.

Causes [1-4, 6-7, 11, 16-17]
- The exact pathophysiology of hiccups is unclear. The hiccup reflex arc includes the afferent pathway (phrenic, vagus, and sympathetic nerves) and efferent pathway (phrenic and accessory nerves) to the diaphragm and intercostal muscles. Dopamine and GABA are the primary neurotransmitters involved.
- Other causes of hiccups may involve structural, metabolic, inflammatory, and infectious diseases.
- Causes of persistent (2-30 days) or intractable (>1 month) hiccups may differ from the more common benign (minutes to hours) hiccup causes (Table 1 & 2).

Table 1. Causes of Benign, Self-limiting Hiccups

Category	Examples
Gastric	Distention, excessive food, alcohol or carbonated beverage intake, reflux, aerophagia, gastric insufflation, sudden changes in gastric temperature
Toxins	Tobacco use, alcohol intoxication

Table 2. Causes of Persistent or Intractable Hiccups

Categories	Examples
Central nervous system	Stroke, cerebral contusion, hematoma, encephalitis, meningitis, hydrocephalus, neoplasm, head trauma, anxiety, neurosyphilis, multiple sclerosis
Medications	CNS stimulants, sulfonamides, corticosteroids, benzodiazepines, barbiturates, antibiotics, analgesics
Metabolic	Hyponatremia, hypocalcemia, hypocapnia, hyperuricemia, gout, fever, renal failure, infection
Peripheral nervous system	Head or neck tumors, mediastinal or lung masses, goiter
Surgical	Inadequate ventilation, intubation, hyperextension of neck, laparotomy, thoracotomy, craniotomy, manipulation of diaphragm

Clinical Characteristics [1]
- Hiccups are classified based on duration of episode:
  - Acute and self-limiting: less than 48 hours
  - Persistent or chronic: between 48 hours and 1 month
  - Intractable hiccups: more than 1 month

Non-Pharmacological Treatment [2, 8-9]
- Respiratory maneuvers (holding breath, re-breathing in a bag, Valsalva maneuver, compression of the diaphragm, or induction of a sneeze or cough).
- Nasal and pharyngeal stimulation (pressure on the nose, traction of the tongue, gargling, drinking water, eating sugar).
- Gastric distension relief (fasting, naso-gastric (NG) tube, lavage, induction of vomiting).
- Vagal maneuvers (digital rectal massage, ocular compression or carotid massage)

Pharmacotherapy [1-7, 10-17]

- Treatment of hiccups is based on the underlying cause if identifiable. For example, proton pump inhibitors or metoclopramide (Reglan) can be used if reflux is thought to be contributing.
- In most situations, a cause is not identifiable; non-pharmacological therapies are usually initiated first line. Medications are typically reserved for persistent or intractable hiccups.
- Chlorpromazine (Thorazine) is the only drug with an FDA-approved indication for hiccups in adults; however, numerous reports are available regarding the use of baclofen (Lioresal) and gabapentin (Neurontin). Baclofen and gabapentin provide a more gradual response and may be useful for prolonged episodes of hiccups.[3,11]

Clinical Pearls

- Individual patients may respond differently to various therapies, so multiple drug trials are often necessary to find an effective therapy.
- Polypharmacy may be useful if a patient has failed several attempts with monotherapy. Combinations have been used including omeprazole and metoclopramide with baclofen, gabapentin, or both.
- Palliative sedation may be acceptable for patients with severe, intractable hiccups depending on patient and family goals of care.

Pharmacological Management of Hiccups

Generic Name (Trade Name)	Adult Starting Dose	Routes	Common Strengths and Formulations	Comments
Centrally-Mediated Hiccups				
Baclofen (Lioresal®)	10 mg PO TID	PO	**Tablets:** 10 mg, 20 mg	• May cause drowsiness, delirium. • Also provides muscle relaxation of diaphragmatic spasm.
Chlorpromazine (Thorazine®)	25 mg PO TID	PO IV IM PR	**Tablets:** 10 mg, 25 mg, 40 mg, 100 mg, 200 mg **Injection:** 25 mg/mL	• More sedating than haloperidol. • Risk of orthostatic hypotension. • *Only* drug with FDA-approved indication for hiccups.
Gabapentin (Neurontin®)	300 mg PO TID	PO	**Capsules:** 100 mg, 300 mg, 400 mg **Tablets:** 600 mg, 800 mg **Oral solution:** 250 mg/5 mL	• Adjunct therapy for centrally-mediated hiccups. • Immediate release tablets may be split in half. • Reduce dose in renal failure.
Haloperidol (Haldol®)	0.5 mg PO Q6H PRN	PO SL SC IM IV	**Tablets:** 0.5 mg, 1 mg, 2 mg, 5 mg **Injection:** 5 mg/mL **Oral solution:** 2 mg/mL	• Less sedating than chlorpromazine. • More versatile dosing than chlorpromazine.
Gastric Distension or Gastric Reflux-Mediated Hiccups				
Metoclopramide (Reglan®)	10 mg PO TID	PO SC	**Tablets:** 5 mg, 10 mg **Injection:** 5 mg/mL **Oral solution:** 5 mg/5 mL	• Promotes gastric emptying; also has anti-emetic properties.

Continued

Generic Name (Trade Name)	Adult Starting Dose	Routes	Common Strengths and Formulations	Comments
Gastric Distension or Gastric Reflux-Mediated Hiccups, *continued*				
Omeprazole (Prilosec®)	20 mg PO Daily	PO	**Capsules:** 10 mg, 20 mg, 40 mg **Tablets:** 20 mg	• Omeprazole is most cost-effective. • All PPIs will have similar effectiveness. • Capsules may be opened and contents added to a bite of applesauce.
Famotidine (Pepcid®)	20 mg PO BID	PO		• Tablets may be crushed if needed. • All H2RAs will have similar effectiveness.
Simethicone (Gas-X®, Phazyme®)	125 mg PO QID	PO SL	**Capsules:** 125 mg, 180 mg **Tablets:** 80 mg, 125 mg **Oral suspension:** 40 mg/0.6 mL	• Adjunct to metoclopramide. • Administer after meals.
Other				
Lidocaine (Xylocaine®)	Nebulize 5 mL Q4H PRN	Inh	**Injection:** 1%, 2%	• Nebulize injectable diluted with normal saline. • Inhalation will numb mouth and throat. Advise patients not to eat or drink for 30 minutes after nebulizer treatment to reduce risk of aspiration.
Methylphenidate (Ritalin®)	10 mg-20 mg QAM	PO	**Tablets:** 5 mg, 10 mg, 20 mg	• C-II controlled substance. • May be of use in patients with comorbid depression or opioid-induced sedation.
Midazolam (Versed®)	5-15 mg loading dose followed by continuous infusion	IV SC	**Injection:** 1 mg/mL, 5 mg/mL	• Used for palliative sedation in severe, intractable hiccups. • See *Palliative Sedation* chapter for additional information.
Nifedipine (Procardia®)	10 mg PO Q8H	PO	**Capsules, IR:** 10 mg, 20 mg	• Risk of severe hypotension especially in hypovolemic patients; monitor blood pressure.
Normal Saline	Nebulize 3 mL over 5 minutes PRN	Inh	**Solution for nebulization (0.9%):** 3 mL, 5 mL	• Suspected phrenic or vagal stimulation induced hiccups.

See *Drug Dosing for Liver and Renal Disease* for additional drug information.

References

1. Woelk CJ. Managing hiccups. *Can Fam Physician*. 2011;57:672-675.
2. Marinella MA. Diagnosis and management of hiccups in the patient with advanced cancer. *J Support Oncol*. 2009;7:122-127,130.

3. Calsina-Berna A, Garcai-Gomez G, Gonzalez-Barboteo J, Porta-Sales J. Treatment of chronic hiccups in cancer patients: a systematic review. *J Palliat Med.* 2012;15(10):1142-1150.

4. Smith HS, Busracamwongs A. Management of hiccups in the palliative care population. *Am J Hospice Palliat Med.* 2003;20(2):149-154.

5. Dunst MN, Margolin K, Horak D. Lidocaine for severe hiccups [letter]. *New Engl J Med.* 1993;329(12):890-891.

6. Tegeler ML, Baumrucker SJ. Gabapentin for intractable hiccups in palliative care. *Am J Hospice Palliat Med.* 2008;25(1):52-54.

7. Neuhaus T, Ko Y-D, Stier S. Successful treatment of intractable hiccups by oral application of lidocaine. *Support Care Cancer.* 2013:20:2009-3011.

8. Ohen M, Olivan A. Hiccups and digital rectal massage [letter]. *Arch Otolaryngol Head Neck Surg* 1993;119:1383

9. Fesmire FM. Termination of intractable hiccups with digital rectal massage [letter]. *Ann Emerg Med.* 1988;17(8):872.

10. Hernandez JL, Pajaron M, Garcia-Regata O, Jimenez V, et al. Gabapentin for intractable hiccup [letter]. *Am J Med.* 2004;117:279-280.

11. Mirajello A, Addolorato G, D'Angelo C, Ferrulli A, et al. Baclofen in the treatment of persistent hiccup: a case series. *Int J Clin Pract* 2013;67(9):918-912

12. Macris SG. Methylphenidate for hiccups [letter]. *Anesthesiology.* 1971;34(2):200.

13. Gregory GA, Way WL. Methylphenidate for hiccups [letter]. *Anesthesiology.* 1971;34(2):200-201.

14. Marechal R, Berghmans T, Sculier JP. Successful treatment of intractable hiccup with methylphenidate in a lung cancer patient. *Support Care Cancer.* 2003;11:126-128.

15. Sanchack KE: Hiccups: When the diaphragm attacks. *J Palliat Med. 2004;*7(6):870-874.

16. Viera AJ, Sullivan SA. Letter to the editor: remedies for prolonged hiccups. *Am Fam Physician.* 2001;63(9):1684-1685.

17. Rizzo C, Vitale C, Montagnini M. Management of intractable hiccups: an illustrative case and review. *Am J Hosp Palliat Med.* 2014;31(2):220-224.

Treatment Algorithm for Hiccups

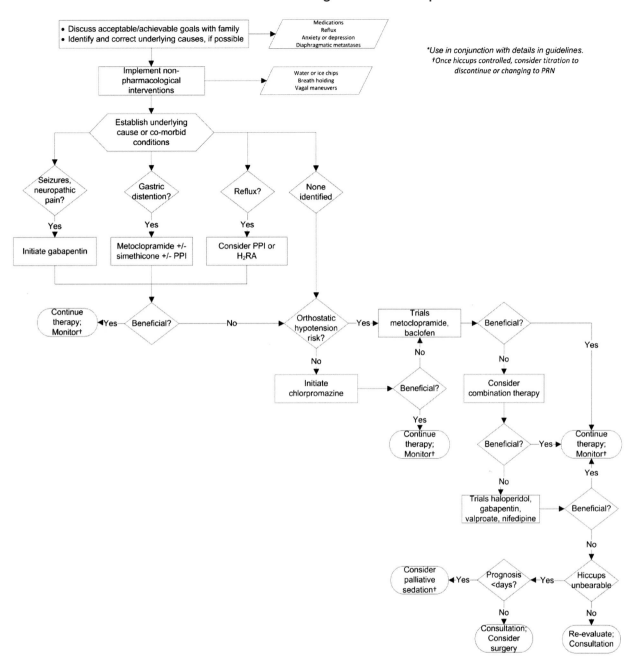

Infections

Introduction and Background[1,2]

- At hospice admission, and periodically after, discuss goals for antimicrobial (antibiotics and antifungals) therapy with the patient and family or caregivers. Patients may choose to seek continued antimicrobial therapy including parenteral antibiotics, to receive antimicrobials for symptom relief only, or to refuse further antimicrobial therapy.
- Potential adverse effects of treatment, the need for laboratory monitoring, and the patient's comfort and convenience are crucial considerations for developing an individualized regimen.
- Symptom response generally occurs in less than half of patients treated with antibiotic therapy. Urinary tract infections (UTI) are the exception, with symptomatic response in 79 – 90% of patients.
- Guide antibiotic therapy by culture and sensitivity (C&S) when available or empiric therapy. If empiric therapy, consider referring to the antibiogram of your local hospital for information regarding regional patterns of infectious organisms and antibiotic resistance. C&S reports minimum inhibitory concentration (MIC) and a qualitative interpretation of the tested drugs ability to treat the infection by inhibiting growth of the organism.
  - *Resistance*: bacteria/organism present in sample is NOT likely to respond to treatment regardless of dosage of drug or location of infection.
  - *Susceptible*: bacteria/organism present in sample is likely to respond to treatment at the recommended dosage; bacterial resistance is clinically insignificant.
  - *Intermediate*: bacteria/organism present in sample is inhibited with uncertain therapeutic effect; successful treatment may be possible if the antimicrobial if it tends to concentrate at the site of infection (e.g., urinary tract) or if higher end of the dosage range is used.

Prevalence[3,4]

- Although the exact rate of infections complicating hospice care is unknown, some studies indicate that approximately 40% of patients with cancer contract an infection at the end of life.
- Frequently, the presence of fever is the leading factor to a clinical diagnosis of infection despite the fact that non-infectious causes of fever may be the source (e.g., drug-induced fever, fever secondary to underlying malignancy).
- Infection, specifically pneumonia, may be the cause of death in one-third to two-thirds of patients with advanced dementia.

Causes[1,5]

- For patients receiving hospice care, infections may result from alteration in physical defense mechanisms (mucositis), decreased immune response (neutropenia), catheter-related (urinary, venous, or parenteral), and aspiration.
- Other contributing factors to infection include malnutrition, asthenia, decreased level of consciousness, and immobility.
- The most common types of infection in patients who are terminally ill include:
  - Upper and lower respiratory tract infections
  - Bloodstream infections
  - Urinary tract infection
  - *Clostridium difficile* diarrhea
  - Oral or pharyngeal candidiasis
  - Intraabdominal infection
  - Skin or subcutaneous infection

Clinical Characteristics

- General signs and symptoms of an infection include a fever higher than 100.5 degrees, chills, pain, ache, malaise, confusion, delirium, and night sweats.

Pharmacotherapy[6]

- Before *initiating* antimicrobial therapy:
  - o Evaluate likely outcomes of antibiotic therapy and potential for symptom control.
  - o Consider if recovery from infection with continued quality of life is likely, or if antibiotic therapy may only extend the patient's suffering.
  - o Define the goals of treatment with the patient and family.
  - o Identify risks and benefits; establish monitoring parameters for reassessment of benefit.
  - o Predefine boundaries for time limited trial, if one is being used by identifying start and stop date.
- Before *continuing* antimicrobial therapy:
  - o Evaluate the continued utility of the antimicrobial medication based on site of infection, patient's Palliative Performance Scale (PPS) score, C&S data.
  - o If antimicrobial therapy was initiated prior to start of hospice care, determine how many days the patient has been on the current therapy and the remaining duration of therapy.
  - o Assess response to therapy: decrease in white blood cell count; fever resolution; improvement in symptoms based on site of infection (dyspnea, painful urination); identify patient/family goals for antibiotic therapy if patient doesn't respond to current therapy or develops a recurrent infection.
  - o Transition parenteral antimicrobial therapy to oral antimicrobial alternatives, if available.

Table 1. Factors Influencing Antibiotic Selection for Home Care

Consideration	Comment
Spectrum & profile of activity	Empiric therapy is chosen based on most likely organism and patterns of local antibiotic resistance; consider C&S for recurrent infections or apparent treatment failure. C&S may suggest microbe susceptibility but antibiotic must be able to penetrate the site of infection for clinical benefit.
Dosage regimen	Antibiotics may be scheduled 1 to 4 times/day dependent on the type of antibiotic and duration of activity, continuous IV infusion, or daily IM injection. Less frequent dosing usually improves patient adherence; stress importance of completing entire course of prescribed antibiotics.
Mode of administration	Oral is preferred; IM can be painful and difficult for patients with low body weight or low muscle mass; IV infusion usually requires line placement and nursing care and monitoring during the length of infusion.
Duration of therapy	Depends on site, severity of infection, usually range: 3 to 14 days; relief of symptoms of infection usually begins within the 2-3 days of antibiotic start but active infection won't resolve without completing the antibiotic course.
Safety & tolerability	Consider side effects of antibiotic (nausea, headache, diarrhea); renal toxicity if improperly dosed; pain at injection site, especially for IM; antibiotic interactions with other concomitant medications (increased PT/INR with warfarin, decreased antibiotic activity with calcium or iron supplements).
Stability & sterility	Some oral solutions may require refrigeration for stability and palatability, others must be stored at room temperature; injectable antibiotics must be stable for a reasonable period of time (preparation to administration); injectable preparations must also remain sterile until administration.
Cost	Newer, branded antibiotics tend to be more expensive than older, generic antibiotics; however local resistance patterns and antibiotic susceptibility must drive selection, not cost of therapy.

Pneumonia and Pneumonitis

Introduction and background[7-11]

- Upper and lower respiratory tract symptoms may be an indication of an infectious process (e.g., aspiration pneumonia, community-acquired pneumonia (CAP), viral infection, etc.) or pneumonitis. Pneumonitis is an inflammation of the lung tissue secondary to chemical or particle aspiration, hypersensitivity reaction, or a consequence of radiation.
- Pneumonia is the second most common infection in nursing home residents, but has the highest rate of morbidity and mortality.
- Oropharyngeal dysphagia is most common in patients with neurological disorders such as Alzheimer's disease, Parkinson's disease, or stroke. Other contributing factors include head and neck cancer, tooth loss, diabetes, and xerostomia.
- Patients generally lose the ability to swallow before they develop deficiencies in the cough reflex. Once the cough reflex is impaired, the risk of aspiration and aspiration pneumonia significantly increases.
- **Aspiration pneumonitis** occurs following the aspiration of sterile gastric contents.
  - A pH of < 2.5 and a volume of gastric aspirate more than 0.3 mL/kg body weight (20-25 mL in most adults) is required for the development of aspiration pneumonitis.
  - Aspiration of particulate food matter may cause severe pulmonary injury even if pH is > 2.5.
  - There are two phases involved in aspiration pneumonitis, immediate phase tissue injury (peaks 1-2 hours after aspiration) and acute inflammatory response (peaks 4-6 hours after aspiration).
  - Cellular regeneration takes 3-7 days.
- **Aspiration pneumonia** is an infectious process caused by the inhalation of oropharyngeal fluids that are colonized by bacteria.

Causes[8]

- Viral pneumonias are more common among children, infants, and immunocompromised adults. Viral pneumonias typically occur during specific times of year.
- Several risk factors have been identified for aspiration pneumonia and pneumonitis.

Table 1. Predictors of Aspiration Pneumonia in Older Adults

Condition	Examples
Comorbidities	Multiple comorbidities, COPD, CHF, CVA, delirium, UTI, obesity, neurological or neuromuscular diseases (Alzheimer's, Parkinson's, ALS)
Gastrointestinal complications	Dysphagia , GERD, mechanically altered diet, dependence for eating, feeding tube, decrease salivary flow, malnutrition
Airway complications	Suctioning, tracheostomy care, poor pulmonary clearance,
General decline	Decreased locomotion, bedfast/immobility, weight loss, advanced age, decreased activities of daily living, decreased immune response
Other	Polypharmacy, poor oral hygiene, chronic use of proton pump inhibitors

Clinical Characteristics[8,12,13]

- Distinguishing between types of pneumonia or pneumonitis based on clinical presentation may be very difficult for clinicians; many symptoms may be present in all conditions.
- Documentation of gastric content aspiration may be helpful in determining when antibiotic therapy may not be necessary to manage upper respiratory symptoms (aspiration pneumonitis) and if symptom-based medications rather than antimicrobial therapy might be more appropriate.

Table 2. Clinical Presentations of Respiratory Tract Infections[8,11-13]

Condition	Symptoms
Aspiration pneumonitis	• Patients may be asymptomatic or present with symptoms including severe dyspnea, wheezing, cyanosis, hypoxia, cough, low grade fever, hypotension, pulmonary edema, and acute respiratory distress syndrome. • In almost 60% of cases, symptoms resolve within 2-4 days
Aspiration pneumonia	• Tachypnea, +/- cough, dyspnea, abnormal breath sounds • Fever & cough are present in about 50% of older patients with aspiration pneumonia. Other symptoms include decline in functional status, altered mental status, weakness, and decreased appetite
Community-acquired pneumonia	• Cough, expectoration, fever, dyspnea, pleuritic pain, altered mental status, pulmonary consolidation, leukocytosis • Altered mental status may be more common, and chest pain may be less common in patients > 65 years of age.
Viral pneumonia	• Fever, chills, nonproductive cough, rhinitis, myalgia, headache, fatigue • Symptoms often being slowly and may start out less severe in contrast to influenza, which usually presents with sudden onset fever. • Studies have shown a lower probability of having chest pain and rigors with viral pneumonia as compared to bacterial.

Table 3. Common Bacteria Associated with Respiratory Infections

Community-acquired	Institutions (LCTF, Hospital)
S. aureus *S. pneumoniae* *H. influenzae* *Enterobacteriaceae*	*Methicillin-resistant S. aureus (MRSA)* *H. influenzae* *P. aeruginosa* *Enterobacteriaceae* Gram negative bacilli *Klebsiella spp.* *E. coli*

Non-Pharmacological Treatment

- Supplemental oxygen, if hypoxia is present.
- Humidified air may be more comfortable and soothing for patients with cough.
- Consult with speech pathologist and dietician for diagnostic evaluation of dysphagia and recommendations for safe feeding practices and nutrition advice.
- Maintain a moderate temperature environment, avoiding drafts and extreme temperature variations.

Pharmacotherapy[8,10,13-15]

- Since aspiration pneumonitis is not an infectious process, use of antibiotics is not recommended.
    - Aspiration of gastric contents does not generally have bacterial involvement because bacteria cannot grow at the normal gastric pH.
    - In about 25% of cases, symptoms initially improve, but then worsen, indicating a secondary bacterial infection. If a secondary infection develops, then consider antibiotic therapy.
    - Antibiotics at onset of symptoms of pneumonitis do not appear to alter clinical outcome, death rate, or subsequent development of infection.
- Empiric antibiotic therapy following an aspiration event may be appropriate in patients with risk factors for bacterial growth in their gastric content (enteral feedings, gastroparesis, small bowel obstruction, or chronic use of acid-suppressing medications).
- Base antibiotic selection on C&S (when available), most common infectious organisms, local resistance patterns, antimicrobial spectrum, and available routes of administration.

- Antimicrobials with anaerobic spectrum are only indicated for patients with severe periodontal disease, putrid sputum, and evidence of necrotizing pneumonia or lung abscess.
- Antibiotics and not indicated for the treatment of suspected viral infection. If influenza is suspected, oseltamivir (Tamiflu®) and zanamivir (Relenza®) should be initiated within 48 hours of the onset of symptoms.
- Mucolytics, cough suppressants, or bronchodilators may provide symptomatic relief to patients experiencing upper respiratory symptoms. See also *Cough GEMS.*
- There is insufficient evidence to support the use of corticosteroids for the treatment of pneumonia or pneumonitis. Patients treated with systemic corticosteroids tend to have more adverse effects and a higher risk of superinfection.

Clinical Pearls[16-19]

- Transition from parenteral antibiotic treatment to an appropriate oral antibiotic as soon as the patient is clinically stable and able to tolerate oral administration.
- The swallowing function of elderly people seems to be temperature sensitive. The swallowing reflex is delayed most around normal body temperature. Delay in the swallowing reflex trigger increases the risk of aspiration. Food served at hot or cold temperatures increases sensory input in the pharynx and larynx and improves swallowing reflex.
- One month of daily oral care significantly improved both cough and swallow reflexes in elderly nursing home patients by stimulating sensory nerves in the oral cavity.
- Chronic use of proton pump inhibitors and subsequent gastric acid suppression may lead to overgrowth of bacteria in GI tract and an increased risk of pneumonia.

Antibiotic Therapy for Respiratory Infections

Generic Name (Trade Name)	Adult Dose	Routes	Common Strengths and Formulations	Comments
Beta Lactam				
Amoxicillin (Amoxil®)	875mg Q12H for 7-10 days	PO	**Tablets:** 500 mg, 875 mg **Capsules:** 250 mg, 500 mg **Oral solution:** 125 mg/5 mL	• Reduce dose to 500mg Q12H in renal impairment (CrCL<30 mL/min). • May mix oral solution with water, milk, juice, or ginger ale; administer immediately after mixing. • CAP use only; resistant organisms in institutionalized patients
Amoxicillin-Clavulanate (Augmentin®)	875mg-125mg Q12H for 7-10 days	PO	**Tablets:** 250-125 mg, 500-125 mg, 875-125 mg **Oral solution:** 250 mg/5 mL, 400 mg/5 mL	• For mixed, aspiration pneumonia. • Reduce dose to 500mg Q12H in renal impairment (CrCL<30 mL/min). • Other formulations and strengths available.
Ceftriaxone (Rocephin®)	1g daily for 7-14 days	IM IV	**Injection:** 500 mg, 1 g, 2 g	• 3rd generation cephalosporin. • Inject deep IM; large muscle mass. • Can be diluted 1:1 with lidocaine 1% for IM administration.

Continued

Generic Name (Trade Name)	Adult Dose	Routes	Common Strengths and Formulations	Comments
Beta Lactam				
Cefuroxime (Ceftin®)	750mg Q8H for 7-10 days	PO IM IV	**Tablets:** 250 mg, 500 mg **Oral liquid:** 125 mg/5 mL, 250 mg/5 mL **Injection:** 750 mg, 1.5 mg	• 2nd generation cephalosporin. • Inject deep IM; large muscle mass. • Swallow tablet whole; strong, persistent bitter taste if chewed or crushed.
Cefpodoxime (Vantin®)	200mg Q12H for 14 days	PO	**Tablets:** 100 mg, 200 mg **Oral liquid:** 50mg /5 mL, 100 mg/5 mL	• 3rd generation cephalosporin. • Administer Q24H in renal impairment (CrCL <30mL/min).
Cefepime (Maxipime®)	1g Q8H for 10 days	IV IM	**Injection:** 1 g, 2 g	• 4th generation cephalosporin. • Inject deep IM; large muscle mass.
Macrolide				
Azithromycin (Zithromax®, Z-pak®)	500mg on day 1; 250mg on days 2-5	PO	**Tablets:** 250 mg, 500 mg **Oral liquid:** 100 mg/5 mL, 200 mg/5 mL	• Risk of QTc interval prolongation. • Prolonged use associated with *C. difficile* diarrhea suprainfection.
Clarithromycin (Biaxin®)	250mg Q12H for 7-14 days	PO	**Tablets:** 250 mg, 500 mg **Oral liquid:** 125 mg/5 mL, 250 mg/5 mL	• Risk of QTc interval prolongation. • Prolonged use associated with *C. difficile* diarrhea suprainfection. • Reduce dose 50% if CrCL<30 mL/min.
Fluoroquinolones				
Levofloxacin (Levaquin®)	500mg daily for 7-14 days	PO IV	**Tablets:** 250 mg, 500 mg, 750 mg **Oral liquid:** 25 mg/mL **Injection:** 250 mg/ 50 mL	• Risk of QTc interval prolongation. • Avoid use with calcium, iron, dairy, antacids, sucralfate. • Alternate dosing: 750mg Q24H for 5 days; CrCL<30 mL/min extend to 48H.
Moxifloxacin (Avelox®)	400mg daily for 7-14 days	PO IV	**Tablets:** 400 mg **Injection:** 400 mg/ 250 mL	• Risk of QTc interval prolongation. • Avoid use with calcium, iron, dairy, antacids, sucralfate.
Tetracycline				
Doxycycline (Vibramycin®)	100mg Q12H for 7 days	PO	**Tablets:** 50 mg, 75 mg, 100 mg, 150 mg **Capsules:** 50 mg, 75 mg, 100 mg, 150 mg	• Administer with 8oz. water to reduce risk of esophageal irritation. • Other formulations and strengths available. • Avoid use with calcium, iron, dairy, antacids, sucralfate.
Aminoglycoside				
Gentamicin	7mg/kg/day for 7 days	IM IV	**Injection:** 10 mg/mL, 40 mg/mL	• Inject deep IM; large muscle mass. • Extend dosing interval to 48H if CrCL<60 mL/min.
Amikacin	15mg/kg/day for 7 days	IM IV	**Injection:** 500 mg/2 mL	• Inject deep IM; large muscle mass. • Dosing interval adjustment required based on renal function; consult pharmacist for assistance.
Other				
Clindamycin (Cleocin®)	300mg TID for 7-21 days	PO	**Capsules:** 75 mg, 150 mg, 300 mg **Oral liquid:** 75 mg/5 mL	• Infection involving anaerobic bacteria, aspiration pneumonia. • Risk of *C. difficile* suprainfection.

See Drug Dosing for Liver and Renal Disease for additional drug information.

Urinary Tract Infection

Introduction and Background[2,20]

- For elderly women in the community, urinary tract infections (UTI) are the second most common cause of infection. For residents of long term care facilities, in the hospital setting, or receiving hospice care, UTI is the number one cause of infection.
- *Asymptomatic bacteriuria*: presence of bacteria in the urine with no symptoms of UTI and no indwelling catheter within 7 days of sample collection. Asymptomatic bacteriuria is common in elderly patients and is not "diagnostic" for UTI.
- *Complicated UTI*: occurs when functional or structural abnormalities of the urinary tract interfere with the flow of urine or urinary tract defense mechanisms (e.g., stone formation, cancer, indwelling catheter, prostatic hypertrophy, or neurologic disorders). Male UTI are all considered complicated.
- *Catheter-associated bacteriuria*: asymptomatic presence of bacteria in the urine of patients with an indwelling, suprapubic, or freshly applied condom catheter. After about 30 days almost all patient with a catheter will have asymptomatic bacteriuria.

Causes[21]

- Urinary incontinence represents a significant risk factor for the development of UTI in older or debilitated patients, especially those with a diagnosis of dementia, or caregiving challenges.

Category of Risk Factors	Examples of Risk Factors
Recurrent UTI, but no little to no risk of more severe outcomes	Sexual behavior, hormonal deficiency in postmenopausal women, diabetes
Non-urogenital, with risk of more severe outcome	Male gender, poorly controlled diabetes, immunosuppression, immunocompromised, renal insufficiency/kidney failure, polycystic nephropathy, interstitial nephritis
Urological risk factors, with risk of more severe outcomes	Urinary catheter, urinary obstruction, neurogenic bladder disturbances, malignancy, asymptomatic bacteriuria, nephrostomy tube, ureteral stents

Clinical Characteristics[20,21]

- The presence of nitrates in the urine indicates gram (-) bacteria.
- Positive leukocyte esterase indicates bacterial growth. Use of clavulanic acid may cause a false positive; use of doxycycline, gentamicin, and cephalexin may cause a false negative.
- Patients with recent removal of urinary catheter may also present with symptoms of cystitis secondary to catheterization.

Table 1. Clinical Presentation of Urinary Tract Infections

Condition	Clinical symptoms
Cystitis	Dysuria, frequency, urgency, suprapubic pain, confusion
Mild or moderate pyelonephritis	Fever, flank pain, tenderness, +/- symptoms of cystitis
Severe pyelonephritis	Nausea, vomiting, fever, chills, flank pain, tenderness, +/- symptoms of cystitis, +/- hematuria
Urosepsis	Fever, tachycardia, tachypnea, hypotension, +/- symptoms of cystitis or pyelonephritis
Catheter-associated UTI (CAUTI)	New onset fever, rigors, hypotension, altered mental status, costovertebral angle pain, malaise, lethargy, pelvic discomfort, acute hematuria

Table 2. Common Organisms Associated with UTI

Bacterial	Fungal
E. coli *Proteus mirabilis* *Klebsiella spp.* *Enterobacter spp.* *Pseudomonas spp.* *Enterococcus spp.*	*Candida spp.* (primarily in elderly patient with diabetes)

Non-Pharmacological Treatment

- Encourage regular and complete emptying of bladder.
- Reinforce proper hygiene and catheter maintenance with patient and caregiver.
- Avoid bladder irritants such as carbonated, caffeinated, alcoholic, and acidic foods or drink.
- Drink water; increase hydration.
- Heat packs to lower abdomen may improve bladder pain from spasm.

Pharmacotherapy[20,22]

- Asymptomatic bacteriuria: antibiotic treatment is not recommended. Treatment has not been linked with a decrease in symptomatic UTI, prevalence of bacteriuria, or an effect on overall survival, but increases the risk of resistant infections and antibiotic adverse effects.
- Catheter-associated bacteriuria: antibiotic treatment is not recommended.
- Choice of antibiotics should be based on C&S (when available), most common infectious organisms, local resistance patterns, antimicrobial spectrum, and available routes of administration.
- Duration of therapy for elderly women with uncomplicated UTI should range from 3-7 days.
- In suspected pyelonephritis, the duration of therapy should be extended to 10-14 days for women and at least 14 days for men.
- Duration of therapy for elderly males should range from 7-14 days, but male patients with recurrent UTI through to be secondary to a prostate source may be treated for 6-12 weeks.
- Patients typically show symptomatic improvement within 72 hours of initiation of appropriate therapy. If no improvement is noted, discuss goals of care and consider transitioning to comfort medications (pain, fever, nausea) or investigating complicating factors such as obstruction or intrarenal abscess.
- Phenazopyridine, a urinary analgesic, may provide symptomatic relief of dysuria.

Clinical Pearls[20,22-25]

- Elderly patients are more likely to present with neurologic changes (altered mental status) with the onset of cystitis or pyelonephritis.
- Some clinicians advocate for initiation of prophylactic antibiotics in women who have experienced ≥ 2 symptomatic UTI over a 6 month period or ≥ 3 symptomatic UTI over a 12 month period after an existing infection has been eradicated. Consider only if counseling and behavioral modifications have been attempted and failed to prevent recurrence.
- Prophylactic antibiotics lead to increased antibiotic resistance and antibiotic side effects (e.g., nausea, vomiting, *C. difficile*, oral or vaginal candidiasis). Prophylactic antibiotics are not recommended for routine catheter removal or replacement.
- If a patient displays signs of UTI while on UTI prophylaxis, discontinue the prophylactic antibiotic. The infectious organism will not be susceptible to the prophylactic antibiotic. Do not restart the same prophylactic antibiotic once the acute treatment course is complete.
- Patients in LTCF have a higher risk of resistant organisms; recommend urine C&S for symptoms of a UTI especially if UTI is recurrent.

- Discontinue urinary catheters as soon as clinically indicated; consider patient and family goals of care and the ability of caregivers to either maintain the catheter or toilet and change the patient.
- Topical estrogen products applied to the vagina may reduce the risk of UTI in postmenopausal women.
- Clinical research provides some support for the cranberry supplements to prevent UTI. The amount of the active ingredient responsible for cranberry's therapeutic effect is not standardized.
- Methenamine salts, hippurate (Hiprex) or mandelate (Mandelamine), may be beneficial for the prevention of recurrent UTI in healthy patients, but are contraindicated in renal dysfunction, hepatic dysfunction, and severe dehydration. Use with caution in hospice patients, who tend to be less stable and experience rapid or sudden decreases in organ function or fluid status.
- Although primarily studied in pediatric, single-dose therapy of gentamicin may provide relief of symptoms of UTI at end of life. Single IM dose of gentamicin (2mg/kg); inject deep IM into large muscle.

Pharmacological Therapy of Urinary Tract Infections

Generic Name (Trade Name)	Adult Dose	Routes	Common Strengths and Formulations	Comments
Cephalosporins				
Ceftriaxone (Rocephin®)	1g daily for 7-14 days	IM IV	**Injection:** 500 mg, 1 g, 2 g	• 3rd generation cephalosporin. • Inject deep IM; large muscle mass. • Can be diluted 1:1 with lidocaine 1% for IM administration.
Cefpodoxime (Vantin®)	100mg Q12H for 7 days	PO	**Tablets:** 100 mg, 200 mg **Oral liquid:** 50mg /5 mL, 100 mg/5 mL	• 3rd generation cephalosporin. • Administer Q24H in renal impairment (CrCL <30mL/min). • For uncomplicated UTI.
Sulfonamide				
Trimethoprim-Sulfamethoxazole (Bactrim DS®, Septra®)	1 DS tab Q12H for 3-10 days	PO	**Tablets:** 400-80 mg, 800-160 mg **Oral liquid:** 200-40 mg/5 mL	• Risk factors for resistance include recent hospitalization or antibiotic usage. • Complicated: 7-10 days. • Dosage adjustment required for CrCL<30mL/min.
Fluoroquinolone				
Ciprofloxacin (Cipro®)	250mg Q12H for 3 days	PO IV	**Tablets:** 100 mg, 250 mg, 500 mg, 750 mg **Oral liquid:** 250 mg/5mL **Injection:** 200 mg/100 mL	• Risk factors for resistance include recent hospitalization, prior quinolone usage, urinary catheter use, male, LTCF residents. • Complicated: 500mg Q12H for 7-14 days. • Dosage adjustment required for CrCL<50mL/min. • Other formulations and strengths available.
Aminoglycosides				
Gentamicin	4.5mg/kg daily for 5-7 days	IV IM	**Injection:** 10 mg/mL, 40 mg/mL	• Inject deep IM; large muscle mass. • Extend dosing interval to 48H if CrCL<60 mL/min.
Amikacin	15mg/kg daily for 5-7 days	IV IM	**Injection:** 500 mg/2mL	• Inject deep IM; large muscle mass. • Dosing interval adjustment required based on renal function; consult pharmacist for assistance.

Continued

Generic Name (Trade Name)	Adult Dose	Routes	Common Strengths and Formulations	Comments
Other				
Nitrofurantoin (Macrodantin®, Macrobid®)	*Macrobid*: 100mg Q12H for 7 days *Macrodantin*: 50mg Q6H for 7 days	PO	**Capsules**: 50 mg, 100 mg **Oral liquid**: 25 mg/5 mL	• Avoid in suspected kidney or prostate infection because of poor tissue penetration. • Contraindicated with CrCl< 60 ml/min. • Chronic use of nitrofurantoin has been linked to pulmonary toxicity, hepatic reactions, and neuropathy. • Oral liquid may be mixed with water, milk, or fruit juice.
Fosfomycin (Monurol®)	*Female*: 3g in single dose *Male*: 3g every other day for 3 doses	PO	**Pack:** 3 g	• Mix with 4oz. cool water prior to administering. • Maintains high concentration in urine for up to 48 hours.
Phenazopyridine (Pyridium®)	200mg TID for 2 days	PO	**Tablet:** 95 mg, 100 mg, 200 mg	• Low dose available OTC. • Take after meals. • Does not treat UTI; only acts as analgesic. • Contraindicated with CrCL<50 mL/min. • May discolor urine reddish-orange.

See Drug Dosing for Liver and Renal Disease for additional drug information.

Clostridium difficile Associated Diarrhea

Introduction and background[26-28]

- *Clostridium difficile* causes a particularly virulent form of infectious diarrhea that can causes symptoms escalating from diarrhea to pseudomembranous colitis and death.
- After hospitalization, 15-25% of patients are colonized by *C. difficile;* up to 50% of patients in long-term care facilities are asymptomatic carriers.
- Recurrent *C. difficile* infection occurs in about 20% of patients after being treated with metronidazole or vancomycin, but recurrence rates may reach 50% or higher in elderly patients treated with metronidazole.
- 50% of all recurrences are caused by reinfection, not a relapse of the primary infection.

Causes[27-30]

Risk Factors for Primary *C. difficile* Diarrhea	
Patient factors	age > 65, recent or prolonged hospitalization, malnutrition, multiple comorbidities
Gastrointestinal	rectal transplantation, GI surgery, nasogastric tube feeding
Medication related	recent antibiotic use (clindamycin, fluoroquinolones, 3rd generation cephalosporins), multiple or prolonged antibiotic use, proton pump inhibitors, immunosuppressive drugs, 2nd generation cephalosporins, antineoplastic agents, enemas
Risk Factors for Recurrent *C. difficile* Infection	
Patient factors	age > 65, chronic renal failure, fecal incontinence, WBC count $\geq 15x10^9$, those infected with particular strains of *C. difficile,* history of recurrent *C. difficile*
Medication related	Frequent or chronic antibiotic use, proton pump inhibitors, H$_2$ antagonist treatment, immunosuppressive drugs

Clinical Characteristics[28,31]

- Diarrhea generally presents as a change in normal bowel function including altered bowel consistency, increased water content, volume, and frequency of stools.
- Diarrhea may develop as long as 8 weeks after a course of antibiotics has ended.
- Elderly patients may be less likely to develop fever in response to *C. difficile* infection. Other non-specific symptoms of infection may be present such as weakness, increased falls, altered mental status, weight loss, decreased appetite, or confusion.

Non-Pharmacological Treatments[30,32]

- Discontinue antibiotic therapy to allow the restoration of normal bowel flora.
- Fluid and electrolyte replacement with an oral rehydration therapy solution.
- Fecal transplantation is currently being studied
  - Liquid stool from a healthy donor is instilled into the upper GI tract through a nasogastric tube, nasoduodenal tube, or gastroscopy, or into to colon through colonoscopy or a rectal catheter.
  - Case series studies report 83% of patient experienced resolution of diarrhea following the first fecal transplant with results lasting for several months.
  - An oral, capsulized, and frozen fecal microbiota transplant process reported similar high response rates of up to 90%.

Pharmacotherapy[28,33]

- For patients with confirmed or suspected infectious diarrhea such as *C. difficile*, avoid antidiarrheal agents. Preventing bowel movements may lead to toxic megacolon.
- Metronidazole is not recommended for treatment beyond the first recurrence of *C. difficile*. For subsequent infections, oral vancomycin or an alternative agent should be initiated.
- Consider pulsed or tapered antibiotic treatment in patients with recurrent *C. difficile* infections.
  - Example: vancomycin 125 mg PO QID x 10-14 days; then 125 mg PO BID x 7 days; then 125mg PO daily x 7 days; then 125 mg PO every 2-3 days x 2-8 weeks

Clinical Pearls[33]

- Probiotics are not recommended for the primary prevention of *C. difficile* infection due to the limited amount of clinical evidence, lack of standardization of formulations, and potential risk of blood stream infections in patients who are immunocompromised.
- Advise healthcare providers and family members that hand washing with soap and hot water is required to prevent the spread of *C. difficile*. Alcohol-based gel or foam sanitizers will not kill *C. difficile* spores.
- Routine screening and treatment of asymptomatic *C. difficile* infection is not recommended. Although treatment with oral vancomycin may be effective, patients treated with vancomycin are at a higher risk of reinfection after treatment is stopped.
- Minimize use and duration of all broad spectrum antibiotic therapy to reduce the risk of *C. difficile*.

Pharmacological Therapy of *C. difficile* Diarrhea

Generic Name (Trade Name)	Adult Dose	Routes	Common Strengths and Formulations	Comments
Metronidazole (Flagyl®)	500mg Q8H for 10-14 days	PO IV	**Tablets**: 250 mg, 500 mg **Capsules**: 375 mg **Injection**: 500 mg/100 mL	• Severe or complicated infection may require IV treatment and/or co-treatment with oral vancomycin. • Convert to oral vancomycin if no treatment response within 5-7 days. • Avoid consumption of alcohol during therapy.
Vancomycin (Vancocin®)	125mg Q6H for 10 days	PO	**Capsules**: 125 mg, 250 mg **Compound kit**: 25 mg/mL, 50 mg/mL **Injection**: 1 g, 5 g, 10 g	• Only oral administration is effective for *C. difficile*. • Powder for injection may be compounded for use as an oral solution; oral solution compounding kits are also available for easier preparation.
Fidaxomicin (Dificid®)	200mg Q12H for 10 days	PO	**Tablets**: 200 mg	• Less studied than vancomycin, but may have lower relapse and recurrence rate. • Expensive ($3750/course).
Rifaximin (Xifaxan®)	400mg Q12H for 14 days	PO	**Tablets**: 200 mg, 550 mg	• Best dose and regimen not well studied in clinical trials. • May be beneficial if relapse after vancomycin course. • Rifaximin resistant strains of *C. difficile* reported.
Nitazoxanide (Alinia®)	500mg Q12H for 10 days	PO	**Tablets**: 500 mg **Oral solution**: 100 mg/5 mL	• Off-label use of antiprotozoal agent. • Expensive ($1000/course).

See Drug Dosing for Liver and Renal Disease for additional drug information.

References

1. White PH, Kuhlenschmidt HL, Vancura BG, Navari RM. Antimicrobial use in patients with advanced cancer receiving palliative care. *J Pain Symptom Manage.* 2003;25(5):438-443.

2. Reinbolt RE, Shenk AM, White PH, Navari RM. Symptomatic treatment of infections in patients with advanced cancer receiving hospice care. *J Pain Symptom Manage.* 2005;30(2):175-182.

3. Van der Steen JT, Ooms ME, van der Wal G, Ribbe MW. Withholding or starting antibiotic treatment in patients with dementia and pneumonia: prediction of mortality with physicians' judgment of illness severity and with specific prognosis models. *Med Decis Making.* 2005;25(2):210-221.

4. Van der Steen JT, Meuleman-Peperkamp I, Ribbe MW. Trends in treatment of pneumonia among Dutch nursing home patients with dementia. *J Palliat Med.* 2009;12(9):789-795.

5. Thompson AJ, Silviera MJ, Vitale CA, Malani PN. Antimicrobial use at the end of life among hospitalized cancer patients with advanced cancer. *Am J Hosp Palliat Med.* 2012;29(8):599-603.

6. Leggett JE. Ambulatory use of parenteral antibiotics: contemporary perspectives. *Drugs.* 2000;59(S3):1-8.

7. Mylotte JM. Nursing home-acquired pneumonia: update on treatment options. *Drugs Aging.* 2006;23(5):377-390.

8. Eisenstadt ES. Dysphagia and aspiration pneumonia in older adults. *J Am Acad Nurse Pract.* 2010;22:17-22.

9. Ebihara S, Ebihara T. Cough in the elderly: a novel strategy for preventing aspiration pneumonia. *Pulm Pharmacol Ther.* 2011;24(3):318-323.

10. Graterol JF, Clayton T. Pulmonary aspiration. *Anaesth Intensive Care Med* 2010;11(10):447-448.

11. Marik PE. Aspiration pneumonitis and aspiration pneumonia. *N Engl J Med* 2001;344(9):665-671.

12. Kelly E, MacRedmond RE, Cullen G, et al. Community-acquired pneumonia in older patients: does age influence systemic cytokine levels in community-acquired pneumonia? *Respirology.* 2009;14(2):210-216.

13. Mosenifar Z, Jeng A, Kamangar N, et al. Viral pneumonia clinical presentation. *Medscape Drugs & Diseases.* October 21, 2014. Available at http://emedicine.medscape.com/article/300455-clinical. Accessed October 24, 2014.

14. Daoud E, Guzman J. Are antibiotics indicated for treatment of aspiration pneumonia? *Cleve Clin J Med.* 2010;77(9):573-576.

15. Povoa P, Salluh JI. What is the role of steroids in pneumonia therapy? *Curr Opin Infect Dis.* 2012;25(2):199-204.

16. Watando A, Ebihara S, Ebihara T, et al. Effect of temperature on swallowing reflex in elderly patients with aspiration pneumonia. *J Am Geriatr Soc.* 2004;52(12):2143-2144.

17. El-Solh AA. Association between pneumonia and oral care in nursing home residents. *Lung.* 2011;189(3):173-180.

18. Yoshino A, Ebihara S, Ebihara T, et al. Daily oral care and risk factors for pneumonia among elderly nursing home patients. *JAMA.* 2001;286(18):2235-2236.

19. Watando A, Ebihara S, Ebihara T, et al. Daily oral care and cough reflex sensitivity in elderly nursing home patients. *Chest.* 2004;126(4):1066-1070.

20. Matthews SJ, Lancaster JW. Urinary tract infections in the elderly population. *Am J Geriatr Pharmacother.* 2011;9(5):286-309.

21. Bjerklund Johansen TE, Naber K, Wagenlehner F, Tenke P. Patient assessment in urinary tract infections: symptoms, risk factors, and antibiotic treatment options. *Surgery.* 2011;29(6):265-271.

22. Hooten TM, Gupta K. Acute uncomplicated cystitis and pyelonephritis in women. In: Calderwood SB, ed. *UpToDate.* Waltham, MA: UpToDate; 2014. Available at http://www.uptodate.com. Accessed October 23, 2014.

23. Lichtenberger P, Hooton TM. Antimicrobial prophylaxis in women with recurrent urinary tract infections. *Int J Antimicrob Agents.* 2011;38(suppl):36-41.

24. Wang C, Fang CC, Chen NC, et al. Cranberry-containing products for prevention of urinary tract infections in susceptible populations: a systematic review and meta-analysis of randomized controlled trials. *Arch Intern Med.* 2012;172(13):988-996.

25. Bailey RR. What evidence is there for the use of single-dose therapy for urinary tract infections in children? *Infection.* 1994;22(suppl1):S14-S15.

26. Mullane KM, Miller MA, Weiss K, et al. Efficacy of fidaxomicin versus vancomycin as therapy for *Clostridium difficile* infection in individuals taking concomitant antibiotics for other concurrent infections. *Clin Infect Dis.* 2011;53(5):440-447.

27. Tal S, Gurevich A, Guller V, et al. Risk factors for recurrence of *Clostridium difficile*-associated diarrhea in the elderly. *Scand J Infect Dis.* 2002;34(8):594-597.

28. Kee VR. *Clostridium difficile* infection in older adults: a review and update on its management. *Am J Geriatr Pharmacother.* 2012;10(1):14-24.

29. Tattevin P, Buffet-Bataillon S, Donnio PY, et al. *Clostridium difficile* infections: do we know the real dimensions of the problem? *Int J Antimicrob Agents.* 2013;42(suppl):S36-S40.

30. Guo B, Harstall C, Louie T, et al. Systematic review: faecal transplantation for the treatment of Clostridium difficile-associated disease. *Aliment Pharmacol Ther.* 201235(8):865-875.

31. Zilberberg MD, Shorr AF, Micek ST, et al. *Clostridium difficile*-associated disease and mortality among the elderly critically ill. *Crit Care Med.* 2009;37(9):2583-2589.

32. Youngster I, Russell GH, Pindar C, et al. Oral, capsulized, frozen fecal microbiota transplantation for relapsing *Clostridium difficile* infection. *JAMA.* 2014;Oct 11. epub ahead of print. doi:10.1001/jama.2014.13875

33. Cohen SH, Gerding DN, Johnson S, et al. Clinical practice guidelines for *Clostridium difficile* infection in adults: 2010 update by the Society for Healthcare Epidemiology of America (SHEA) and the Infectious Disease Society of America (ISDA). *Infect Control Hosp Epidemiol.* 2010;31(5):431-455.

34. *Sanford Guide to Antimicrobial Therapy.* Sanford Guide Web Edition. Sperryville, VA: Antimicrobial Therapy, Inc. Available at http://webedition.sanfordguide.com/ Accessed October 26, 2014.

Treatment Algorithm for Infections

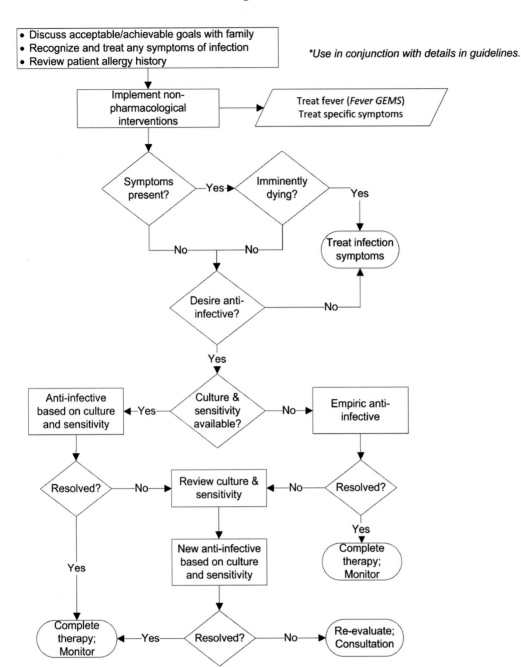

- Discuss acceptable/achievable goals with family
- Recognize and treat any symptoms of infection
- Review patient allergy history

*Use in conjunction with details in guidelines.

Implement non-pharmacological interventions

Treat fever (*Fever GEMS*)
Treat specific symptoms

Symptoms present? —Yes→ Imminently dying? —Yes→ Treat infection symptoms

No — No

Desire anti-infective? —No→ Treat infection symptoms

Yes

Culture & sensitivity available?

Anti-infective based on culture and sensitivity ←Yes— | —No→ Empiric anti-infective

Resolved? —No→ Review culture & sensitivity ←No— Resolved?

Yes — Yes

Complete therapy; Monitor

New anti-infective based on culture and sensitivity

Complete therapy; Monitor

Resolved?

Complete therapy; Monitor ←Yes— Resolved? —No→ Re-evaluate; Consultation

Insomnia

Introduction and Background [1-2, 4-5]

- Insomnia is a common symptom that contributes to suffering at the end of life.
- Insomnia syndrome has been defined as the occurrence of difficulty with initiating or maintaining sleep 3 or more days per week to a degree that impairs daytime function.
- Patients receiving hospice care may not meet formal criteria for insomnia syndrome, yet they experience symptoms that contribute to their total suffering.
- Insomnia may be described as a disruption of previous sleep patterns, difficulty falling asleep, frequent waking, non-restorative sleep, or some combination of these problems.
- Insomnia diminishes quality of life for people at the end of life, and may intensify feelings of isolation and loneliness. Lack of sleep and decreased tolerance to physical symptoms contributes to caregiver distress and fatigue.
- Effective control of this symptom requires a comprehensive assessment of contributing factors and a combination of behavioral and pharmacologic approaches to restore a restful pattern of sleep.
- Treatment goals for insomnia include restful, restorative sleep as reported by the patient. Perception of sleep quality may not correlate with the duration of time spent sleeping.

Prevalence [1, 4]

- Prevalence of insomnia in the hospice population is not well studied but may be as high as 70%.
- Patients with cancer are 2 to 3 times more likely than the general population to suffer from insomnia symptoms.
- Women are twice as likely as men to experience insomnia.

Causes [3-4]

- Poorly controlled physical symptoms are common underlying factors of insomnia:
  - Pain, shortness of breath, nausea, hot flashes, involuntary limb movements, headaches, and frequent urination are also likely to contribute to sleep disturbance.
- Diagnostic criteria for psychological disorders often include insomnia, which can be caused by and a symptom of psychiatric illness.
- Daytime fatigue, waking before desired time, and difficulty returning to sleep after night waking are signs of insomnia syndrome as well as depression.
- Anxiety, depression, and insomnia are more common at the end of life than in the general population.
- Cancer may increase the incidence of sleep difficulty, though it is not clear if malignancy is a cause or an aggravating factor. Patients with cancer are also more likely to have involuntary limb movements during sleep, which often results in an increased frequency of night waking.
- Apparent insomnia may be a prodrome of the day/night reversal of delirium. Assessing for and treating underlying causes of delirium can help reduce symptoms insomnia.
  - Delirium prevalence increases as patients approach end of life.
  - Pharmacotherapy used to manage insomnia, especially benzodiazepines, may worsen symptoms of delirium.
  - Improvement of reversible underlying factors will improve both delirium and insomnia.
- Medication regimens can contribute to insomnia, either from medication side effects or disturbed night time routine from administration (Table 1).
- When pharmacokinetics, nutritional status, hepatic or renal function change, medications that were previously tolerated may cause insomnia due to increased free blood levels. Regularly review patient medication profiles, assess patients for possible adverse effects, and discontinue non-essential medications

Table 1. Medications Contributing to Insomnia

Medication	Disturbance
Antihistamines	Paradoxical excitation possible
albuterol, levalbuterol (Xopenex)	Stimulates CNS
Caffeine	Stimulates CNS
Corticosteroids	Sleep disturbance
Diuretics	Night wakening to urinate
lamotrigine (Lamictal)	Irritability, sleep disturbance, dream abnormality
methylphenidate (Ritalin)	Stimulates CNS
nicotine (smoking cessation products)	Stimulates CNS
Non-steroidal anti-inflammatory (NSAIDs)	Dyspepsia symptoms
Selective serotonin reuptake inhibitors (SSRIs)	Increase sleep onset latency, decrease sleep efficiency, exacerbate preexisting periodic limb movements
Tricyclic antidepressants (TCAs)	Exacerbate restless leg syndrome or periodic limb movements

Clinical Characteristics [1,3-4]

- Insomnia symptoms include difficulty with sleep initiation, decreased duration of sleep intervals, and early morning wakening.
- The presence of daytime fatigue, headache, diarrhea, gastrointestinal upset, palpitations, and generalized pain are all increased in patients who report insomnia symptoms.
- Patients may appear to sleep an adequate number of hours at night, but report that their sleep is not restful or restorative.
- Undertreated pain, dyspnea, and intrusive thoughts may be exacerbating factors to unsatisfying sleep.
- While optimization of pain and symptom management is a necessary component of the treatment plan for insomnia, treatment of insomnia as a symptom should not be delayed in this process.
- Patients are often hesitant to report the symptom of insomnia, and it is important to be vigilant about screening for it throughout decline.

Non-Pharmacological Treatment [1-2, 4]

- Behavioral interventions take 4-6 weeks to see effect, but improvement does not diminish over time.
- Sleep may improve substantially with attention to good sleep hygiene.
    - Wake up at the same time of day.
    - Minimize caffeine and nicotine use, especially late in the day or during nighttime awakenings.
    - Avoid alcohol use late at night.
    - Avoid heavy meals late at night, though a light bedtime snack may promote sleep.
    - Avoid excessive fluids before bedtime.
    - Consider moderate regular exercise (if tolerated), but not close to bedtime.
    - Minimize noise, light, and extremes of temperature in the bedroom.
    - Try simple relaxation techniques.
    - Consider a bedtime ritual (e.g., warm bath, reading) to help relax.
- Hospice patients may not have the energy or attention to adhere to all standard sleep hygiene recommendations, but even a minimal modification of behavior to reinforce a normal day/night sleep pattern can yield dramatic symptomatic improvements.
- Relaxation therapy may involve progressive muscle relaxation (avoid in persons with painful bony metastases due to risk of pain exacerbation) or guided imagery, and is most helpful in reducing in intrusive thoughts and promoting sleep onset.
- Establishing a comforting bedtime routine may be helpful for the patient and allow the caregiver to participate by reading, listening to music, massage, or holding hands.

Pharmacotherapy [3-4, 6-12]

- Evaluation of the sleep disturbance is helpful when choosing therapy.
  - Sleep onset (falling asleep) difficulty: may benefit from a shorter acting agent, such as lorazepam.
  - Maintenance (staying asleep) difficulty: evaluate for possible causes of wakening; may benefit from a longer acting agent, such as trazodone.
  - Circadian rhythm dysfunction (biological daily cycle), common in patients with neurocognitive disorders or blindness may benefit from melatonin. Melatonin has minimal risk and side effects.
- While benzodiazepines and GABA receptor agonists improve insomnia symptoms quickly, they are FDA-approved for a only short term use. With chronic use, GABA receptors are down-regulated and tolerance develops to their effects. Rapid discontinuation of long-term benzodiazepine use has been shown to have a low risk of mild withdrawal symptoms and improvement in sleep quality after the washout period.
- Melatonin may modestly improve sleep latency and quality. At best, there is a minimal effect on sleep duration. Results are dose dependent and no signs of tolerance or significant adverse effects were seen.
- Elderly patients with insomnia are likely to be melatonin deficient. Immediate-release melatonin preparations improve sleep latency after 1 week of chronic use. Extended-release formulations are preferred to mimic the natural cycle of melatonin levels and effect, but improvement in sleep latency can take up to 2 months.
- Routine use of diphenhydramine, diazepam, and tricyclic antidepressants is not recommended due to the risk of accumulating active metabolites, anticholinergic adverse effects, and increased daytime fatigue or confusion.

Clinical Pearls

- Behavioral therapy is the most effective long-term intervention to improve symptoms of insomnia.
- The effects of most medications prescribed to improve sleep will decrease rapidly with routine use.
- If melatonin therapy is initiated, recommend extended-release preparations and routine dosing. Maximum effect many not be seen for 8 weeks.
- While addressing insomnia as an independent symptom, also continue to improve the management of other physical and psychological contributing factors, e.g. pain, dyspnea, nocturnal urination, nausea, anxiety, and depression.
- Insomnia is a common prodrome of acute delirium. Benzodiazepines can worsen symptoms of delirium, but may be appropriate adjunct therapy to cause sedation.
- Patient specific co-morbid symptoms should influence pharmacotherapy decisions.
- Chloral hydrate was withdrawn from the US market by the manufacturer in 2012 (oral solution) and early 2013 (capsules).

Pharmacological Management of Insomnia

Generic Name (Trade Name)	Adult Starting Dose	Routes	Common Strengths and Formulations	Comments
Benzodiazepines				
Lorazepam (Ativan®)	0.5 mg QHS	PO SL	**Tablets**: 0.5 mg, 1 mg, 2 mg **Oral solution**: 2 mg/mL	• Tolerance to sedating effects may develop with longer use. • No active metabolites.
Temazepam (Restoril®)	15 mg QHS	PO	**Capsules**: 7.5 mg, 15 mg, 22.5 mg, 30 mg	• 7.5 mg and 22.5 mg strengths are expensive. • Avoid duplication of therapy if patient using other benzodiazepine for anxiety or dyspnea.

Continued

Generic Name (Trade Name)	Adult Starting Dose	Routes	Common Strengths and Formulations	Comments
Antidepressants				
Trazodone (Desyrel®)	50-100 mg QHS	PO	**Tablets:** 50 mg, 100 mg, 150 mg	• Unlikely to have significant anti-depressant effect at doses used for sleep. • Daytime sedation common at higher doses. • Orthostasis at higher doses.
Mirtazapine (Remeron®)	7.5-15 mg QHS	PO	**Tablets:** 15 mg, 30 mg	• May lose sedating effect at higher doses. • May also stimulate appetite.
GABA Receptor Agonists				
Zolpidem (Ambien®)	5-10 mg QHS	PO	**Tablets:** 5 mg, 10 mg **ER Tablets:** 6.25 mg, 12.5 mg	• Little to no anxiolytic effect. • No clear advantage over benzodiazepines. • Monitor for excess sedation, falls, and confusion especially in elderly patients. • Alternate dosage forms available but expensive.
Zaleplon (Sonata®)	5-10 mg QHS	PO	**Capsules:** 5 mg, 10 mg	• No clear advantage over benzodiazepines. • Very short duration of action.
Eszopiclone (Lunesta®)	1 mg QHS	PO	**Tablets:** 1 mg, 2 mg, 3 mg	• Monitor for excess sedation, falls, and confusion especially in elderly patients.
Melatonin Receptor Agonist				
Ramelteon (Rozerem®)	8 mg QHS	PO	**Tablets:** 8 mg	• Mechanism of action similar to melatonin. • Associated with taste perversion in some patients.
Complementary & Alternative Medicine (CAM)				
Melatonin	5-10 mg QHS *or* 2 mg ER QHS	PO	IR & SR products available in doses ranging from 0.1-10 mg from various manufacturers	• Not FDA tested or approved. • Limited efficacy and specific dosing data. • Favorable safety profile. • No rebound effect seen when discontinued. • Administer 1-2 hours before bedtime.

See Drug Dosing for Liver and Renal Disease for additional drug information.

References
1. Savard J, Morin CM. Insomnia in the context of cancer: a review of a neglected problem. *J Clin Oncol.* 2001;19:895-908.
2. Morin C, Colecchi C, Stone J, Sood R, Brink D. Behavioral and pharmacological therapies for late-life insomnia. *JAMA.* 1999; 281:991-999.
3. Hugel H, Ellershaw J, Cook L, Skinner J, Irvine C. The prevalence, key causes, and management of insomnia in palliative care patients. *J Pain Symptom Manage.* 2004;27: 316-321.
4. Kvale EA, Shuster JL. Sleep disturbance in supportive care of cancer: a review. *J Palliat Med.* 2006;9:437-450.

5. Katz DA, McHorney CA. The relationship between insomnia and health-related quality of life in patients with chronic illness. *J Fam Pract*. 2002;51(3):229-235.

6. Bruera E, Fainsinger RL, Schoeller, Ripamonti C. Rapid discontinuation of hypnotics in terminal cancer patients: a prospective study. *Ann Oncol*. 1996;7:855-856.

7. Krystal AD, Walsh JK, Laska E, et al. Sustained efficacy of eszopiclone over 6 months of nightly treatment: results of a randomized, double-blind, placebo controlled study in adults with chronic insomnia. *Sleep*. 2003;26(7):793-799.

8. Poyares D, Guilleminault C, Ohayon MM, Tufik S. Chronic benzodiazepine usage and withdrawal in insomnia patients. *J Psych Research*. 2003; 38(2004):327-334.

9. Ferracioli-Oda E, Qawasmi A, Bloch MH. Meta-Analysis: Melatonin for the treatment of primary sleep disorders. *PLoS ONE*. 2013;8(5):e63773.

10. Cajochen C, Krauchi K, Wirz-Justice A. Role of melatonin in the regulation of human circadian rhythms and sleep. *J of Neuroendocrin*. 2003;15:432-437.

11. Haimov I, Lavie P, Laudon M, et al. Melatonin replacement therapy of elderly insomniacs. *Sleep*. 1995;18(7):598-603.

12. Natural Medicines Comprehensive Database. Stockton, CA: Therapeutic Research Faculty; 2013. http://naturaldatabase.therapeuticresearch.com/. Accessed October 21, 2013.

13. U.S. Food & Drug Administration (FDA). Drugs to be discontinued. Accessed October 21, 2013. Available at http://www.fda.gov/drugs/drugsafety/drugshortages/ucm050794.htm

Treatment Algorithm for Insomnia

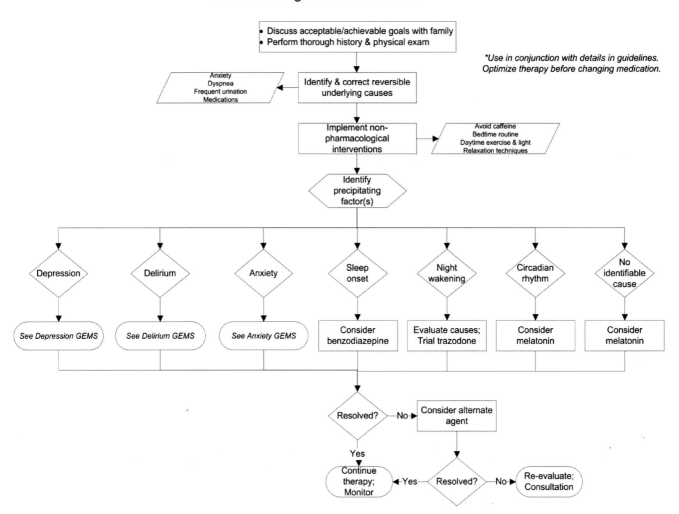

*Use in conjunction with details in guidelines.
Optimize therapy before changing medication.*

Muscle Spasms

Introduction and Background[1,2]

- *Muscle spasms* are a quick, painful, spontaneous contraction of either a single muscle or group of muscles (often used interchangeably with the term muscle cramps) caused by involuntary repetitive firing of motor unit action potentials at high frequency, which can impair mobility and cause pain.
- *Tremor* is an involuntary, rhythmic, oscillating movement of any body part caused by contractions of reciprocally innervated antagonist muscles.
- *Myoclonus* is a brief, involuntary jerking of a muscle or group of muscles caused by neuronal discharges, often seen at the end of life and can be due to accumulation of opioid metabolites. Myoclonus may progress to seizures if left untreated. See also *Seizure GEMS*.
- *Muscle spasticity* is a muscle control disorder that is characterized by tight or stiff muscles and an inability to control those muscles. Reflexes may persist for too long and may be too strong (hyperactive reflexes).

Prevalence[1,2]

- The prevalence of muscle spasms in hospice and palliative care is not well documented, but can be a symptom seen in patients approaching end of life.
- Patients with malignancies, heart failure, HIV/AIDs, and advanced neuromuscular disease may be at highest risk.

Causes[1-7]

- *Muscle spasms* may occur in patients due to overexertion, strain, or overuse of certain muscle groups or holding muscles in one place for extended periods.

Table 1. Underlying Causes of Muscle Spasm by Disease State

Disease	Cause
Cancer, advanced stages	direct neural or muscle invasion, along with biochemical abnormalities, such as hypomagnesemia
AIDS-related neuropathies	spasms due to underlying nerve pathology or inflammation
Heart failure	muscle spasms and cramps, commonly due to hypokalemia
Peripheral arterial disease	inadequate blood flow
Neuromuscular & neurodegenerative diseases (multiple sclerosis, Parkinson's disease, Alzheimer's disease, or Creutzfeldt-Jakob disease)	myoclonus and spasticity

Table 2. Causes of Muscle Spasm and Spasticity and Related Conditions

Cause	Examples
Lower motor neuron disorders	Amyotrophic lateral sclerosis (ALS), post-poliomyelitis, radiculopathy, neuropathy
Metabolic disorders	Uremia, cirrhosis, hypothyroidism, hypoadrenalism
Acute extracellular volume depletion	Perspiration ("heat cramps"), hemodialysis, diarrhea, vomiting
Medications	Diuretics (e.g., furosemide, bumetanide, torsemide, metolazone, hydrochlorothiazide), donepezil, neostigmine, nifedipine, raloxifene, terbutaline, albuterol, tolcapone, statins (e.g. rosuvastatin, atorvastatin, pravastatin, simvastatin)

- Nocturnal muscle spasms or "leg cramps" are poorly understood but are likely due to muscle fatigue and nerve dysfunction. Nocturnal leg spasm may respond well to massage.

- Spasticity is caused by an imbalance of signals from the central nervous system (brain and spinal cord) to the muscles. This imbalance is often found in people with cerebral palsy, traumatic brain injury, stroke, multiple sclerosis, and spinal cord injury.
- Although muscle spasms often occur with spasticity, they are not caused by spasticity.

Clinical Characteristics [1,2,4,5-8]

- Muscle spasms are unpredictable. Spasms range from rare to very frequent and can last for variable lengths of time, but usually not longer than several minutes.
- As with any painful condition, patient description can be wide ranging depending on the muscle group affected and the degree of muscle contraction.
- A series of contractions or a prolonged muscle spasm can lead to residual tenderness and hypersensitivity in the muscle group.
- Myoclonus is a brief, involuntary muscle jerk or group of muscle contractions caused by neuronal discharges that is transient and not sustained as a spasm. A single muscle discharge occurs but can reoccur in repetitive fashion. Myoclonus occurs spontaneously or with sensory stimulation, arousal, or initial movement (action myoclonus). Myoclonus may be a symptom of opioid-induced neurotoxicity. The incidence of opioid-induced myoclonus varies between 2.7% and 87%. See also *Pain GEMS*.
- Muscle spasticity may present as increased muscle tone, overactive reflexes, involuntary movements which may include:
  - Spasms - brisk or sustained involuntary muscle contraction
  - Clonus - series of fast involuntary contractions
  - Contractures - permanent contraction of the muscle and tendon due to severe persistent stiffness and spasms, and bone and joint deformities
- Muscle spasticity can result in pain, decreased functional abilities, difficulty with care and hygiene, and abnormal posture.

Non-Pharmacological Treatment [1,2,6,7]

- Gentle massage and stretching of affected muscle groups and activating the antagonist muscles can prevent cramps during exercise and treat nocturnal leg cramps.
- For nocturnal cramps, foot splints may provide passive stretch of the calf muscle.
- Positioning and repositioning can provide comfort for immobile patients or those with paralysis.
- Apply mild heat to affected muscle groups; do not apply heat for longer than 20 minutes at a time. Ice application may be beneficial in acute spasms.
- Evaluate and treat dehydration if contributing to spasms. Add sodium with fluid replacement or add salt to food to help replace fluid losses.
- Patients may benefit from physical, occupational, or aquatic therapy.
- *Spasticity* treatment may include occupational and physical therapy programs, involving muscle stretching, range of motion exercises, and braces, may help prevent tendon shortening. Rehabilitation may help reduce or stabilize the severity of symptoms and improve functional performance.

Pharmacotherapy [1-12]

- Treatment must be patient specific and focused on individual goals of therapy, relieving pain, and improving activities of daily living.
- If there are elements of underlying pain, tenderness, or inflammation in the affected muscle groups, patients may benefit from acetaminophen, NSAIDs, or opioids.
- Over the counter topical agents may provide localized relief. These agents usually include menthol or trolamine salicylate, causing a heating or cooling sensation when applied. Some patients may find these sensations unpleasant.
- Capsaicin cream may provide relief, but can cause irritation and burning at the application site. Capsaicin may take 2 to 4 weeks of continuous use (applied 3 to 4 times per day) for full effect.
- Diazepam acts at the GABA receptor within the CNS on inhibitory neurons, producing receptor stabilization leading to muscle relaxation and decreased spasticity.
- Baclofen acts at the GABA receptor to inhibit transmission reflexes at the spinal cord level, resulting in relief of muscle spasticity.

- Gabapentin acts at receptors throughout the brain at the presynaptic calcium voltage-gated channels to modulate the release of excitatory neurotransmitters.
- Muscle relaxants cause common side effects of sedation, dry mouth, drowsiness, and dizziness.
- Depending on severity and frequency of spasms, the initial starting dose should be low, with as needed use. Medication selection, dosage, and schedule should be individually titrated to meet patient's goals for symptom relief with minimal side effects. Most of these medications require tapered withdrawal.
- Trigger point injections can be used to treat painful areas containing trigger points or knots of muscle that form when muscles do not relax. The procedure includes injecting a local anesthetic and corticosteroid into the trigger point.
- Medications used to treat muscle spasms potentiate effects of other central nervous system medications such as antidepressants, anxiolytics, and opioids. Use caution when prescribing these medications together.
- Medications for spasticity may include baclofen, tizanidine, dantrolene, diazepam, or clonazepam.
  - Antispasmodic agents, clonidine and tizanidine, are both centrally acting alpha-2 adrenergic agonists which decrease spasticity by increasing presynaptic inhibition of spinal neurons to reduce facilitation of spinal motor neurons.
  - Dantrolene blocks the release of calcium ions in skeletal muscle and can cause muscle weakness.

Clinical Pearls [1,7,9,13]

- The primary focus for patients with advanced illness is comfort and symptom control. Non-pharmacological treatments are important in combination with medications.
- Avoid duplication of therapy. If a patient is already using a benzodiazepine for other symptoms, the same benzodiazepine can be used for muscle spasms.
- Botulinum toxins (A or B) can be injected into individual spastic muscles. This procedure is usually reserved for treatment of cervical dystonia, although there may be benefit for other contractures.
- Cannabis and cannabinoids have been used for muscle relaxation and may relieve some forms of spasticity, especially in patients with multiple sclerosis or spinal cord injury. However, there is very limited clinical evidence to support the use of cannabinoids for any medical purpose.
- All skeletal muscle relaxants can cause drowsiness and dizziness. Use cautiously in elderly patients due to increased risk of falls. Lower doses may be better tolerated but are less likely to be therapeutically effective.
- Because of limited distribution of baclofen from the spinal column when administered by intrathecal (IT) pump or injection, higher spinal concentrations may be tolerated with fewer peripheral side effects.

Pharmacological Management of Muscle Spasms

Generic Name (Trade Name)	Adult Starting Dose	Routes	Common Strengths and Formulations	Comments
Benzodiazepines				
Clonazepam (Klonopin®)	0.25mg BID	PO SL PR	**Oral disintegrating tablets:** 0.125 mg, 0.25 mg, 0.5 mg, 1 mg, 2 mg **Tablets:** 0.5 mg, 1 mg, 2 mg	• C-IV controlled substance. • Tabs may be crushed for SL or PR administration. • ODT tabs are expensive.
Diazepam (Valium®)	2mg Q8H	PO SL PR IM IV	**Oral solution:** 1 mg/mL, 5 mg/mL **Tablets:** 2 mg, 5 mg, 10 mg **Injection:** 5 mg/mL	• C-IV controlled substance. • Active metabolite can accumulate in patients with renal insufficiency. • Tabs may be crushed for SL or PR administration.

Continued

Generic Name (Trade Name)	Adult Starting Dose	Routes	Common Strengths and Formulations	Comments
Skeletal Muscle Relaxants				
Cyclobenzaprine (Flexeril®, Amrix®)	5 mg TID	PO	**Tablets:** 5 mg, 7.5 mg, 10 mg **ER capsules:** 15 mg, 30 mg	• Structurally similar to tricyclic antidepressants; Do not use within 14 days of MAOIs. • Not effective in cerebral palsy (CP) or spinal cord disease. • ER capsules are expensive.
Metaxalone (Skelaxin®)	800 mg TID	PO	**Tablets:** 800mg	• No direct effect on skeletal muscle; likely benefit from general CNS depressant effect. • Tablets are scored and can be split.
Methocarbamol (Robaxin®)	500 mg QID	PO IV	**Tablets:** 500 mg, 750 mg **Injection:** 100 mg/mL	• Skeletal muscle relaxation caused by general CNS depressant effect. • Short duration of action requires frequent, multiple daily dosing. • Injection use limited to 3 day intervals.
Antispasmodic				
Tizanidine (Zanaflex®)	2mg Q8H	PO	**Capsules:** 2 mg, 4 mg, 6 mg **Tablets:** 2 mg, 4 mg	• Structurally related to clonidine; may cause orthostatic hypotension. • Taper off medication over 1-2 weeks; do not discontinue abruptly. • Capsules may be opened and sprinkled on food.
Baclofen (Lioresal®)	10mg TID	PO IT	**Tablets:** 10 mg, 20 mg **Injection, IT:** 50 mcg/mL, 500 mcg/mL, 1,000 mcg/mL, 2,000 mcg/mL	• Avoid abrupt withdrawal due to risk of seizures. • May be as beneficial for spasticity as diazepam with less sedation. • Tolerance may develop over time; dosage adjustment may be required to maintain clinical benefit.
Dantrolene (Dantrium®)	25mg daily for 7 days, with titration of dose every 7 days.	PO	**Capsules:** 25 mg, 50 mg, 100 mg	• Doses must be individualized; titrate slowly to lowest effective dose. • Each dose level should be maintained for 7 days to determine response. • Stop therapy if benefits are not evident within 45 days. • Limited to treatment of spasticity with upper motor neuron disorders.

Continued

Generic Name (Trade Name)	Adult Starting Dose	Routes	Common Strengths and Formulations	Comments
Miscellaneous				
Clonidine (Catapres®, Duraclon®)	PO: 0.1mg BID *or* TD: 0.1 mg every 7 days	PO TD Epidural	**Tablets:** 0.1 mg, 0.2 mg, 0.3 mg **ER tablets:** 0.1 mg **Transdermal patch:** 0.1 mg, 0.2 mg, 0.3 mg **Injection:** 100 mcg/mL, 500 mcg/mL	• Oral tablets and transdermal patches have been used in for the treatment of spasticity in children. • Epidural reserved for cancer patients with severe, refractory pain as opioid adjuvant. • Orthostatic hypotension, dizziness, drowsiness are common.
Gabapentin (Neurontin®, Gralise®)	300mg QHS	PO	**Capsules:** 100 mg, 300 mg, 400 mg **Tablets:** 600 mg, 800 mg **Oral solution:** 250 mg/5 mL **ER tablets:** 300 mg, 600 mg	• May be effective for painful tonic spasms (PTS) in multiple sclerosis. • Slowly titrate to effect based on patient's tolerance to sedation and CNS effects. • Dose adjustments required in renal insufficiency.

See Drug Dosing for Liver and Renal Disease for additional drug information.

References

1. Khoshknabi DS. Muscle Spasms. In: Walsh DT, Caraceni AT, Fainsinger R, et al, editors. *Palliative Medicine.* Philadelphia, PA: Elsevier; 2009. http://www.expertconsultbook.com; Accessed June 25, 2014.
2. Gelber D, Jeffery D. *Clinical Evaluation and Management of Spasticity* [e-book]. Totowa, N.J.: Humana Press; 2002. Available from: eBook Collection (EBSCOhost), Ipswich, MA. Accessed August 28, 2014.
3. Lussier, D, Huskey, AG, Portenoy, RK. Adjuvant analgesics in cancer pain management. *Oncologist.* 2004;9:571-591.
4. See S, Ginzburg R. Skeletal muscle relaxants. *Pharmacother J Human Pharmacol Drug Ther.* 2008;28(2):207–213.
5. Smith, HS, Barton, AE. Tizanidine in the management of spasticity and musculoskeletal complaints in the palliative care population. *Am J Hospice Palliat Care.* 2000;17(1): 50-58.
6. Allen RE, Kirby KA. Nocturnal leg cramps. *Am Fam Physician.* 2012;86(4):350-355.
7. Nair KPS, Marsden J. Management of spasticity in adults. *BMJ.* 2014;349:g4737.
8. Montané E, Vallano A, Laporte JR. Oral antispastic drugs in nonprogressive neurologic diseases: a systematic review. *Neurology* 2004;63(8):1357.
9. Chou, R, Peterson, K, Helfand, M. Comparative efficacy and safety of skeletal muscle relaxants for spasticity and musculoskeletal conditions: a systematic review. *J Pain Symptom Manage.* 2004;28(2): 140-175.
10. Wheeler A, Smith, HS. Botulinum toxins: mechanisms of action, antinociception and clinical applications. *Toxicology.* 2013;306:124-146.
11. Solaro C, Messmer Uccelli M. Pharmacological management of pain in patients with multiple sclerosis. *Drugs.* 2010;70(10):1245-1254.
12. Lexi-Comp Online, Lexi-Drugs Online, Hudson, Ohio: Lexi-Comp, Inc; June 23, 2014.
13. Miller RD, Katzung BG. Skeletal muscle relaxants. In: Katzung BG, editor. *Basic and Clinical Pharmacology.* 8th ed. New York: Lange Medical Books/McGraw-Hill; 2001.

Treatment Algorithm for Muscle Spasms

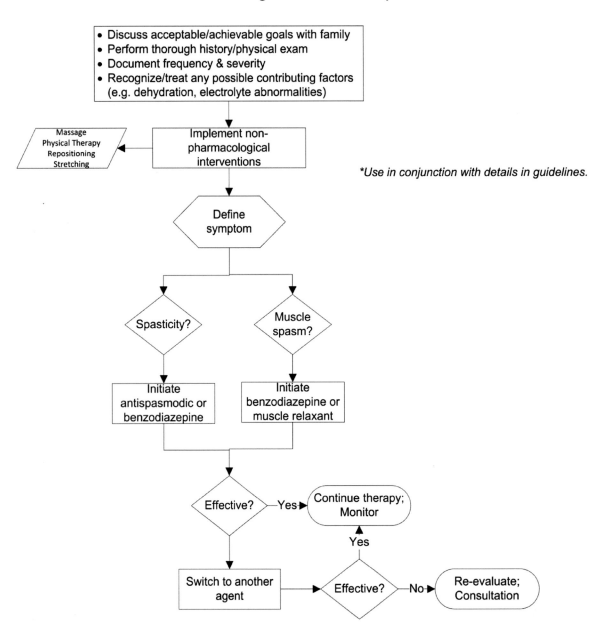

- Discuss acceptable/achievable goals with family
- Perform thorough history/physical exam
- Document frequency & severity
- Recognize/treat any possible contributing factors (e.g. dehydration, electrolyte abnormalities)

Massage
Physical Therapy
Repositioning
Stretching

Implement non-pharmacological interventions

*Use in conjunction with details in guidelines.

Define symptom

Spasticity?

Muscle spasm?

Initiate antispasmodic or benzodiazepine

Initiate benzodiazepine or muscle relaxant

Effective? —Yes▶ Continue therapy; Monitor

Yes

Switch to another agent

Effective? —No▶ Re-evaluate; Consultation

Nausea and Vomiting

Introduction and Background[1-3]

- Nausea is the unpleasant sensation of feeling the need to vomit, which may be accompanied by abdominal discomfort, sweating, or tachycardia. Nausea can be acute, anticipatory, delayed, or chronic. Vomiting is the process of ejection of gastric contents through the mouth as a result of prolonged contraction of the diaphragm and abdominal muscles. Retching presents as spasmodic movements of the esophagus and gastric muscles, without vomiting.
- Nausea and vomiting involves both the GI tract and the brain. In these two organ systems, dopamine, histamine, acetylcholine, and serotonin ($5HT_3$) are the primary neurotransmitters that mediate symptoms of nausea and vomiting.
- The pathology of nausea and vomiting is complex. The brain's vomiting center receives input from various areas in the brain as well as from the gastrointestinal tract. Figure 1 below indicates the four major mechanisms for stimulation of the vomiting center.

Figure 1. Mechanisms Involved in Nausea & Vomiting

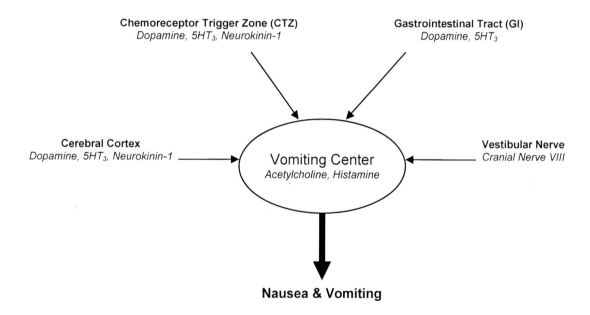

Prevalence[1,4,5]

- Nausea and vomiting is common in end-of-life care; up to 71% of palliative care patients will develop nausea and vomiting, with approximately 40% of patients experiencing these symptoms in the last six weeks of life. Of patients with advanced cancer, roughly 20-30% experience nausea, with 70% reporting nausea in the last week of life.
- Nausea and vomiting is more likely to occur in female patients and those younger than 50 years of age.
- Patients often complain of nausea and vomiting in combination with other symptoms. Studies of patients with cancer report that approximately 25% of those being treated for pain also report nausea.

Causes[2-4]

- Major causes of nausea include:
  - Anxiety
  - Autonomic dysfunction
  - Bowel obstruction
  - Constipation
  - Increased intracranial pressure
  - Infection
  - Medications: Antibiotics, chemotherapy, NSAIDs, opioids
  - Metabolic abnormalities: renal or hepatic failure, hypercalcemia
  - Peptic ulcer disease
  - Radiation therapy

Clinical Characteristics[1,3,4,6]

- *Chemoreceptor trigger zone* (CTZ) is located in the area postrema of the medulla and receives emetogenic stimulation via the blood and cerebrospinal fluid. Chemotherapeutic agents, bacterial toxins, metabolic products (e.g., uremia), opioids and other medications can stimulate the CTZ. This stimulation causes nausea with or without vomiting. Dopamine (D_2), serotonin ($5HT_3$) and neurokinin-1 (NK_1) are the primary neurotransmitters involved in this process. Therapy is based on blocking D_2 with dopamine antagonists such as a butyrophenone (haloperidol), phenothiazines (prochlorperazine, promethazine, chlorpromazine), or metoclopramide. Serotonin ($5HT_3$) antagonists (e.g., ondansetron) are mainly used for chemotherapy-induced nausea and vomiting (CINV) or radiotherapy-induced nausea and vomiting.
- *Cerebral cortex*-induced nausea and vomiting can be caused by meningeal irritation, anxiety, taste, and smell as well as increased intracranial pressure from brain tumors or metastases. Dexamethasone is used to decrease intracranial pressure while methylprednisolone or dexamethasone may be given as an adjuvant anti-emetic with chemotherapy. Benzodiazepines (e.g., lorazepam) are used to manage anticipatory and anxiety-related nausea.
- *Vestibular* nausea and vomiting is triggered by motion or vertigo. Opioids can sensitize the vestibular center, resulting in movement-induced nausea. Ambulatory patients may be more susceptible to vestibular nausea and vomiting then those who are bedbound. Since histamine and acetylcholine are the predominant neurotransmitters in vestibular nausea, antihistamines (e.g., meclizine) and anticholinergics (e.g., glycopyrrolate) are the drugs of choice for movement-induced nausea and vomiting.
- *Gastrointestinal (GI) tract* stimulation occurs via vagal, sphlanchnic, glossopharyngeal nerves, and sympathetic ganglia. These pathways can be triggered by stimulation of either mechanoreceptors or chemoreceptors found in the GI tract, serosa, and viscera. Drugs, bacterial toxins, chemotherapeutic agents, and irradiation can lead to nausea and vomiting. Anticholinergic agents (e.g., dicyclomine) block the action of acetylcholine in smooth muscle of the GI tract, decreasing GI spasticity and motility, thus relieving nausea.
- *Gastroparesis*, or gastric stasis, presents as nausea, vomiting, early satiety, and postprandial fullness. Abdominal pain may also occur. Delayed gastric emptying is frequently observed in patients with diabetes mellitus and autonomic failure from neurological disorders. Pro-kinetic agents (metoclopramide) are preferred to manage gastric stasis.
- *Hyperacidity* is often accompanied by gastroesophageal reflux (GERD) and may cause nausea, heartburn, or bitter taste. Vomiting may occur in response to acid reflux. Hyperacidity is best managed with antacids (e.g., calcium carbonate), H_2 receptor antagonists (e.g., famotidine, ranitidine), or proton pump inhibitors (e.g., omeprazole, lansoprazole).

Non-Pharmacological Treatment[4,8]

- Relaxation techniques, acupressure, or acupuncture
- Avoid strong odors, foods, or other triggers
- Eliminate offending medications if possible
- Promote good oral care
- Offer clear liquids
  - Sip liquids slowly
  - Sipping off a spoon may prevent gulping
- Provision of small, frequent meals chosen by the patient
  - Cold foods may be better tolerated
  - Promote bland foods: mashed potatoes, apple sauce, sherbet, crackers, toast
  - Avoid greasy, fried, or spicy foods
- Oral Rehydration Therapy (ORT) if prolonged vomiting (see *Diarrhea GEMS*)

Pharmacotherapy[2,4,8-16]

- Use of D_2 antagonists (e.g., haloperidol, prochlorperazine) is recommended first-line for many cases of end-of-life nausea and vomiting.
- Corticosteroids (e.g., dexamethasone) have a role in non-specific nausea and vomiting in addition to their usefulness in reducing intracranial pressure. The mechanism of action has not been fully elucidated, but several methods have been considered: reduction in tryptophan levels (a precursor of serotonin),

prevention of serotonin release in the GI tract, decrease in inflammation caused by radiation or chemotherapy, or return of the body to a normal physiological state during times of stress.

- If nausea is due to gastritis, hiatal hernia, gastroesophageal reflux disease (GERD), or peptic ulcer disease, administer histamine$_2$ (H$_2$) antagonists or proton pump inhibitors (PPIs) to reduce gastric acidity and reflux symptoms.
- Refractory cases of nausea and vomiting often require judiciously selected combinations of medications from different classes (e.g., various combinations of haloperidol, metoclopramide, diphenhydramine, lorazepam, dexamethasone).
- 5HT$_3$ antagonists such as ondansetron (Zofran) have limited usefulness for nausea and vomiting at end of life. They are indicated for prevention and treatment of CINV or radiation induced-nausea and vomiting and are very neurotransmitter-selective. Most effectiveness for 5HT$_3$ antagonists is gained with use for antiemetic prophylaxis appropriate to the planned chemotherapy regimen.
- Olanzapine (Zyprexa) may be an effective option for CINV, both prophylaxis and breakthrough treatments. Olanzapine has been found as effective as aprepitant as an adjuvant antiemetic for highly emetic chemotherapy. The National Comprehensive Cancer Network (NCCN) and the American Society of Clinical Oncology (ASCO) include olanzapine as an alternative agent to aprepitant in antiemetic clinical practice guidelines.
- Aprepitant (Emend) is an NK$_1$ antagonist indicated for the treatment of nausea from highly emetogenic chemotherapy, blocking NK$_1$ receptors both in the CNS and GI tract. Aprepitant is only approved for use in combination with a 5-HT$_3$ antagonist and corticosteroid, not as a sole agent.
- Cannabinoids (dronabinol) have shown antiemetic activity in studies, but generally less activity than traditional agents when using for generalized nausea and vomiting. Cannabinoid receptors are found widespread throughout the brain and periphery, so patients frequently report side effects such as dizziness, sedation, hypotension, and dysphoria. Cannabinoids are not recommended for CINV either by ASCO or NCCN.

Clinical Pearls[1-4,8,11,15]

- Always assess the patient for underlying or potentially reversible causes of nausea and vomiting (e.g., constipation, anxiety, pain, medications).
- Patients with cancer can experience nausea and vomiting from a variety of causes: bowel obstruction, brain tumor, gastroparesis, chemotherapy, anxiety, organ failure, etc. Attempt to identify the cause of nausea in order to optimize the antiemetic regimen.
- Many patients develop tolerance to nausea and vomiting caused by opioids. If symptoms remain burdensome, rotation to an alternate opioid may alleviate symptoms.
- Chemotherapy regimens are identified by their emetogenic potential from low and minimal emetic risk, moderate emetic risk, and high emetic risk. Additionally, acute and/or delayed emesis onset is considered when choosing antiemetic therapy to control CINV.
- Prior to the development of safer and more effective 5HT$_3$ antagonists and combination antiemetic regimens, limited options were available for control of CINV. At that time, cannabinoids (dronabinol and nabilone) were used for refractory CINV symptoms. Therapeutic benefit from cannabis (marijuana) use remains controversial for clinicians and patients. Legal challenges at the state and federal level continue.
- Effective and ongoing communication between the clinician and patient is critical to ensure optimal symptom management, including regular assessment of frequency and severity of nausea or vomiting episodes, ability of prescribed medications to control symptoms, and adverse effects reported by the patient.

Pharmacological Management of Nausea and Vomiting

Generic Name (Trade Name)	Adult Starting Dose	Routes	Common Strengths and Formulations	Comments
Chemoreceptor Trigger Zone: Dopamine Antagonists				
Haloperidol (Haldol®)	0.5mg Q4H PRN	PO PR SC IM IV	**Tablets:** 0.5 mg, 1 mg, 2 mg, 5 mg, 10 mg, 20 mg **Oral solution:** 2 mg/mL **Injection:** 5 mg/mL	• Potent D_2 antagonist. • Extrapyramidal symptoms (EPS) rare in low doses. • Parenteral route may cause less EPS than oral. • Less sedation than other antiemetics.
Prochlorperazine (Compazine®)	10mg PO Q6H PRN 25mg PR Q12H PRN	PO PR IM IV	**Tablets:** 5 mg, 10 mg **Injection:** 5 mg/mL **Suppositories:** 25 mg	• More sedation than haloperidol. • May cause EPS. • Deep IM to gluteal muscle recommended; do not give IV bolus, push slowly or infuse. • Suppositories are expensive.
Chlorpromazine (Thorazine®)	10mg Q6H PRN	PO PR SL IM IV	**Tablets:** 10 mg, 25 mg, 50 mg, 100 mg, 200 mg **Injection:** 25 mg/mL	• More sedation than haloperidol. • Risk of orthostatic hypotension. • May cause EPS. • 100 mg/mL oral solution may be compounded for SL administration.
Promethazine (Phenergan®)	25mg Q6H PRN	PO PR IM IV	**Tablets:** 12.5 mg, 25 mg, 50 mg **Oral solution:** 6.25 mg/5 mL **Injection:** 25 mg/mL, 50 mg/mL **Suppositories:** 12.5 mg, 25mg, 50 mg	• More sedating than haloperidol • May cause EPS. • Deep IM to gluteal muscle recommended; avoid IV administration if possible; risk of extravasation. • Antiemetic of choice for patients with Parkinson's disease or Lewy Body Dementia. • More antihistamine effect than dopamine blockade. • Suppositories are expensive.
Gastric Stasis: Pro-Kinetic Agents				
Metoclopramide (Reglan®)	5mg QID, 30 minutes prior to meals and at bedtime	PO PR IV IM SC	**Tablets:** 5 mg, 10 mg **Oral solution:** 5 mg/5 mL **Injection:** 5 mg/mL	• D2 antagonist. • $5HT_4$ agonist activity in GI tract and weak $5HT_3$ antagonist activity in CTZ. • May cause sedation, confusion, EPS. • Higher risk of tardive dyskinesia in elderly patients and diabetics. • Oral dissolving tablets are expensive.
Erythromycin (E-Mycin®)	250mg TID before meals	PO	**Tablets:** 250 mg, 400 mg, 500 mg **Capsules:** 250 mg **Suspension:** 200 mg/5 mL	• Beneficial if patient cannot tolerate metoclopramide due to EPS. • Tachyphylaxis may occur with duration of therapy > 4 weeks.
Vestibular Nausea: Antihistamines, Anticholinergics				
Meclizine (Antivert®)	25mg Q6H PRN	PO	**Tablets:** 12.5 mg, 25 mg	• Sedating, anticholinergic side effects. • Available OTC. • Drug of choice for vertigo.

Continued

Generic Name (Trade Name)	Adult Starting Dose	Routes	Common Strengths and Formulations	Comments
Vestibular Nausea: Antihistamines, Anticholinergics, *continued*				
Scopolamine (Transderm Scop®)	1 patch Q72H 0.4mg SC Q6H PRN	TD	**Transdermal patch:** 1.5 mg	• Sedating, anticholinergic side effects. • Do not cut transdermal patches. • Injectable product withdrawn from market in early 2015.
Glycopyrrolate (Robinul®, Cuvposa®)	0.2mg SC Q6H PRN	PO SC IV	**Tablets:** 1 mg, 2 mg **Oral solution:** 1 mg/ 5mL **Injection:** 0.2 mg/mL	• Use as adjuvant to control symptoms of malignant bowel obstruction. • Fewer CNS effects (sedation, confusion) but more xerostomia than other anticholinergics. • Oral bioavailability is low (< 15%). • Oral solution is expensive.
Cerebral Cortex Nausea: Anxiolytics, Corticosteroids				
Lorazepam (Ativan®)	0.5 mg Q6H PRN	PO SL PR SC IV IM	**Tablets:** 0.5 mg, 1 mg, 2 mg **Oral solution:** 2 mg/mL **Injection:** 2 mg/mL, 4 mg/mL	• C-IV controlled substance. • For anxiety-induced nausea or anticipatory nausea only. • No direct antiemetic effect. • All benzodiazepines equally effective for this indication; select based on patient-specific factors.
Hydroxyzine (Atarax®, Vistaril®)	25mg Q6H PRN	PO IM	**Tablets:** 10 mg, 25 mg, 50 mg **Capsules:** 25 mg, 50 mg, 100 mg **Oral solution:** 10 mg/5 mL **Injection:** 25 mg/mL, 50 mg/mL	• Antihistamine with weak anxiolytic properties. • Sedating, anticholinergic side effects. • IM injection is painful. • Do not give IV or SC. • Atarax® (hydroxyzine HCl) and Vistaril® (hydroxyzine pamoate) are different salt forms of same active ingredient. • There is no clinical difference between HCl and pamoate products.
Dexamethasone (Decadron®)	4mg Daily	PO PR SC IV	**Tablets:** 1 mg, 2 mg, 4 mg, 6 mg **Oral solution:** 1 mg/ mL **Injection:** 4 mg/mL, 10 mg/mL	• Higher doses (10mg) given on chemotherapy treatment days. • Useful when nausea is due to increased intracranial pressure. • Daily or BID dosing preferred; no added benefit to Q6H dosing.
Chemotherapy and Radiation: 5HT₃ Antagonists, NK₁ Antagonists				
Ondansetron (Zofran®)	8mg prior to chemotherapy or radiotherapy, then 8mg Q12H for 2 more days.	PO PR SL SC IV IM	**Tablets:** 4 mg, 8 mg **Oral film:** 4 mg, 8mg **Oral solution:** 4 mg/5 mL **Injection:** 4 mg/2 mL	• Risk of QT prolongation, especially with doses greater than 16mg. • Off-label uses other than pediatric gastroenteritis not been studied. • Use traditional antiemetics as first line before 5HT3 antagonists for acute nausea and vomiting. • Effective when scheduled, not PRN.

Continued

Generic Name (Trade Name)	Adult Starting Dose	Routes	Common Strengths and Formulations	Comments
Chemotherapy and Radiation: 5HT₃ Antagonists, NK₁ Antagonists, *continued*				
Granisetron (Kytril®, Sancuso®)	2mg prior to chemotherapy or radiotherapy and up to 48 hours post-treatment.	PO IV TD	**Tablets:** 1 mg **Transdermal patch:** 3.1 mg/24H **Oral solution:** 2 mg/10 mL **Injection:** 0.1 mg/mL, 1 mg/mL	• Risk of QT prolongation. • Use traditional antiemetics as first line before 5HT3 antagonists for acute nausea and vomiting. • Cover patch and avoid exposure to sunlight. • Do not cut patch; apply 24H prior to chemotherapy. • Not effective for breakthrough nausea and vomiting; no PRN use. • Patch is expensive.
Dolasetron (Anzemet®)	100mg prior to chemotherapy	PO IV	**Tablets:** 50 mg, 100 mg **Injection:** 20 mg/mL	• Risk of QT prolongation. • Use traditional antiemetics as first line before 5HT3 antagonists for acute nausea and vomiting. • Not effective for breakthrough nausea and vomiting; no PRN use.
Aprepitant (Emend®)	125mg prior to chemotherapy combined with 5HT₃ antagonist + dexamethasone.		**Capsules:** 40 mg, 80 mg, 125 mg	• Neurokinin-1 antagonist • Only use in combination with 5HT₃ antagonist and dexamethasone. • Nausea and GI distress is a significant side effect. • Expensive; limit use only to highly emetogenic chemotherapy regimens.
Miscellaneous Antiemetics				
Dronabinol (Marinol®)	5mg prior to chemotherapy	PO	**Capsules:** 2.5 mg, 5 mg, 10 mg	• C-III controlled substance. • Less effective than traditional antiemetics and higher risk of adverse effects. • Expensive.
Olanzapine (Zyprexa®)	10mg prior to chemotherapy, then 10mg daily for 3-8 more days.	PO	**Tablets:** 2.5 mg, 5 mg, 7.5 mg, 10 mg, 15 mg, 20 mg **Injection:** 10mg	• As effective as aprepitant as adjuvant for CINV prophylaxis. • Oral dosing preferred for CINV although IM injection is available.
Trimethobenz-amide (Tigan®)	300mg TID PRN IM: 200mg TID PRN	PO IM	**Capsules:** 300 mg **Injection:** 100 mg/mL	• Alternative antiemetic for patients with Parkinson's disease or Lewy Body Dementia. • Less effective than promethazine. • Suppositories withdrawn from US market in 2007.

See Drug Dosing for Liver and Renal Disease for additional drug information.

References
1. Nausea and Vomiting (PDQ®). National Cancer Institute. http://www.cancer.gov/cancertopics/pdq/supportivecare/nausea/HealthProfessional/. Accessed December 17, 2013.
2. Glare PA, Dunwoodie D, Clark K, et al. Treatment of nausea and vomiting in terminally ill cancer patients. *Drugs.* 2008;68(18):2675-2590.
3. Ferris FD, von Gunten CF, Emanuel LL. Ensuring competency in end-of-life care: controlling symptoms. *BMC Palliat Care.* 2002;1(5). http://www.biomedcentral.com/1472-684X/1/5. Accessed December 17, 2013.
4. Wood GJ, Shega JW, Lynch B, et al. Management of intractable nausea and vomiting in patients at the end of life. *JAMA.* 2007;298(10):1196-1208.
5. Gordon P, LeGrand SB, Walsh D. Nausea and vomiting in advanced cancer. *Eur J Pharmacol.* 2014;722(5):187-191.
6. Camilleri M, Parkman HP, Shafi MA, et al. Clinical guideline: management of gastroparesis. *Am J Gastroenterol.* 2013;108(1):18-38.
7. Tyler LS. Nausea and vomiting in palliative care. In: *Evidence Based Symptom Control in Palliative Care.* Binghampton, NY: The Haworth Press, Inc., 2000:163-181.
8. Gralla RJ, Osoba D, Kris MG, etc al. Recommendations for the use of antiemetics: evidence-based, clinical practice guidelines. *J Clin Oncol.* 1999;17(9):2971-2994.
9. Rojas C. Raje M. Tsukamoto T, et al. Molecular mechanisms of 5-HT3 and NK1 receptor antagonists in prevention of emesis. *Eur J Pharmacol.* 2014;722(5):26-37.
10. Chu CC, Hsing CH, Shieh JP, et al. The cellular mechanisms of the antiemetic action of dexamethasone and related glucocorticoids against vomiting. *Eur J Pharmacol.* 2014;722(5):48-54.
11. Smith HS, Laufer A. Opioid induced nausea and vomiting. *Eur J Pharmacol.* 2014;722(5):67-78.
12. Sharkey KA, Darmani NA, Parker LA. Regulation of nausea and vomiting by cannabinoids and the endocannabinoid system. *Eur J Pharmacol.* 2014;722(5):134-146.
13. Prommer E. Role of haloperidol in palliative medicine: an update. *Am J Hosp Palliat Med.* 2012;29(4):295-301.
14. Hocking C, Kichenadasse G. Olanzapine for chemotherapy-induced nausea and vomiting: a systematic review. *Support Care Cancer.* 2014;22(4):1143-1151.
15. Basch E, Prestrud A, Hesketh P, et al. Antiemetics: American Society of Clinical Oncology clinical practice guideline update. *J Clin Oncol.* 2011;29(31):4189-4198.
16. Todaro B. Cannabinoids in the treatment of chemotherapy-induced nausea and vomiting. *J Natl Compr Canc Netw.* 2012;10(4):487-492.
17. Reichmann JP, Kirkbride MS. Reviewing the evidence for using continuous subcutaneous metoclopramide and ondansetron to treat nausea and vomiting during pregnancy. *Managed Care* 2012;21(5):44-47.

Treatment Algorithm for Nausea & Vomiting

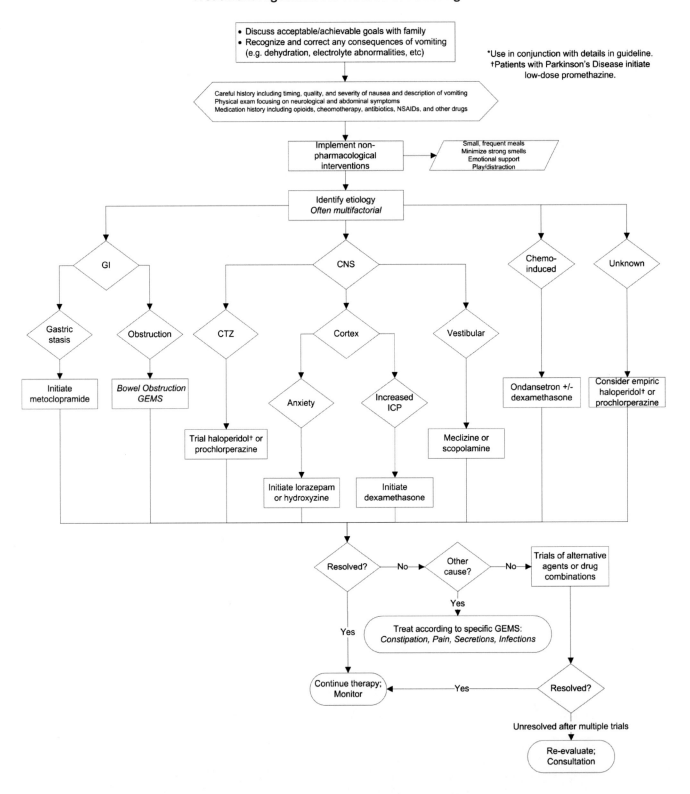

- Discuss acceptable/achievable goals with family
- Recognize and correct any consequences of vomiting (e.g. dehydration, electrolyte abnormalities, etc)

*Use in conjunction with details in guideline.
†Patients with Parkinson's Disease initiate low-dose promethazine.

Careful history including timing, quality, and severity of nausea and description of vomiting
Physical exam focusing on neurological and abdominal symptoms
Medication history including opioids, cheomotherapy, antibiotics, NSAIDs, and other drugs

Implement non-pharmacological interventions

Small, frequent meals
Minimize strong smells
Emotional support
Play/distraction

Identify etiology
Often multifactorial

GI

CNS

Chemo-induced

Unknown

Gastric stasis

Obstruction

CTZ

Cortex

Vestibular

Initiate metoclopramide

Bowel Obstruction GEMS

Anxiety

Increased ICP

Ondansetron +/- dexamethasone

Consider empiric haloperidol† or prochlorperazine

Trial haloperidol† or prochlorperazine

Meclizine or scopolamine

Initiate lorazepam or hydroxyzine

Initiate dexamethasone

Resolved? — No → Other cause? — No → Trials of alternative agents or drug combinations

Yes

Treat according to specific GEMS:
Constipation, Pain, Secretions, Infections

Yes

Continue therapy; Monitor ← Yes — Resolved?

Unresolved after multiple trials

Re-evaluate; Consultation

Pain Overview

Introduction and Background[1-4]

- Medical Definition: "An unpleasant sensory and emotional experience associated with actual or potential tissue damage, or described in terms of such damage.", or described in terms of such damage... Pain is always subjective... It is unquestionably a sensation in a part or parts of the body, but it is also always unpleasant and therefore also an emotional experience." *International Association for the Study of Pain (IASP)*
- Subjective Definition: "Pain is what the person says it is and exists whenever he or she says it does" (McCaffery, 1968)

Ideal Analgesia = Pain Control + Improved Function

- **Pain as a Symptom:** Clinicians must acknowledge the presence of and treat both physical pain and nonphysical factors. Nonphysical pain increases perception of physical pain often leading to inappropriately high opioid requests.
- Both chronic and acute pain can cause or exacerbate collateral symptoms which then can lead to increased pain perception. See Table 1 below.

Table 1. Non-Physical Pain and Collateral Pain Symptoms

Non-physical pain symptoms (suffering)	Psychological or emotional pain Behavioral pain Cognitive pain Spiritual/existential pain Cultural or sociological pain
Collateral pain symptoms	Insomnia Fatigue Malaise Loss of appetite Anorexia Depression Anxiety

Prevalence[1,4-6]

- The prevalence of pain at the end of life had been estimated at 51%. The prevalence 4 months before death (28%), then it increased, reaching 46% in the last month of life. The prevalence of pain in the last month of life was 60% among patients with arthritis versus 26% among patients without arthritis and did not differ by terminal diagnosis category (cancer [45%], heart disease [48%], frailty [50%], sudden death [42%], or other causes [47%]).
- Bone metastases are considered the most common causes of pain in cancer patients.
- Visceral pain due to tumor invasion of hollow viscera, with or without pleural or peritoneal involvement, is the second most common type of pain of cancer.
- An estimated 30% of cancer patients experience neuropathic pain at some point in their disease (usually advanced disease).
- Headache and lower back pain are the most common cause of chronic non-malignant pain.
- Abdominal pain is a common complaint in all health care settings ranging from benign underlying conditions, such as constipation and irritable bowel syndrome (IBS), to life-threatening illnesses such as pancreatic cancer.

Figure 1. Classification of Common Pain Types based on Pathophysiology

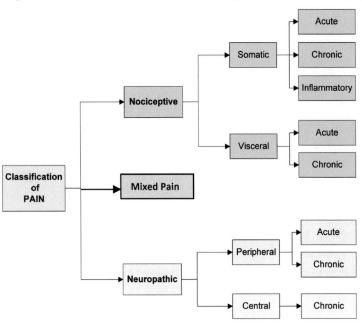

Table 2. Classification of Acute versus Chronic Pain

Acute pain	Identified event Resolves within days to weeks Usually nociceptive
Chronic pain	Cause not often easily identifiable, multifactorial Indeterminate duration (typically >3 months) Nociceptive and/or neuropathic Typically pain free intervals
Chronic persistent pain	Near constant pain Nociceptive and/or neuropathic Pain that cycles, or remits and recurs (e.g., migraine)

Pain Assessment[4,7]

- Before initiating therapy, conduct a thorough, whole person assessment.
- A complete physical exam can help establish a relationship between the pain and the disease process.
- Considerations when assessing pain include:
    - Chronological age
    - Type of pain (acute, chronic, procedural, neuropathic)
    - Underlying cause(s) of pain
    - Neurologic impairment
    - Chronic illness
    - Language barriers
    - Emotional, psychosocial, cultural and spiritual components
- Behavioral observation may be useful in nonverbal patients. However, interpret behaviors carefully; there may be other causes of distress besides pain.
- When assessing pain, assess *each site* of pain individually.
- Review the patient's complete medical history for comorbid conditions, social history, or medication use that might impact decision-making on pain treatments.
    - History of gastritis, ulcers, GI bleeding, or thrombocytopenia
    - Presence of liver or renal dysfunction (medications may need dosage adjustment)

- o Disease progression
- o Associated symptoms: nausea, anorexia, sleep disturbances, anxiety, depression
- o Sources of pain: neuropathic, somatic, bone, visceral, intracranial pressure, muscle spasms
- o Medication allergies
- o Potential drug interactions with current medications
- o History of medication misuse or substance abuse in patient or family
  - Risk assessment tools such as the *Opioid Risk Tool* (ORT) or *Screener and Opioid Assessment for Patients with Pain* (SOAPP)
  - Refer to section on drug misuse and addiction at the end of this chapter
- Ease and appropriateness of dosing schedule
  - Ability to adhere to dosage regimen
- Ease and appropriateness of route

Table 3. PQRST Model for Pain Assessment

P	Provokes	*Aggravating or alleviating factors* What causes pain? What makes pain better? What makes pain worse?
Q	Quality	*Patient describes the pain depending on developmental and communication level.* What does it feel like? Is it sharp, dull, stabbing, burning, crushing, etc?
R	Radiates	*Patient describes any sensation of pain "traveling", "wrapping", or "shooting" from its origin.* Does the pain go anywhere? Where does it start and where does it go (e.g. shoulder to hand)? Is it in one place? Does it go anywhere else? Did it start elsewhere and now is localized in one spot?
S	Severity	*Use pain scale (e.g., 0-10, words , colors, FACES, PAIN-AD))* What is your pain currently, in the last 24 hours on average, at its worse and least? At rest and with activity or stimulation
T	Time	*Onset and duration* What time and date did the pain start? How long does it last? Is it worse in morning or evening, or is it constant all day?

Pain Assessment Severity Tools

- Assessment tools are intended to help care providers assess pain based on the individual patient need.
- Neonatal, infant, and child pain scales[8-11]
  - o Crying, Requires increased oxygen, Increased vital signs, Expression, Sleeplessness (CRIES) Scale for Neonatal Pain for 32 weeks gestation to 6 months
  - o Face, Legs, Activity, Cry, Consolability (FLACC) Behavior Pain Assessment Scale for Young Children from 0-18 years
  - o Wong-Baker FACES Pain Rating Scale 4-18 years
- Pain scales for adults[12]
  - o 0-10 numeric ruler
  - o Color Scale
  - o Verbal Descriptor Scale
  - o Activity Tolerance Scale
- Pain scales for non-verbal or cognitively impaired adults[13-15]
  - o Pain Assessment in Advanced Dementia (PAIN-AD)
  - o IASP Faces Pain Scale – Revised
  - o Pain Assessment Check List for Seniors with Limited Ability to Communicate (PACSLAC)
- Helpful assessment questions:
  1. *"What does your pain keep from doing that you would like to do if you had less pain?"*
  2. *"Do you feel you could cope better if you are a little more relaxed or sleepy, or would you rather be more alert? There is no wrong answer."*

- With the second question if the patient is using opioid pain medications to help them relax or sleep, re-enforce that the pain medication is just used to help control pain. The sleepiness is a side effect that goes away after a while. Other medications are more appropriate to help with relaxation or insomnia.

Figure 2. 0-10 Numeric Scale, Color Scale, and Word Descriptor Scale[12]

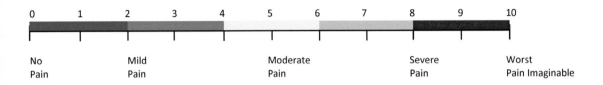

Figure 3. Activity Tolerance Scale

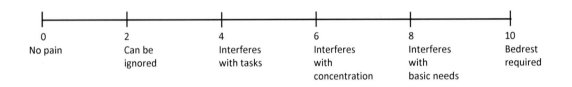

Figure 4. Wong-Baker FACES® Pain Rating Scale[11]

Wong-Baker FACES® Pain Rating Scale

0	2	4	6	8	10
No Hurt	Hurts Little Bit	Hurts Little More	Hurts Even More	Hurts Whole Lot	Hurts Worst

Figure 5. Pain Assessment in Advanced Dementia (PAINAD)[13]

Items*	0	1	2	Score
Breathing independent of vocalization	Normal	Occasional labored breathing. Short period of hyperventilation.	Noisy labored breathing. Long period of hyperventilation. Cheyne-Stokes respiration.	
Negative vocalization	None	Occasional moan or groan. Low-level speech with a negative or disapproving quality.	Repeated troubled calling out. Loud moaning or groaning. Crying.	
Facial expression	Smiling or inexpressive	Sad. Frightened. Frown.	Facial grimacing.	
Body language	Relaxed	Tense. Distressed pacing. Fidgeting.	Rigid. Fists clenched. Knees pulled up. Pulling or pushing away. Striking out.	
Consolability	No need to console.	Distracted or reassured by voice or touch	Unable to console, distract. or reassure.	
			Total**	

*Five-item observational tool
**Total scores range from 0-10, with a higher score indicating more severe pain (0=no pain, 10=severe pain)

Complete instructions and explanations of the observational assessment process are available at http://www.amda.com/publications/caring/may2004/painad.cfm

Figure 6. IASP Faces Pain Scale – Revised[14]

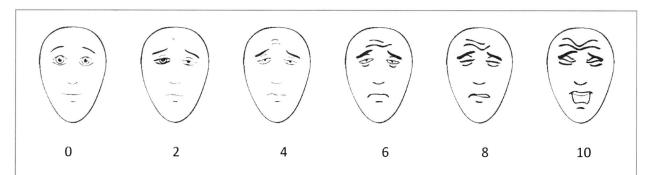

0   2   4   6   8   10

*Score the chosen face **0**, **2**, **4**, **6**, **8**, or **10**, counting left to right, so "0" = "no pain" and "10" = "very much pain". Do not use words like "happy" or "sad".*

Complete instructions and explanations of the observational assessment process are available from IASP at http://www.iasp-pain.org/Education/

Table 4. Description of Pain Types[16]

Type of Pain	Pathology	Description
Nociceptive pain	<ul><li>Pain is a normal symptom and serves a protective function.</li><li>Nociceptors stimulated following injury or tissue damage.</li><li>Nerve impulse is generated and conveyed by neurons to the brain.</li><li>Pain is C-fiber and Aδ-fiber mediated.</li><li>Generally opioid sensitive.</li></ul>	***Somatic Pain*** arises from bone, joints, muscles, skin, and connective tissue, is well localized.<ul><li>Pain presents as sharp, pressure-like, throbbing, or aching.</li><li>Bone pain is an inflammatory type of somatic pain.</li></ul>***Visceral Pain*** arises from smooth muscle internal organs. Pain is usually less well defined and poorly localized or referred. Visceral pain can be further subdivided into two major categories:<ul><li>Pain resulting from tumor involvement within the organ capsule; causing stretching, aching, fairly well localized.</li><li>Pain resulting from obstruction of a hollow organ (e.g., stomach, esophagus, colon), presenting as intermittent cramping, poorly localized.</li></ul>
Neuropathic pain	<ul><li>*Abnormal* processing of nerve impulses caused by a lesion or dysfunction within the nervous system.</li><li>Pain is pathological.</li><li>Spontaneous or evoked by activity.</li><li>Develops in days or months.</li><li>May be associated with inflammation.</li><li>Pain outlasts duration of the stimulus.</li><li>Pain sensed in non-injured areas.</li><li>Mediated by Aβ-fibers, C-fibers, and Aδ-fibers.</li><li>Generally opioid insensitive.</li></ul>	***Peripherally-generated neuropathy*** is the result of abnormalities in processing of peripheral pain sensations with no clear nerve injury or lesion.<ul><li>Mononeuropathy: one or several nerves; entrapment syndromes, phantom limb pain, post-herpetic neuralgia.</li><li>Polyneuropathy: if diffuse and bilateral; diabetes mellitus, HIV neuropathy, toxin neuropathies (arsenic, thallium, vinca alkaloids, isoniazid, etc.).</li></ul>***Centrally-generated neuropathy*** is due to processing abnormalities within the CNS.<ul><li>Spinal cord injury, brain or spinal infarction, multiple sclerosis, stroke.</li></ul>

Non-Pharmacological Therapy[4,17,18]

- Non-pharmacological therapies are essential in chronic pain management and may be beneficial in acute pain management.
- Physical, complementary, and cognitive behavioral interventions reduce the perception of pain and can decrease the dosage requirements of medication.
  - Active/passive movement
  - Acupressure, acupuncture, healing touch
  - Art, music, aromatherapy, or pet therapy
  - Biofeedback
  - Distraction, guided imagery, relaxation
  - Environmental modification, explanations, familiar objects
  - Heat/cold application
  - Humor
  - Hypnosis
  - Journaling
  - Positioning
  - Massage or therapeutic touch
  - Physical or occupational therapy
  - Progressive muscle relaxation
  - Storytelling
  - Transcutaneous electrical stimulation (TENS)

Pharmacotherapy[19-21]

- Pain management should be:
  - based on the patient's reported or observed pain level using an assessment scale
  - given around the clock for chronic pain
  - given by the least invasive route; oral is preferred

- o   tailored to the individual's circumstance and needs
- Base opioid doses on patient-specific factors and titrated if needed to adequately control pain. Adjuvant medications can be initiated at any point during therapy.
- The WHO stepladder approach to cancer pain management is appropriate for most nociceptive somatic and visceral pain, including non-cancer chronic pain.
- Certain opioids (e.g., codeine, meperidine, tramadol, tapentadol) are not recommended due to the uncertainty of response, potentially higher risk of adverse effects, and drug interactions.

Clinical Pearls

- Patient/family/caregiver involvement in assessment, interventions, evaluation, and treatment plans is essential for success.
- Neuropathic pain
  - o   Although most neuropathic pain cannot be eliminated. Symptomatic treatment usually produces a marked reduction in pain.
  - o   Multiple medications may be necessary to control neuropathic pain.
- Pain can cause or exacerbate collateral symptoms such as insomnia, fatigue, malaise, loss of appetite, anorexia, depression, and anxiety.
- Medications should be used in conjunction with non-pharmacological therapies, which can reduce the perception of pain and decrease medication requirements.
- The doctrine of double effect supports the aggressive palliation of pain as different from the active hastening of death and is ethically justifiable as long as the caregiver's primary intent is to alleviate suffering. During the dying process, appropriate doses of opioids or other medication which may cause respiratory depression, but are given to alleviate suffering, do not typically cause death. The terminal disease is the cause of death.

Nociceptive Pain: Somatic, Visceral, Bone

Introduction and Background[1,22,23]
- Somatic pain is a subset of nociceptive pain arising from afferent nerve stimulation from bone, joint, muscle, skin, or connective tissues. Somatic nociceptive pain can be either acute or chronic in nature.

Causes[1,22,23]
- Nociceptors are stimulated following injury or tissue damage.
- Nociceptive pain involves 4 processes: transduction, transmission, perception, and modulation.

Figure 1. Four Processes of Nociception[22]

Transduction occurs when mechanical, thermal, or chemical stimuli cause tissue damage resulting in the release of substances that either sensitize (leukotrienes, prostaglandins, substance P) or stimulate (bradykinin, histamine, serotonin, potassium, norepinephrine) pain fibers.	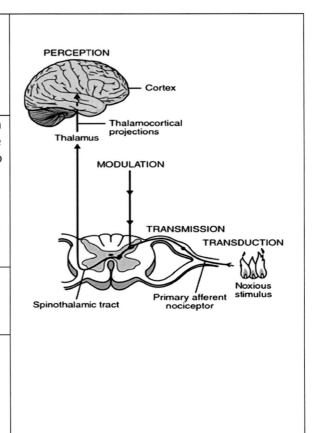
Transmission occurs when the stimulation is great enough that the nerve generates an impulse transmitted from the site of injury to the spinal cord, through the brain stem, to the thalamus and cortex. The nerve impulses are generated and conveyed to the brain via C-fibers and Aδ-fibers. The N-methyl-D-aspartate (NMDA) receptor is one of many receptors that facilitate pain transmission. When this receptor is blocked, pain transmission is blunted or inhibited.	
Perception occurs when the pain impulse reaches the brain. The somatosensory cortex identifies the location and character of the pain while the limbic system assigns emotional and behavioral responses to pain.	
Modulation is the final process. The descending pathway from the brain through the dorsal horn of the spinal cord releases substances that moderate or inhibit pain transmission. These substances include endogenous opioids such as dynorphins and enkephalins, serotonin, norepinephrine, gamma-aminobutyric acid (GABA), neurotensin, and alpha-2 adrenergic substances.	

Somatic Pain
- Nociceptive somatic pain can be caused by "mechanical" (e.g., incisional pain, sprains, broken bones, crushing, tearing, shearing, etc.), "thermal" (e.g., heat (burns) or cold (frostbite), and "chemical" (e.g., alcohol in a cut, chili powder in the eye).
- Nociceptive somatic pain due to soft tissue involvement may include headache and facial pain, ear and eye pain, pleural pain, or muscle cramps.

Bone Pain
- Bone pain is a subset of somatic, nociceptive pain.
- Examples of nociceptive somatic pain due to bone metastases are multifocal bone pain, vertebral pain syndrome in epidural spinal cord compression, pain syndrome related to pelvis and hip, base of skull.
  - Bone pain can be due to primary bone cancer (stretching of the periosteum as tumor size increases) or more commonly due to bone metastases.
  - Solid tumors or osteosarcoma can contribute to bone pain.

Visceral Pain

- Both mechanical (stretching, distension, contraction, and compression) and chemical (substance P, serotonin, prostaglandins, and hydrogen ions) stimuli can activate visceral nociceptors.
- Pathological causes of visceral pain may include irritable bowel syndrome, pancreatic cancer, ovarian cancer, lung cancer, hepatomegaly, midline retroperitoneal syndrome, chronic intestinal obstruction, peritoneal carcinomatosis, and obstruction of ureter.
- Examples of visceral pain due to malignancy are hepatic distention syndrome, chronic bowel obstruction, midline retroperitoneal syndrome, malignant perineal pain, ureteric obstruction.
- Visceral pain can be caused by Crohn's disease, ulcerative colitis, celiac disease, inflammatory bowel disease, irritable bowel syndrome, carcinoid syndrome, pancreatitis, gallstones, lactose intolerance.

Clinical Characteristics[4,24-26]

- Nociceptive pain is typically opioid sensitive.

Somatic Pain

- Somatic pain arises from bone, joints, muscles, skin, and connective tissue, and is localized to the area of tissue damage.
  - Pain presents as sharp, pressure-like, throbbing or aching.
  - Swelling, cramping and bleeding may exist with somatic pain.

Bone Pain

- Bone pain is an inflammatory subset of somatic pain.
- Cancer cells cause bone destruction by stimulating osteoclast activity.
  - As tumors increase in size, the pain often becomes continuous and achy with sharp exacerbations. However, some patients may experience continuous pain early in the disease process.
- Vertebral bone lesions can cause neuropathic pain due to spinal cord compression. Both anti-inflammatory and neuropathic analgesics are usually needed in such cases.
- Symptoms of bone pain may be intermittent, but increase and may become persistent with standing or walking on weight-bearing bones.

Visceral Pain

- Visceral nociceptors are fewer in number in the primary somatosensory cortex than their somatic counterparts. However, their presence in the secondary somatosensory cortex leads to intense perception and psychological processing of visceral pain, though not well localized.
- Visceral pain arises from smooth muscle internal organs; pain is usually less well defined, poorly localized, or referred.
- The two major categories of visceral pain include:
  - Pain resulting from tumor involvement within the organ capsule, which causes stretching, aching, and is fairly localized.
  - Pain resulting from obstruction of a hollow viscus (e.g., stomach, esophagus, colon), which presents as intermittent cramping and is poorly localized.
- Visceral pain produces nonspecific regional or whole-body motor responses, strong autonomic responses, leads to sensitization of somatic tissues, and produces strong affective responses.
- Patients describe visceral nociceptive pain as gnawing, cramping, diffuse, and poorly localized. Colic occurs with obstruction of a hollow viscus as an achy, sharp or throbbing pain with internal organ capsule invasion or mesenteric infiltration. Nausea, vomiting, and diaphoresis often accompany visceral pain.
- Referred pain is a common characteristic of visceral pain occurring when visceral pain and somatic pain converge upon the same area of the dorsal horn. The intensity of the referred pain is a reflection of the severity of the visceral involvement. Visceral pain can also be referred to the skin and present as cutaneous hyperalgesia. Referred pain is often misdiagnosed as musculoskeletal pain due to its somatic presentation.

Non-Pharmacological Therapy

- *See **Pain Overview** above.*

Pharmacotherapy[19-21,24-27]

- The World Health Organization (WHO) Cancer Pain Relief Ladder has provided a stepwise intervention approach to cancer pain management. The WHO Ladder is widely accepted and effective and is currently in revision to reflect updates in the clinical approach to pain management.
- In end-of-life care, opioid/non-opioid combination products are often omitted in favor of a low-dose pure opioid (e.g., morphine, hydromorphone, oxycodone). This allows for greater dosing flexibility and more available routes of administration.
- Non-pharmacologic comfort measures and adjuvant medication should always be considered, and especially when there are signs of neuropathic pain.

Figure 2. Pain Management Continuum

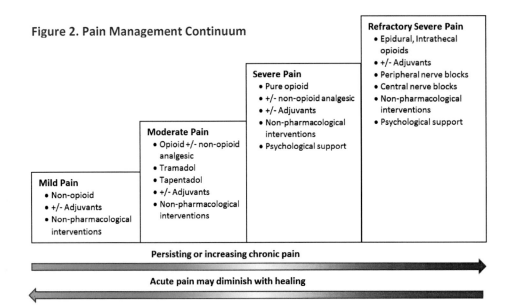

Figure 3. WHO's Method for Use of Analgesics[27]

By mouth	Oral administration is preferred; cost-effective and widely available dosage forms.
By the clock	Schedule doses of analgesics at fixed intervals to provide continuous pain control; add rescue doses for breakthrough pain on an as needed basis.
By the ladder	Sequential use of drugs for progressing pain; jump to pure opioids if needed for patients presenting with severe pain.
For the individual	Do not assume standard doses; the right dose is the one that relieves the patient's pain.
Attention to detail	Discuss the pain regimen and pain relief expectations with the patient and caregiver. Do not assume understanding with first conversation; provide a written pain management plan.

- Initiate opioids conservatively; titrate based on patient response.
- If pain is constant, around-the-clock dosing of analgesics is preferred. Scheduled opioid doses are administered based on their duration of action.
- Breakthrough (as needed) opioid dosing is based on expected time to peak effect. Breakthrough doses are generally calculated as 10-15% of the daily maintenance dose.
- If the patient is experiencing unrelieved pain, or receiving 3-4 breakthrough doses per day, the maintenance dose may be increased by 25-50%.
- In a severe pain crisis, or when the opioid dose is very low, the dose may be increased by 100%.
- Frequency of breakthrough dosing depends on route of administration and opioid pharmacology. Example: Morphine, oxycodone, and hydromorphone breakthrough dose frequencies → IV: 6-10min; SC: 15-20min; Oral: 60-90min
- Do not order extended-release opioids for "as needed" use.
- Assess effectiveness of pain management regimen on a regular basis.
- All opioids have black box warnings:
  - o Do not crush or chew extended- or sustained-release dosage forms.

- Long-acting opioids are indicated for the management of moderate to severe pain when around the clock pain control is needed.
- Use opioids with caution when administered with medications that may cause respiratory depression. Do not use alcohol with opioids.
- Healthcare providers must remain alert to potential abuse, misuse, or diversion of opioids and other drugs of abuse. See *Symptom Management with Co-Morbidity of Drug Misuse and Addiction* section.

Nociceptive Somatic Bone Pain Special Considerations[26,27]

- Acetaminophen does *not* have peripheral anti-inflammatory effects and can be a dose limiting factor when opioid-acetaminophen combinations are used. Management of bone pain may fail when opioids are used exclusively or in combination with acetaminophen rather than an anti-inflammatory medication.
- Anti-inflammatory agents are first line therapy and provide a high rate of response. As the bone involvement of disease progresses, or when adequate pain relief is not achieved with anti-inflammatory medications alone, an opioid should be *added* to the regimen.
- All non-selective, non-steroidal anti-inflammatory drugs (NSAIDs) have similar efficacy. Ibuprofen and naproxen are cost effective choices in hospice care if there are no contraindications. Risk factors such as GI bleeding, recent GI ulcers, pre-existing cardiovascular concerns, or renal insufficiency (especially in the elderly) must be assessed prior to initiation.
- COX-II selective NSAID (celecoxib) and COX-II preferential NSAID (meloxicam) cause less GI problems than non-selective NSAIDs however, they carry the same risk of renal toxicity and cardiovascular events.
- Adding a proton pump inhibitor (PPI) to non-selective NSAIDs provides a level of GI protection similar to COX II selective NSAIDs.
- For bone pain, corticosteroids in combination with opioids may be preferred over NSAIDs unless contraindicated (e.g., unstable diabetes) particularly if the patient is experiencing anorexia or fatigue. See *Anorexia GEMS* and *Fatigue GEMS*.
- Higher doses of corticosteroids, usually in combination with opioids, may improve the severe pain of spinal cord compression within several hours.
- Bisphosphonates may be used for diffuse metastatic bone pain. Bisphosphonate-related osteonecrosis of the jaw has been strongly correlated with the amino-bisphosphonates pamidronate and zoledronic acid, especially with chronic use (longer than 12-24 months). Dental evaluation is recommended.
- Palliative external beam radiation therapy is highly effective in treating pain due to localized bone lesions and may greatly reduce or eliminate the need for analgesics. However, analgesics are generally needed for several days after treatment until the radiation effect is maximized. Single fraction radiation may be more expedient than multiple fractions administered over days to weeks.
- Systemic radionuclide therapy has been used to provide pain relief from bone cancer for up to three to six months. This therapy might be considered when patients have multiple, remote bone metastases, a life expectancy of at least six months, and are unable to tolerate systemic analgesics. However, the results have not been promising.

Nociceptive Somatic Visceral Pain Special Considerations[4,26,28]

- Corticosteroids may reduce visceral pain associated with pleuritic chest pain, capsular organ stretching, and inflammatory processes.
- Visceral pain not adequately managed using the stepladder approach and presenting as colicky or cramping pain may be better managed by anticholinergic medication either alone or in combination with opioid and adjuvant analgesics.

Clinical Pearls

- Nociceptive pain (somatic, visceral, bone)
  - Assess patient and family understanding of pain interventions and provide education regarding pain management myths, especially opioids.
- Visceral pain
  - Although anticholinergic agents such as hyoscyamine and scopolamine effectively treat colic, they can worsen constipation. Encourage patients to drink plenty of fluids and increase their fiber intake to balance benefits and the constipating effects of these agents.

- o Anti-inflammatory effects of corticosteroids make them a beneficial adjuvant to opioids in the treatment of pain that results from visceral stretching and also bone pain.
  - o In pancreatic disease or steatorrhea (fatty stool), consider providing pancreatic lipase enzymes (pancrelipase) with meals, celiac plexus block, or jejunal feeding below the sphincter of Oddi for pain control.
- Benzodiazepines alone (e.g., alprazolam, diazepam, lorazepam) do not have analgesic properties not demonstrated except for some instances of neuropathic pain or as muscle relaxants.
- Sedation caused by anxiolytics may compromise neurological assessment in patients receiving opioids.
- Sedative/hypnotic drugs alone (barbiturates, benzodiazepines) do not have analgesic properties.
  - o Added sedation from sedative/hypnotic drugs limits opioid dosing.
- Anaphylactic opioid reactions are the only true opioid allergies (incidence 1:200,000)
  - o Urticaria (hives) with diffuse rash can be an allergic reaction and part of an anaphylactic reaction; careful assessment is needed.
- Provide education to patient, caregivers and family about opioid adverse effects; anticipate and aggressively treat them.
- Both opioid tolerance and physical dependence are common with chronic opioid use; these are not synonymous with addition, psychological dependence, or pseudoaddiction.

Pharmacological Management of NOCICEPTIVE Pain - ANALGESICS

Generic Name (Trade Name)	Adult Starting Dose	Routes	Common Strengths and Formulations	Comments
Non-Opioid Analgesics				
Acetaminophen (Tylenol®, Ofirmev®)	650mg Q6H PRN	PO PR IV	**Tablets:** 325 mg, 500 mg, 650 mg **Capsules:** 500 mg **Oral solution:** 160 mg/5 mL **Suppository:** 120 mg, 325 mg, 650 mg **Injection:** 10 mg/mL	• Maximum daily dose: 4000 mg. • Caution in hepatic and renal impairment. • May be used in conjunction with NSAIDs or opioids. • Weigh risk vs benefit in patients with severe liver dysfunction. • FDA now recommends 325mg or less per dosage unit. • Injection (Ofirmev®) is expensive; hospital use only. • Chewable tablets available.
Non-Steroidal Anti-Inflammatory Drugs (NSAID)				
Ibuprofen (Motrin®, Advil®)	400mg Q6H PRN	PO IV	**Tablets:** 200 mg, 400 mg, 600 mg, 800 mg **Oral suspension:** 100 mg/5 mL **Injection:** 100 mg/mL	• Maximum daily dose: 3200mg. • Take with food or milk to lessen stomach upset. • Weigh vs risk benefit in patients with renal insufficiency. • Chewable tablets available. • Patients must be well hydrated prior to IV ibuprofen use.
Ketorolac (Toradol®, Sprix®)	IV: 30mg Q6H PRN PO: 10mg Q6H PRN	PO IV IM IN	**Tablets:** 10 mg **Intranasal:** 15.75 mg/spray **Injection:** 15 mg/mL, 30 mg/mL	• Maximum combined duration of therapy is 5 days total for any route of administration. • Oral tablets intended only for continuation of IV or IM therapy. • Warnings: ulceration, bleeding, renal impairment.
Meloxicam (Mobic®)	7.5mg daily	PO	**Tablets:** 7.5 mg, 15 mg **Oral suspension:** 7.5 mg/5 mL	• Maximum daily dose: 15mg. • More COX-II selective than other non-selective NSAIDs. • More cost effective to use 1/2 of 15mg tablets for lower dose than 7.5mg tablets.

Continued

Generic Name (Trade Name)	Adult Starting Dose	Routes	Common Strengths and Formulations	Comments
Non-Steroidal Anti-Inflammatory Drugs (NSAID), *continued*				
Naproxen (Naprosyn®, Aleve®)	250mg Q8H PRN	PO	**Tablets:** 220 mg, 250 mg, 375 mg, 500 mg **ER tablets:** 375 mg, 500 mg, 750 mg **Capsules:** 220 mg **Oral suspension:** 125 mg/5 mL	• Maximum daily dose: 1250mg (naproxen base). • Naproxen sodium (OTC) 220mg = naproxen base 200mg + 20mg sodium. • Weigh risk vs benefit in patients with renal insufficiency. • Take with food or milk to lessen stomach upset.
Opioid Combination Products				
Hydrocodone + acetaminophen (Lortab®, Norco®, Vicodin®)	5-325mg Q6H PRN	PO	**Tablets:** 5-300 mg, 5-325 mg, 7.5-300 mg, 7.5-325 mg, 10-300 mg, 10-325 mg **Oral solution:** 7.5-325 mg/15 mL, 10-325 mg/ 15 mL	• C-II controlled substance. • Monitor acetaminophen intake from all sources. • Hydrocodone dosage forms containing > 325mg acetaminophen were discontinued in early 2014.
Oxycodone + acetaminophen (Percocet®, Endocet®)	5-325mg Q6H PRN	PO	**Tablets:** 2.5-325 mg, 5-325 mg, 7.5-325 mg, 10-325 mg, 5-300 mg, 7.5-300 mg, 10-300 mg **Oral solution:** 5-325 mg/5 mL	• C-II controlled substance. • Monitor acetaminophen intake from all sources. • Oxycodone dosage forms containing > 325mg acetaminophen were discontinued in early 2014.
Atypical Opioid-Monoamine Reuptake Inhibitor Analgesics				
Tramadol (Ultram®, Ultram ER®)	50mg Q6H PRN	PO	**Tablets:** 50 mg **ER tablets:** 100 mg, 200 mg, 300 mg	• C-IV controlled substance. • Maximum daily dose, IR: 400mg • Maximum daily dose, ER: 300mg • Not recommended in patients with renal or hepatic impairment. • ER tablets are dosed once daily. • Increased seizure risk even with recommended dosage. • Opioid agonist with serotonin reuptake inhibition. • Risk of serotonin syndrome when used with other serotonergic medications. • Avoid abrupt discontinuation; withdrawal symptoms. • Also available with acetaminophen.
Tapentadol (Nucynta®, Nucynta ER®)	50mg Q6H PRN	PO	**Tablets:** 50 mg, 75 mg, 100 mg **ER tablets:** 50 mg, 100 mg, 150 mg, 200 mg, 250 mg	• C-II controlled substance. • Increased seizure risk. • Opioid agonist with norepinephrine reuptake inhibition. • Not recommended in renal or hepatic impairment. • Do NOT split, crush, or chew ER tablets. • Avoid abrupt discontinuation; withdrawal symptoms.

Continued

Generic Name (Trade Name)	Adult Starting Dose	Routes	Common Strengths and Formulations	Comments
Opioid Mixed Agonist-Antagonist				
Buprenorphine (Buprenex®, Butrans®)	**TD:** 5 mcg/H every 7 days	TD IV IM SL	**Transdermal:** 5 mcg/H, 7.5 mcg/H 10 mcg/H, 15 mcg/H, 20 mcg/H **SL tablets:** 2 mg, 8 mg **Injection:** 0.3 mg/mL	• C-III controlled substance. • Maximum TD dose is 20mcg/H; risk of QTc prolongation at higher doses. • Taper dose of previous opioid to OME 30mg/day before initiating buprenorphine TD. • Not appropriate for patients requiring > OME 80mg/day. • SL tablets only FDA-approved for treatment of opioid dependence, not pain management.
Pure Opioids				
Fentanyl (Duragesic®)	**TD:** 25 mcg/H every 72 hours *Opioid-tolerant patients only.*	TD IV SC Buccal SL IN	**Transdermal:** 12.5 mcg/H, 25 mcg/H, 50 mcg/H, 75 mcg/H, 100 mcg/H **Injection:** **TIRF:** *refer to product chart*	• C-II controlled substance. • Potentially erratic absorption in cachectic or debilitated patients. • Difficult to titrate; wait 6 days (2 TD cycles) between dose increases. • TIRF = transmucosal immediate release fentanyl
Hydrocodone (Zohydro ER®, Hysingla ER®)	**ER capsules:** 10mg Q12H **ER tablets:** 20mg Q24H	PO	**ER capsules:** 10 mg, 15 mg, 20 mg, 30 mg, 40 mg, 50 mg **ER tablets:** 20 mg, 30 mg, 40 mg, 60 mg, 80 mg, 100 mg, 120 mg	• C-II controlled substance. • Do NOT open, crush, or chew ER tablets or capsules. • Dosages above 40mg per unit are for opioid-tolerant patients only. • Dose titrations may occur every 3-7 days.
Hydromorphone (Dilaudid®, Exalgo®)	**IR tablets:** 2mg Q4H PRN **Parenteral:** 0.2mg Q2H PRN *ER tablets for opioid-tolerant patients only.*	PO SL PR IV SC IM	**Tablets:** 2 mg, 4 mg, 8 mg **ER tablets:** 8 mg, 12 mg, 16 mg, 32 mg **Oral solution:** 1 mg/mL **Injection:** 1 mg/mL, 2 mg/mL, 4 mg/mL, 10 mg/mL	• C-II controlled substance. • Dose titrations may occur every 3-4 days. • Less risk of neurotoxicity than morphine, however myoclonus and seizures have been reported with high doses. • Do NOT crush or chew ER tablets. • ER tablets are dosed every 24H. • Suppository formulation available.
Methadone (Dolophine®)	2.5mg Q12H	PO SL PR IV SC IM	**Tablets:** 5 mg, 10 mg **Oral solution:** 5 mg/5 mL, 10 mg/5 mL, 10 mg/mL **Injection:** 10 mg/mL	• C-II controlled substance. • Refer to *Methadone* section in this chapter for more information. • Provides both short-acting and long-acting opioid analgesia. • Tablets may be crushed or given SL. • QTc prolongation and multiple drug interactions. • Methadone 40mg tablet use restricted to facilities authorized for detoxification and maintenance treatment of opioid addiction.

Continued

Generic Name (Trade Name)	Adult Starting Dose	Routes	Common Strengths and Formulations	Comments
Pure Opioids, *continued*				
Morphine (Roxanol®, Avinza®, Kadian®, MSContin®)	**Oral:** 5mg Q4H PRN **Parenteral:** 2mg Q2H PRN	PO SL PR IV SC IM	**Tablets:** 15 mg, 30 mg **ER tablets:** 15 mg, 30 mg, 60 mg, 100 mg, 200 mg **ER capsules:** 10 mg, 20 mg, 30 mg, 45 mg, 50 mg, 60 mg, 75 mg, 80 mg, 90 mg, 100 mg, 120 mg **Oral solution:** 10 mg/5 mL; 20 mg/5 mL; 20 mg/mL **Injection:** 1 mg/mL, 2 mg/mL, 4 mg/mL, 5 mg/mL, 8 mg/mL, 10 mg/mL, 15 mg/mL, 25 mg/mL, 50 mg/mL	• C-II controlled substance. • Use caution in renal impairment. • Metabolite (M3G) can accumulate and cause neurotoxicity. • Avinza® and Kadian® dosed Q24H • Do NOT crush or chew ER tablets. • ER capsules (Avinza® and Kadian®) may be opened and sprinkled on applesauce and eaten immediately without chewing. • Reserve higher doses (>30mg/dose) for opioid-tolerant patients only. • Additional strengths of ER capsules available; generic products listed. • Suppository formulation available.
Oxycodone (Roxicodone® OxyContin®, OxyFast®)	5mg Q4H PRN	PO	**Tablets:** 5 mg, 10 mg, 15 mg, 20 mg, 30 mg **Capsules:** 5mg **ER tablets:** 10 mg, 15 mg, 20 mg, 30 mg, 40 mg, 60 mg, 80 mg **Oral solution:** 5 mg/5 mL, 20 mg/mL	• C-II controlled substance. • Consider for patients with renal dysfunction. • Do NOT crush or chew ER tablets. • Reserve higher doses (>40mg/dose) for opioid-tolerant patients only. • ER tablets are not indicated for PR administration. • Abuse deterrent formulations have not been studied for PR administration.
Oxymorphone (Opana®, Opana ER)	5mg Q6H PRN	PO SC IV IM	**Tablets:** 5 mg, 10 mg **ER tablets:** 5 mg, 7.5 mg, 10 mg, 15 mg, 20 mg, 30 mg, 40 mg **Injection:** 1 mg/mL	• C-II controlled substance. • Administer on empty stomach, 1 hour before or 2 hours after a meal. • Do NOT crush or chew ER tablets. • Avoid use in moderate to severe hepatic impairment. • Similar structure to hydromorphone.

See Drug Dosing for Liver and Renal Disease for additional drug information.

Pharmacological Management of NOCICEPTIVE Pain - ADJUVANTS

Generic Name (Trade Name)	Adult Starting Dose	Routes	Common Strengths and Formulations	Comments
Colicky/Cramping Visceral Pain				
Dicyclomine (Bentyl®)	20mg Q6H PRN	PO IM	**Capsules:** 10 mg **Tablets:** 20 mg **Oral solution:** 10 mg/5 mL **Injection:** 10 mg/mL	• Avoid long-term use of antispasmodics in the elderly; risk of adverse events is greater than the potential benefit. • Anticholinergic effects may not be well tolerated in the elderly.
Glycopyrrolate (Robinul®, Cuvposa®)	**Oral:** 1mg Q8H PRN **Parenteral:** 0.2mg Q6H PRN	PO SC IM IV	**Tablets:** 1 mg, 2 mg **Oral solution:** 1 mg/5 mL **Injection:** 0.2 mg/mL	• Primarily used to control symptoms of malignant bowel obstruction. • Fewer CNS effects but more xerostomia than other anticholinergic agents. • Oral solution is expensive.
Hyoscyamine (Levsin®, Hyomax-SL®)	0.125mg Q4H PRN	PO SL SC IV IM	**Tablets:** 0.125 mg **ER tablets:** 0.375 mg **Oral disintegrating tablets:** 0.125 mg **Oral solution:** 0.125 mg/mL, 0.125 mg/5 mL **Injection:** 0.5 mg/mL	• SL tablets may leave chalky residue. • Do not exceed 12 tablets per 24 hours. • Avoid long-term use of antispasmodics in the elderly; risk of adverse events is greater than the potential benefit. • Oral solution and injection are expensive.
Scopolamine (Transderm Scōp®)	**TD:** 1 patch Q72H **Parenteral:** 0.4mg Q6H PRN	TD SC IV IM	**Transdermal:** 1.5 mg **Injection:** 0.4 mg/mL	• Approximately 6-8 hours from patch placement to onset of effect. • Apply patch to hairless area behind one ear; wash hands before and after application. • Do NOT cut patches.
Bone Pain OR Stretching/Capsule Visceral Pain				
Dexamethasone (Decadron®)	4mg daily *Burst and taper recommended for faster pain control.*	PO PR SC IV IM	**Tablets:** 0.5 mg, 0.75 mg, 1 mg, 1.5 mg, 2 mg, 4 mg, 6 mg **Oral solution:** 1 mg/mL **Injection:** 4 mg/mL, 10 mg/mL	• Give with food or milk to decrease GI upset. • Avoid administering later in the day due to insomnia. • Minimal mineralocorticoid activity lessens risk of peripheral edema. • Taper gradually after long-term therapy. • Rapid IV administration associated with perineal discomfort.

Continued

Generic Name (Trade Name)	Adult Starting Dose	Routes	Common Strengths and Formulations	Comments
Bone Pain OR Stretching/Capsule Visceral Pain, *continued*				
Methylprednisolone (Medrol®)	8mg daily *Burst and taper recommended for faster pain control.*	PO IV IM	**Tablets**: 2 mg, 4 mg, 8 mg, 16 mg, 32 mg **Injection:** 40mg, 125 mg	• Give with food or milk to decrease GI upset. • Avoid administering later in the day due to insomnia. • Taper gradually after long-term therapy. • Consider use when injectable dexamethasone is unavailable or in shortage.
Prednisone (Deltasone®)	10mg daily *Burst and taper recommended for faster pain control.*	PO	**Tablets:** 1 mg, 2.5 mg, 5 mg, 10 mg, 20 mg, 50 mg **Oral solution:** 1 mg/mL, 5 mg/mL	• Give with food or milk to decrease GI upset. • Avoid administering later in the day due to insomnia. • Taper gradually after long-term therapy. • Risk of peripheral edema especially with higher doses.
Bowel Obstruction Colic Pain *(see Bowel Obstruction GEMS)*				
Octreotide (Sandostatin®)	100mcg Q8H	IV SQ	**Injection:** 50 mcg/mL, 100 mcg/mL, 200 mcg/mL, 500 mcg/mL, 1,000 mcg/mL	• May require concomitant administration with an anticholinergic and corticosteroid. • May also be given as continuous infusion: 10-40 mcg/H. • Drug of choice for symptom management of carcinoid or VIPoma (cramping, diarrhea, flushing). • IM depot available; expensive.

See Drug Dosing for Liver and Renal Disease for additional drug information.

Neuropathic Pain: Peripheral and Central

Introduction and Background[1,23,29]

- Neuropathic pain is chronic pain resulting from injury to the nervous system, either the central nervous system (brain and spinal cord) or the peripheral nervous system (nerves outside the brain and spinal cord). It typically occurs weeks to months after an acute nerve injury has occurred.

Causes[1,23,29]

- Neuropathic pain is pain due to direct *damage* to the primary afferent nociceptive nerve fibers (axons) (not the nociceptors, *per se*) in either the peripheral or central nervous system.

Table 1. Causes of Neuropathic Pain

Peripheral pain syndromes	• Tumor invasion of nerve • Nerve ischemia due to impaired blood supply • Mechanical damage of nerve due to pathological fracture • AIDS neuropathy (HIV invasion of nerve) • Diabetic peripheral neuropathy and amyotrophy • Connective tissue disease (vasculitis) • Postherpetic neuralgia (herpes zoster) • Vascular compression • Painful scars • Amputation (phantom pain) • Traumatic nerve damage • Surgical nerve damage
Generalized (polyneuropathies)	• Metabolic or nutritional • Drug-related • Toxin-related • Hereditary • Malignant • Infective or post-infective, immune
Central pain syndromes	• Post-stroke pain syndrome • Vascular lesions in the brain and spinal cord • Nerve demyelination (multiple sclerosis, amyotrophic lateral sclerosis) • Spinal cord injury • Traumatic brain injury • Tumors • Abscesses • Neurosyphilis • Epilepsy • Parkinson's disease
Complex painful neuropathic disorders	• Complex regional pain syndrome type I (reflex sympathetic dystrophy) • Complex regional pain syndrome type II (causalgia)
Mixed pain syndromes	• Chronic low back pain with radiculopathy • Cancer pain with malignant plexus invasion • Complex regional pain syndromes

Clinical Characteristics[1,26, 29]

- Neuropathic and nociceptive pain tends to present differently.
- Neuropathic pain may be continuous (deep, burning, aching) or paroxysmal (sudden, lancinating, electric shocks or sharp stabs) and can occur concurrently with nociceptive pain. Common descriptors include "pins and needles" or "creepy-crawly" (paresthesias).
- Acute nerve injury pain is called neuralgia.

- o Examples: acute herpes zoster neuralgia ("shingles"), traumatic neuralgia (nerve damage due to pathological fracture), and neuralgia due to acute nerve inflammation (neuritis).
        - o Acute neuralgias are treated as other acute pains (e.g. opioids, ice, heat, nerve blocks).
- Neuropathic pain can be a secondary pain occurring weeks to months after an acute nerve injury even though the acute injury has begun to resolve.
- Patients may describe their neuropathic pain as a "new pain" that is different in presentation than the acute nerve injury pain.
- Stimulus-evoked neuropathic pain
    - o Allodynia: a condition in which pain arises from a stimulus that would not normally be experienced as painful (e.g., light touch from clothing or bedding, hot or cold temperatures).
    - o Hyperalgesia: a greater-than-normal sensitivity to pain that may result from a painful stimulus or a lowered pain threshold.
- Spontaneous neuropathic pain may be constant, intermittent, or paroxysmal and described as "shooting," "electric," or "shock-like."
- Paresthesia: An abnormal sensation, spontaneous or evoked; having no objective cause and usually associated with injury or irritation of a sensory nerve or nerve root. Described as pricking, tingling, or creeping skin.
- Dysesthesia: An unpleasant, abnormal sensation, spontaneous or evoked; caused by lesions of the peripheral or central sensory pathways.

Non-Pharmacological Therapy
*See **Pain Overview** above.*

Clinical Pearls
- Management of underlying causes may be attempted:
    - o Vaccination to prevent herpes zoster
    - o Glycemic control in diabetic neuropathy
    - o Reduce tumor burden impinging nerves (e.g., radiation therapy, surgical debulking of tumor, palliative chemotherapy). These relatively invasive approaches often are impractical when life expectancy is very limited or palliative performance status is low.
    - o Most neuropathic pain in the hospice setting cannot be eliminated and must be treated symptomatically. Symptomatic treatment often provides marked reduction in pain.

Pharmacotherapy[4,20,26,29-33]
- Consider patient and family goals of care to determine appropriateness of interventions to manage underlying causes of neuropathic pain.
- Both systemic and topical drugs can be useful in managing neuropathic pain.

Antidepressants
- All antidepressants have a black box warning for worsening depression and suicidal ideation in children and young adults.
- Both norepinephrine and serotonin levels must be increased for neuropathic pain efficacy.
    - o Serotonin selective reuptake inhibitor (SSRI) antidepressants are not as effective as TCAs and are not indicated to treat neuropathic pain.
    - o Serotonin norepinephrine reuptake inhibitors (SNRI) are as effective as TCAs for most patients and will treat depression and pain at equivalent doses.
- Tricyclic antidepressants (TCAs) are well-studied and often selected as drugs of choice for neuropathic pain in adults.
    - o Desipramine and nortriptyline are equally effective and better tolerated than amitriptyline.
    - o TCAs can cause or exacerbate anticholinergic problems; use caution in patients with severe benign prostatic hyperplasia (BPH), urinary retention, constipation, or cardiac arrhythmias.
    - o If used in higher risk patients, start at lower than normal dose (e.g., 10 mg HS), and monitor for exacerbation of underlying condition.

- - Usual dosing for TCAs for neuropathic pain is 25mg at bedtime with a titration by 25 mg every three days to a maximum of 100 mg at bedtime. Maximum benefit for neuropathic pain takes 2 to 3 weeks.
  - TCA doses for neuropathic pain are generally much lower than doses used for depression.
  - Not all patients receive adequate pain relief with TCAs alone; additional drugs are often needed. If TCA therapy alone is insufficient, add an antiepileptic drug (AED), rather than another antidepressant.
- Serotonin-norepinephrine reuptake inhibitors (SNRIs) are well-studied and well-tolerated for neuropathic pain. Recommend an SNRI, preferably duloxetine, if a patient is unable to tolerate a TCA or an AED.
  - Duloxetine (Cymbalta) is FDA-approved for diabetic peripheral neuropathy, fibromyalgia, chronic muscoluskeletal pain, as well as generalized anxiety disorder and depression.
  - Milnacipran (Savella) is FDA-approved for fibromyalgia only.
  - Venlafaxine (Effexor) has produced variable results for neuropathic pain and is only FDA-approved for anxiety and depressive disorders. Venlafaxine is associated with withdrawal symptoms with missed doses and an increased risk of hypertension.

Antiepileptic drugs (AEDs)

- Both epilepsy and neuropathic pain are associated with spontaneous, ectopic discharges of motor neurons; therefore it is not surprising that all AEDs have some effectiveness in neuropathic pain.
- An AED may be used as first line therapy in patients unable to tolerate a TCA; when used as second line therapy, add the AED to the TCA.
- Gabapentin (Neurontin) and pregabalin (Lyrica) are most widely used AEDs for neuropathic pain.
  - Gabapentin dosing usually starts at 100mg to 300mg at bedtime; increased by the same dose to twice daily and then three times daily at three to five day intervals. Most patients respond at when total daily doses reach 900 and 1800 mg.
  - Three times a day dosing is necessary due to gabapentin's short half-life. Patients with renal insufficiency require only twice daily or once daily dosing.
- Pregabalin has good efficacy data in neuropathic pain and is effective with twice daily dosing.
- Other AEDs, such as topiramate (Topamax) and carbamazepine (Tegretol), have been used in neuropathic pain but do not seem to be as effective as gabapentin or pregabalin.

Lidocaine

- Topical lidocaine patches (Lidoderm) are FDA-approved for postherpetic neuralgia but have been used successfully for other types of localized neuropathic pain. Systemic absorption from lidocaine patches is very low and side effects are rare. Minor local irritation at the application site can be managed with hydrocortisone cream.
  - Patches (up to 3) are placed directly over the painful area and left in place for 12 hours/day and then removed for 12 hours before another patch is applied.
  - Lidocaine patches might be considered if the neuropathic pain is in a small area of nerve distribution. Patches can be cut before the backing is removed and placed over the precise area.
  - Lidocaine patch therapy may be added to TCAs and/or AEDs. Each of these medications works by different mechanisms; multiple drug use is synergistic in effect.
- IV lidocaine is effective in managing neuropathic pain, but is potentially toxic and inconvenient to administer.

Opioids

- Although higher doses may be needed to treat neuropathic pain, opioids can be effective.
- Opioids used in combination with other therapies, not as a replacement.
- Methadone has the unique property of blocking the NMDA receptor. NMDA receptor blockage is associated with the relief of neuropathic pain. Methadone has been reported to be the most effective opioid for the treatment this type of pain.
- Tramadol is a weak mu opioid agonist and weak norepinephrine-serotonin reuptake inhibitor. The synergistic effects of these two mechanisms contribute to the effectiveness for neuropathic pain.
  - Abrupt withdrawal from chronic or higher dose tramadol can precipitate withdrawal symptoms and seizures.

Capsaicin topical
- Capsaicin depletes the pain-facilitating chemical substance P from sensory nerves.
- Topical capsaicin is potentially useful as an adjuvant to the therapies listed above, but not as primary therapy. Capsaicin requires 2 to 4 weeks continuous use for best results and must be applied at least TID.
- Initially capsaicin causes irritation and a burning sensation at the application site; this effect lessens within a few days to a week of use.
- Instruct patients/families to wear gloves to apply and wash hands carefully after use; touching mucous membranes or eyes can cause severe local pain.
- Capsaicin cream, gel, and lotion are available in low (0.025%) and high (0.075%) strength concentrations. Because benefit of a particular capsaicin product may take weeks to realize, use the entire package of low strength before changing to the high strength.

NMDA antagonists
- This class of medications is associated with significant adverse effects; reserve for use by experienced clinicians treating patients with refractory pain.
- Methadone: see Methadone section in this chapter for complete information on use.
- Ketamine (Ketalar)
  - Anesthetic given IV, SC, PO, or SL; some successful use for refractory neuropathic pain.
  - Adverse effects include hallucinations, confusion, delirium, hyper/hypotension, arrhythmia.
  - Ketamine can be abused; chemically similar to the illegal substance phencyclidine (PCP).
- Dextromethorphan
  - Anti-tussive has been studied for neuropathic pain but placebo-controlled studies have failed to show consistent clinical usefulness.
  - Doses needed for benefit in neuropathic pain are high, producing unacceptable side effects.

Pharmacological Management of Neuropathic Pain

Generic Name (Trade Name)	Adult Starting Dose	Routes	Common Strengths and Formulations	Comments
Tricyclic Antidepressants (TCA)				
Desipramine (Norpramin®)	25mg QHS	PO	**Tablets:** 10 mg, 25 mg, 50 mg, 75 mg, 100 mg, 150 mg	• Used more commonly for neuropathic pain than depression. • Less anticholinergic effects than amitriptyline (Elavil®). • Titrate every 3 days as tolerated. • Associated with QTc prolongation.
Nortriptyline (Pamelor®)	25mg QHS	PO	**Capsules:** 10 mg, 25 mg, 50 mg, 75 mg **Oral solution:** 10 mg/5 mL	• Used more commonly for neuropathic pain than depression. • Less anticholinergic effects than amitriptyline (Elavil®). • Titrate every 3 days as tolerated. • Associated with QTc prolongation.

Continued

Generic Name (Trade Name)	Adult Starting Dose	Routs	Common Strengths and Formulations	Comments
Serotonin-Norepinephrine Reuptake Inhibitor (SNRI)				
Duloxetine (Cymbalta®)	30mg daily	PO	**Capsules:** 20 mg, 30 mg, 60 mg	• FDA-approved for diabetic neuropathy, fibromyalgia, and chronic musculoskeletal pain. • If discontinuing, taper dose gradually to minimize withdrawal symptoms. • Contents of capsule may be sprinkled on applesauce and swallowed without chewing. • No additional benefit in doses >60mg/day.
Venlafaxine (Effexor®, Effexor XR®)	37.5mg BID	PO	**Tablets:** 25 mg, 37.5 mg, 50 mg, 75 mg, 100 mg **ER tablets:** 37.5 mg, 75 mg, 150 mg **ER capsules:** 37.5 mg, 75 mg, 150 mg, 225 mg	• If discontinuing, taper dose gradually to minimize withdrawal symptoms. • Contents of capsule may be sprinkled on applesauce and swallowed without chewing. • May cause hypertension and tachycardia, use cautiously in patients with cardiovascular disease. • ER tablets and capsules are dosed Q24H. • No additional benefit in doses >225mg/day.
Antiepileptic Drugs (AED)				
Carbamazepine (Tegretol®, Carbatrol®)	100mg Q12H	PO PR	**Tablets:** 200 mg **ER tablets:** 100 mg, 200 mg, 400 mg **ER capsules:** 100 mg, 200 mg, 300 mg **Suspension:** 100 mg/5 mL	• Significant drug interactions. • Well absorbed rectally; use IR tablets at PO dose. • Do not crush or chew ER tablets • Sprinkle formulations can clog feeding tubes. • Studied for trigeminal neuralgia.
Gabapentin (Neurontin®, Gralise®)	300mg QHS	PO	**Capsules:** 100 mg, 300 mg, 400 mg **Tablets:** 600 mg, 800 mg **ER Tablets:** 300 mg, 600 mg **Oral solution:** 250 mg/5 mL	• No FDA-approval for neuropathy. • Reduce dose and extend dosing interval in patients with renal impairment. • Titrate slowly, every 3 days as tolerated. • If discontinuing, taper gradually to avoid withdrawal (seizure risk).
Pregabalin (Lyrica®)	50mg BID	PO	**Capsules:** 25 mg, 50 mg, 75 mg, 100 mg, 150 mg, 200 mg, 225 mg, 300 mg **Oral solution:** 20 mg/mL	• C-V controlled substance. • FDA-approved for diabetic neuropathy, pain with spinal cord injury, fibromyalgia, and postherpetic neuralgia. • Reduce dose in renal impairment. • Titrate slowly, every 3 days as tolerated. • If discontinuing, taper gradually to avoid withdrawal (seizure risk).

Continued

Generic Name (Trade Name)	Adult Starting Dose	Routes	Common Strengths and Formulations	Comments
Antiepileptic Drugs (AED), *continued*				
Valproic acid, Divalproex sodium (Depakene®, Depakote®, Depakote ER®)	250mg BID	PO PR	***Valproic acid:*** **Capsules:** 250 mg **ER capsules:** 125 mg, 250 mg, 500 mg **Oral solution:** 250 mg/5mL ***Divalproex sodium:*** **Capsules:** 125 mg **EC tablets:** 125 mg, 250 mg, 500 mg **ER tablets:** 250 mg, 500 mg	• Capsule sprinkles may be mixed with semisolid food and swallowed without chewing. • Sprinkles can clog feeding tubes. • Depakote® & Depakote ER® not bioequivalent. • Oral solution well absorbed rectally, PO and PR doses are equivalent. • If discontinuing, taper gradually to avoid withdrawal (seizure risk). • Due to multiple, similar formulations check and confirm medication order and dose carefully prior to administration.
Opioids				
Methadone (Dolophine®)	2.5mg Q12H	PO SL PR SC IV IM	**Tablets:** 5, 10 mg **Oral solution:** 5 mg/5 mL, 10 mg/mL **Injection:** 10 mg/mL	• C-II controlled substance. • Other opioids may be used as *adjuvant* treatment of neuropathic pain; methadone may be used as monotherapy. • Refer to *Methadone* section in this chapter for more information. • Provides both short-acting and long-acting opioid analgesia. • Tablets may be crushed. • QTc prolongation and multiple drug interactions.
Local Anesthetics				
Lidocaine (Lidoderm®)	Apply patch for up to 12 hours/day.	Top	**Cream:** 3%, 4%, 5% **Gel:** 2%, 3%, 4%, 5% **Ointment:** 5% **Patch:** 5% **Solution:** 2%, 4%	• Lidoderm® FDA-approved for allodynia and postherpetic neuralgia. • Maximum daily dose: 3 patches. • Patches may be cut to size. • Lidocaine ointment or cream may be applied and covered with transparent dressing as alternative to patch. • Viscous 2% lidocaine is designed for mucous membrane application.
Topical Analgesic				
Capsaicin (Zostrix®, Qutenza®)	Apply cream four times/day	Top	***Over the Counter:*** **Cream:** 0.1%, 0.025%, 0.075% **Lotion:** 0.025% **Gel:** 0.025% **Patch:** 0.0375% ***Prescription Only:*** **Patch:** 8%	• Qutenza® 8% patch FDA-approved for postherpetic neuralgia; applied in physician's office or clinic. • Wear gloves to apply topical products; wash hands before and after application. • May cause local redness, burning, and painful sensation. • Other OTC formulations available.

See Drug Dosing for Liver and Renal Disease for additional drug information.

Opioids: Safe and Effective Use

Background[34-37]

- *Opioids* are any substance that produces morphine-like effects that can be blocked by the opioid antagonist, naloxone.
- *Opiates* include only morphine and codeine, compounds found naturally in the opium poppy.
- Narcotic is an older term for opioids, or drugs that induce sleep, but now more commonly refers to drugs of abuse.
- Morphine is a natural derivative of the opium poppy (*Papaver somniferum*) and has been used as medicine for thousands of years.
- Morphine is the model opioid; other opioids are typically compared to morphine in terms of relative potency.
- Since the structure of morphine was determined, semi-synthetic and synthetic opioids have been developed.

Opioid Pharmacology[35-37]

- Opioids are usually categorized by structural class or opioid receptor activity (agonist, partial agonist, mixed agonist-antagonist, antagonist). See Table 1.
- Understanding opioid structural classes assists in selecting opioids when patients report hypersensitivities, or for opioid rotation for patients with opioid intolerances.
- Methadone's pharmacology is unique and includes activity at opioid and NMDA receptors, as well as serotonergic and norepinephrine effects. See section on *Methadone* in this chapter for additional information.
- The three opioid receptors are mu, delta, and kappa.
  - Mu receptors: responsible for most of the analgesic effects of opioids and some of the adverse effects (respiratory depression, euphoria, sedation, dependence).
  - Delta receptors: responsible for some analgesia, but may also lower the seizure threshold when stimulated.
  - Kappa receptors: contribute to analgesia at the spinal level; cause sedation, dysphoria, and hallucinations.

Table 1. Chemical Structural Classes of Opioids

Phenanthrenes	Diphenylheptanes	Phenylpiperidines	Benzomorphans	Miscellaneous
morphine buprenorphine † butorphanol † codeine hydrocodone hydromorphone levorphanol nalbuphine † naloxone * naltrexone * oxycodone oxymorphone	methadone	fentanyl meperidine	pentazocine †	tapentadol ± tramadol ±

± Indicates atypical opioid with monoamine reuptake inhibition
† Indicates agonist-antagonists (aka, partial agonists)
* Indicates antagonists

Opioid Selection in Special Populations[38-41]

- Due to impaired metabolism and elimination processes, patients with end stage liver (ESLD) or renal disease (ESRD) require a more cautious approach to pain management and opioid selection.
- Most opioids are at least partially metabolized by the liver. Patients with ESLD cannot adequately metabolize codeine to the active analgesic form of the drug and will not receive pain relief. Meperidine

also cannot be properly metabolized and clearance of the drug is reduced, leading to an increased risk of seizures.

- For patients with ESRD, accumulation of metabolites can lead to an increased risk of toxicity. The morphine metabolite, morphine-3-glucuronide (M3G), provides no analgesia but contributes to neurotoxicity (confusion, hyperalgesia).
- Table 2 below can help guide opioid selection. In all patients with ESLD or ESRD, consider reducing initial opioid dose by 50% of usual and extend the dosing interval to help balance the increased risk of adverse effects.

Table 2. Opioid Choice Based on Organ Failure

	Preferred	Consider	Avoid
Hepatic Failure	hydromorphone morphine methadone	oxycodone fentanyl	codeine hydrocodone meperidine oxymorphone tapentadol tramadol
Renal Failure	fentanyl methadone oxycodone	hydromorphone hydrocodone	codeine meperidine morphine* tapentadol tramadol
Hepato-renal Syndrome	hydromorphone methadone	fentanyl oxycodone	codeine hydrocodone meperidine morphine* tapentadol tramadol

cautious use at low doses may be acceptable depending on patient need

Management of Opioid Adverse Effects[4,20,42,43]

Table 3. Opioid Adverse Effects

Common		Uncommon	
Constipation† Nausea/vomiting† Pruritus† Sedation	Sweats Xerostomia (dry mouth)†	Bad dreams Hallucinations Dysphoria Delirium† Myoclonus	Seizures† Urticaria Respiratory depression Urinary retention

† *See associated GEMS chapters.*

Constipation
- Patients do not develop tolerance to opioid-induced constipation. All patients should have a preventative bowel regimen in place at initiation of opioids.
  - Initiate stimulant laxatives (e.g., sennosides, bisacodyl) plus a stool softener (docusate) when a patient begins taking an opioid.
  - Methylnaltrexone (Relistor) is a peripherally-acting opioid antagonist indicated for opioid-induced constipation when other laxative regimens have failed. Methylnaltrexone does not cross the blood brain barrier and will not reverse the opioid's analgesic effects.
  - Methylnaltrexone dosing is according to body weight. Administer 1 dose every other day as needed; maximum: 1 dose/24 hours. Onset of action is 30-60min in patients who respond.
- Dietary interventions (e.g., prunes, bran) alone usually not sufficient.
- Avoid bulk-forming agents such as psyllium or cellulose fibers. The peristalsis-inhibiting effects of opioids in combination with patient dehydration and limited mobility increase the risk of impaction and concretion formation.

Nausea and Vomiting
- Nausea and vomiting usually subsides in 5 to 7 days. If it continues, consider decreasing the opioid dose or switching to another opioid.
- To rule out other causes of nausea, watch for a temporal relationship between the opioid dose and the onset of nausea. Nausea may begin about 60 minutes after taking an oral or sublingual opioid dose.
    - Pharmacological treatment for nausea and vomiting may include: haloperidol (off-label use), metoclopramide, prochlorperazine, promethazine, or ondansetron.

Pruritus
- Pruritus is a side effect, not an allergy. Treatment may include antihistamines, topical anti-itch preparations (menthol-camphor lotions), or rotation to a different opioid.
- Morphine is associated with the most complaints of pruritus.

Diaphoresis
- Excessive sweating, dry mouth, and sedation may be alleviated by reducing the opioid dose.
- Opioids cause hyperhidrosis because of mast cell degranulation and histamine release, but may also cause hypohidrosis due to their ability to raise the thermoregulatory set point.
- Opioid rotation or addition of an antihistamine may reduce sweating.

Dysphoria, Delirium, Hyperalgesia
- May be due to opioid-induced hyperalgesia; see *Opioid-Induced Neurotoxicity* section.

Respiratory Depression
- Life-threatening respiratory depression, although uncommon with proper dosing and patient monitoring, may occur if: patient is opioid naïve and the initial opioid dose is too high; another respiratory depressant drug (e.g., barbiturates, benzodiazepines) is combined with opioids; or accidental or deliberate overdose.
- Provide education for the patient, family, and caregivers about safe controlled substance disposal and risks of abuse and dependence. See *Managing Drug Misuse and Diversion in Hospice* and *Disposal of Controlled Substances* sections.

Table 4. Management of Opioid Induced Respiratory Depression *NCCN Guidelines v2.2014*

- If life threatening respiratory depression occurs, administer naloxone (Narcan) cautiously to avoid sudden reversal of analgesia and precipitation of acute opioid withdrawal.
- Suggested orders: naloxone 0.04 to 0.08 mg (40 to 80 mcg) slow IV push; administer bolus dose every 30 to 60 seconds until improvement in respiratory rate.
    - Dilute 0.4 mg/mL (1 mL) ampule into 9 mL of normal saline for a total volume of 10 mL to achieve a final concentration 0.04 mg/mL (40 mcg/mL)
- If no response is observed after 1mg total naloxone dose administered, consider other causes of respiratory depression or persistent sedation.
- Opioids with a long active half-life (methadone, extended-release preparations) consider using a continuous infusion of naloxone.
- Closely monitor the patient for signs of reoccurring pain during reversal. This may require cautious doses of an additional opioid.

Opioid-Induced Neurotoxicity
- Dependent on both the *dose* and *duration* of opioid therapy.
- Other precipitating factors include:
    - Underlying delirium
    - Dehydration
    - Acute renal failure
    - Advanced age
    - Psychoactive medications (benzodiazepines, tricyclic antidepressants)
- Neurotoxicity can occur with *all* opioids at high doses but most commonly with morphine (morphine-3 glucuronide metabolite) and hydromorphone (hydro morphone-3 glucuronide metabolite).

- Patients present with neuro-excitatory side effects and unrelieved pain despite increasing opioid doses; further increase of dose exacerbates excitatory behaviors.
- Risks for opioid-induced neurotoxicity:
  - morphine > hydromorphone > oxycodone > fentanyl > methadone
  - Renal insufficiency > normal renal function
  - High dose > low dose

Signs and Symptoms of Neurotoxicity
- Rapidly escalating dose requirement
- Pain "doesn't make sense"; not consistent with recent pattern or known disease
- Hyperalgesia: increased sensitivity to painful stimuli
- Allodynia: pain from stimuli that are not normally painful
- Myoclonus: twitching of large muscle groups
- Delirium and hallucinations
- Seizures

Treatment of Opioid-Induced Neurotoxicity
- Rotate opioid to a structurally dissimilar opioid with differing receptor affinity profiles and a lower risk for neurotoxicity (fentanyl or methadone).
- Hydrate patient to facilitate elimination of causative metabolites (e.g., 3-glucuronide metabolites).
- Treat delirium, usually with haloperidol. See *Agitation & Delirium GEMS.*
- Treat neuromuscular excitation and myoclonus with a benzodiazepine, baclofen, barbiturate.
- Behavioral excitation will resolve over hours to days depending on the patient's ability to clear the causative metabolites.

Opioid Equianalgesic Dosing[4,44-48]

- Opioid *potency* refers to the intensity of analgesia provided at a specific dose.
- When a specific dose of one opioid provides the same analgesia (is equipotent) to another opioid at a specific dose, they are considered to be equianalgesic.
  - Example: morphine 10mg IV is equipotent, or analgesic equivalent, to hydromorphone 1.5mg IV
- Because of differences in bioavailability of opioids based on the route of administration, an opioid dose by one route may be equianalgesic to a different dose of that opioid given by a different route.
  - Example: morphine 10mg IV is equianalgesic to morphine 30mg PO
  - Morphine bioavailability IV is 100% but ranges from 17-33% with PO dosing.
- Reasons for lack of adequate patient response to an opioid despite appropriate dosage adjustment:
  - Lack of therapeutic response
  - Disease progression
  - Development of tolerance to that specific opioid
  - Unmanageable or intolerable adverse effects
  - Change in patient status
  - If this occurs, switching to a different opioid or changing to a different route of administration may be appropriate.
- In order to determine the appropriate dose of the new opioid, use an opioid equianalgesic dosing chart. Each may have slight variations in dose equivalents because opioid equianalgesic dosing chart values are often estimates based on single-dose parenteral studies. Table 5 provides an example.
- Always use *the same equianalgesic chart* to calculate doses to minimize the risk of dose conversion errors.
- Considerable inter-patient variability in the efficacy and safety response to opioids can be due to:
  - Tolerance and cross-tolerance
  - Pharmacokinetic and pharmacodynamic variability
  - Use of co-analgesics and other CNS-active medications
  - Psychological variables
- When switching patients from one opioid to another, consider decreasing the dose by 30-50% to account for incomplete cross-tolerance to the new opioid.

Table 5. Equianalgesic Dosing Chart

Generic Name Trade Examples	SC, IV	Oral	Rectal	Maximum Recommended Dose
Morphine Sulfate Roxanol®, MS Contin®, Kadian®, Avinza®	10mg	30mg	30mg	No ceiling dose[a]
Hydromorphone Dilaudid®, Exalgo®	1.5mg	7.5mg	7.5mg	No ceiling dose
Oxycodone Roxicodone®, OxyContin®, *or in combination with aspirin or acetaminophen*: Percocet®, Percodan®, Roxicet®, Tylox®	NA	20mg	20mg[c]	No ceiling dose[b]
Hydrocodone Zohydro ER®, Hysingla ER® *or in combination with ibuprofen or acetaminophen*: Vicodin®, Lortab®, Norco®, Vicoprofen®	NA	30mg	30mg[c]	No ceiling dose[b]
Oxymorphone Opana®, Opana ER®	1mg	10mg	10mg[c]	No ceiling dose
Tramadol Ultram®, Ultram ER®	NA	150-300mg	150-300mg	400mg
Tapentadol Nucynta®, Nucynta ER®	NA	75-100mg	No data	600mg
Fentanyl Transdermal System Duragesic®	**Oral Morphine Equivalents (OME)** 12 mcg/H ≈ OME 25 mg/24H 25 mcg/H ≈ OME 50 mg/24H 50 mcg/H ≈ OME 100 mg/24H 75 mcg/H ≈ OME 150 mg/24H 100 mcg/H ≈ OME 200 mg/24H			
Buprenorphine Transdermal System Butrans®	**Oral Morphine Equivalents (OME)** 5 mcg/H ≈ OME 10-15 mg/24H 7.5 mcg/H ≈ OME 15-20 mg/24H 10 mcg/H ≈ OME 20-25 mg/24H 20 mcg/H ≈ OME 45-50 mg/24H			
Methadone Dolophine®	*Experienced clinicians only; refer to Methadone section of this chapter.*			

a. Avinza® capsules contain fumaric acid; serious renal toxicity from fumaric acid may result from Avinza® >1600 mg/day.

b. Opioid combination products with ibuprofen, aspirin, or acetaminophen (e.g. Norco®, Percocet®) are dose-limited due to these adjuvant ingredients.

c. Oxycodone ER tablets (OxyContin®), oxymorphone ER (Opana ER®), and other abuse deterrent formulations have not been studied for rectal administration; immediate release dosage forms have sufficient evidence to support rectal administration.

Figure 1. Equianalgesic Calculation Format

Step 1. Calculate the equivalent dose of the new opioid.

$$\frac{24 \text{ hour total dose of new opioid}}{24 \text{ hour total dose of current opioid}} = \frac{\text{equianalgesic table dose of new opioid}}{\text{equianalgesic table dose of current opioid}}$$

Step 2. Reduce total dose of new opioid by 25-30% to account for incomplete cross-tolerance. Note: this step may not be needed if patient's pain is poorly controlled on current opioid dose. Consider a 50% dose reduction when converting to oral opioids from transdermal fentanyl products.

Step 3. Calculate the scheduled dose and dose interval. Divide the 24 hour total dose by the appropriate dosing interval based on the new drug's duration of action.

Step 4. Calculate the breakthrough (as needed) dose; about 10-15% of the total daily dose
Example:

$$\frac{X \text{ mg, oxycodone}}{100\text{mg, oral morphine}} = \frac{20\text{mg oxycodone}}{30\text{mg morphine}}$$

$$30 \times X = 20 \times 100$$

$$30X = 2000$$

$$X = 66.7\text{mg oxycodone}$$

$$25\% \text{ dose reduction} = 66.7 - (66.7 \times 0.25) = 50.025 \text{ mg oxycodone}$$

Recommend a scheduled dose using commercially available dosages: *oxycodone ER 30mg every 12 hours.*
Recommend a breakthrough dose based on peak effect: *oxycodone IR 5mg every 2 hours as needed for pain.*

Table 6. NOT Recommended for Chronic Pain Management[*]

Generic Name _Trade Examples_	SC, IV[*]	Oral[*]	Rectal[*]	Comments
Codeine	130mg	200mg	200mg	Low potency opioid with high frequency of nausea, vomiting, constipation; 14% of white patients at risk of treatment failure or toxicity due to genotype-associated CYP2D6 activity
Butorphanol Stadol®	2mg	NA	NA	Partial opioid agonist; contraindicated in opioid-dependent patients; may precipitate opioid withdrawal
Levorphanol Levo-Dromoran®	NA	4mg (acute) 1mg (chronic)	4mg	Similar to methadone with NMDA antagonism, but no QTc prolongation risk and fewer drug interactions; limited availability and limited clinician experience contribute to challenging use
Meperidine Demerol®	100mg	300mg	300mg	American Pain Society (APS) and Institute for Safe Medication Practices (ISMP) do not recommend use as analgesic; lowers seizure threshold; avoid in geriatrics; avoid in renal impairment
Nalbuphine Nubain®	10mg	NA	NA	Mixed opioid agonist-antagonist; may precipitate opioid withdrawal; *maximum daily dose: 160mg*
Pentazocine Talwin®	30mg	NA	NA	Mixed opioid agonist-antagonist; may precipitate opioid withdrawal; *maximum daily dose: 360mg*

*Approximate OME based on available clinical literature; use cautiously when converting from mixed or partial agonists.

Table 7. Transmucosal Immediate Release Fentanyl (TIRF) Products

Fentanyl Products	Route of Administration	Dosage	BA*	Time to Peak (median)
Abstral®	Sublingual tablet	100, 200, 300, 400, 600, 800 mcg	54%	30-60 min
Actiq®	Oral lozenge	200, 400, 600, 800, 1200, 1600 mcg	47%	20-40 min
Fentora®	Buccal tablet	100, 200, 400, 600, 800 mcg	65%	45 min
Lazanda®	Intranasal spray	100, 400 mcg/spray	60%	15-20 min
Onsolis®	Buccal film	200, 400, 600, 800, 1200 mcg	71%	1 hr
Subsys®	Sublingual spray	100, 200, 400, 600, 800 mcg	76%	40-90 min

*Bioavailability

Converting between TIRF products[20]

- All TIRF products have REMS components required with prescribing and dispensing. Abstral® and Lazanda® require prescriber and patient enrollment, with limited pharmacy distribution channels.
- Substantial differences exist in the pharmacokinetic profile of immediate release fentanyl products.
- TIRF products are NOT equivalent microgram to microgram and are NOT interchangeable.
- Do not switch patients on a mcg per mcg basis between any other oral transmucosal or intranasal fentanyl product, unless specific conversion advice provided in package insert.
- Published directions for conversion between TIRF are limited and unidirectional:

Conversion Chart for Actiq® to Fentora® ONLY	
Actiq® 200-400mcg	Fentora® 100mcg
Actiq® 600-800mcg	Fentora® 200mcg
Actiq® 1200-1600mcg	Fentora® 400mcg

Conversion Chart for Actiq® to Subsys® ONLY	
Actiq® 200-400mcg	Subsys® 100mcg
Actiq® 600-800mcg	Subsys® 200mcg
Actiq® 1200-1600mcg	Subsys® 400mcg

Converting from TIRF products to other opioids

- Cautious equianalgesic dose conversions are possible from TIRF products to other immediate release opioids (see conversion chart). Start conservatively and titrate carefully to adequate pain relief.
- If converting to TIRF products from other immediate release opioids, always use the initial dose recommendations in the TIRF product chart or individual TIRF product prescribing information. Generally, initiate all patients at the lowest available dosage of selected TIRF (e.g., 100mcg or 200mcg), regardless of prior opioid use.

Conservative Equianalgesic Dosing for Select Immediate Release Opioids

Opioid	Form (Route)	Equivalent Dose
Hydromorphone	Oral solution or tablets (SL, PO, PR)	2 – 4 mg
	Injectable (SC, IV, IM)	0.4 – 1 mg
Morphine	Oral solution or tablets (SL, PO, PR)	10 – 15 mg
	Injectable (SC, IV, IM)	2 – 5 mg
Oxycodone	Oral solution or tablets (SL, PO, PR)	7.5 – 10 mg
Fentanyl	Buccal tablet (Fentora®)	100 mcg
	Intranasal (Lazanda®)	100 mcg

Methadone[20,33,49-60]

General Considerations
- Methadone is a safe and effective option for hospice pain management when opioid analgesics are needed and the prescriber is an experienced practitioner.
- Factors which are important when considering the use of methadone include appropriate patient selection, knowledge of methadone pharmacology, dosing and titration, adverse drug reactions, drug and disease interactions, and a commitment to ongoing patient monitoring.
- Prior to initiation of methadone, discuss the risks and benefits of the drug with the patient and family or healthcare advocate.

Consider Methadone for Patients with:
- Neuropathic pain as well as nociceptive pain
- Rapidly escalating opioid requirements
  - Oral morphine equivalent > 200mg /day
- Renal insufficiency or end stage renal disease
  - Dosage adjustment needed only when CrCl <10mL/min
- Dose-limiting side effects from other opioids (e.g., nausea, constipation)
  - Neurotoxicity – hyperalgesia, hallucinations, myoclonus

Methadone and Neuropathic Pain
- Methadone may be the most effective opioid for the treatment of neuropathic pain due to unique pharmacology.

Figure 1. Methadone Pharmacology[33]

OPIOID	N-Methyl-D-aspartate (NMDA)	MONOAMINES
• μ agonist • δ agonist	Blocking NMDA receptor prevents: • Central sensitization • Cross tolerance • Hyperalgesia • Wind-up • Opioid tolerance	Inhibits reuptake of: • serotonin • norepinephrine (Similar to tricyclic antidepressants)

Patient Evaluation
- Conduct a complete assessment of the patient's pain, medication history, and co-morbid conditions.
- Evaluate patient's ability to adhere to prescribed methadone dosing regimen.
- Assess patient's expectation of analgesia.
- Determine if a responsible, capable, and willing caregiver is available to assist the patient.
- Evaluate ability of caregiver to successfully monitor patient pain control and methadone use.
- Review current medications for potential drug interactions (see Table 1); consult pharmacist.
- Determine psychological impact of prior opioid CNS effects, especially sedation, euphoria.
- Assess for cardiac risk factors (QTc interval prolongation).
- Determine if opioid use is for pain, dyspnea, or both.

Safety Considerations (select FDA boxed warnings for methadone):
- The following are verbatim boxed warnings placed by the U.S. Food and Drug Administration for the use of methadone between November 2006 and August 2014. Refer to the methadone's full prescribing information for complete boxed warnings list.
  - Methadone exposes patients and other users to the risks of opioid addiction, abuse, and misuse, which can lead to overdose and death. Assess each patient's risk prior to prescribing

methadone, and monitor all patients regularly for the development of these behaviors or conditions.
- o Serious, life-threatening, or fatal respiratory depression may occur with use of methadone. Monitor for respiratory depression, especially during initiation of methadone or following a dose increase.
- o QT interval prolongation and serious arrhythmia (*torsades de pointes*) have occurred during treatment with methadone. Most cases involve patients being treated for pain with large, multiple daily doses of methadone, although cases have been reported in patients receiving doses commonly used for maintenance treatment of opioid addiction. Closely monitor patients for changes in cardiac rhythm during initiation and titration of methadone.
- o Accidental ingestion of even one dose of methadone, especially by children, can result in a fatal overdose of methadone.

Methadone and Cardiac Arrhythmias
- Case reports suggests patients taking methadone have experienced ventricular arrhythmias (*torsades de pointes*): primarily in doses > than 200mg daily and parenteral (IV) use.
- Avoid use of methadone in patients with predisposing cardiac arrhythmias or concomitant use of multiple medications that impact QT interval.
    - o Drugs that can prolong the QT interval (See *Appendix*)
    - o Patients with predisposing clinical conditions
        - known cardiac arrhythmias
        - bradycardia (<50 beats/minute)
        - electrolyte disturbances: hypokalemia, hypomagnesemia, hypocalcemia
        - have congenital QT interval prolongation
    - o If cardiac history is unclear, consider a baseline ECG prior to initiation of methadone, with a follow-up ECG in 30 days. Ideally, QTc interval remains < 450 ms.
- If QTc interval prolongation is a concern *and* the benefit of using methadone for pain management outweighs the potential risks, some clinicians may choose to obtain a baseline electrocardiogram prior to initiating methadone therapy and periodically while on methadone.
- QTc monitoring guidelines:
    - o Obtain ECG to evaluate QTc interval for all patients receiving methadone (baseline, within 30 days of initiation, and annually thereafter).
    - o Increase ECG monitoring if patient receiving >100mg/day or if unexplained syncope or seizure occurs while on methadone.
- Risk stratification:
    - o **QTc >450-499 ms:** Discuss potential risks and benefits; monitor QTc more frequently
    - o **QTc ≥500 ms:** Consider discontinuation or reducing methadone dose *or* eliminate factors promoting QTc prolongation (e.g., potassium-wasting drugs)

Methadone and Drug Interactions
- Methadone is metabolized in the liver by the cytochrome P450 system:
    - o Substrate, major: CYP2B6, CYP3A4
    - o Substrate, minor: CYP2C19 ,CYP2C9, CYP2D6
    - o Inhibitor, moderate: CYP2D6
    - o Inhibitor, weak: CYP3A4
- Assess patient's complete medication profile for drugs that interact with methadone CYP450 metabolism
- Always consult a pharmacist for assistance with medication profile review and risk factor identification.

Table 1. Examples of Drug Interactions with Methadone[20,59]

Drugs that INCREASE Methadone Levels/Effects	Drugs that DECREASE Methadone Levels/Effects
• Cimetidine (Tagamet®) • Ciprofloxacin (Cipro®) • Clarithromycin (Biaxin®) • Doxycycline (Vibramycin®) • Erythromycin (Erytab®) • Fluconazole (Diflucan®) • Fluoxetine (Prozac®) • Fluvoxamine (Luvox®) • Grapefruit Juice • Ketoconazole (Nizoral®) • Paroxetine (Paxil®) • Sertraline (Zoloft®) • Verapamil (Isoptin®)	• Carbamazepine (Tegretol®) • Chronic Alcohol ingestion • Pentobarbital (Nembutal®) • Phenobarbital • Phenytoin (Dilantin®) • Resperidone (Risperdal®) • Rifampin (Rifadin®) • Ritnavir (Norvir®) • Secobarbital (Seconal®) • Spironolactone (Aldactone®)

Note: *list not comprehensive. Consult clinical pharmacist for complete medication profile review prior to initiating methadone or before initiating any other medications after methadone has been started.*

Avoiding Problems with Methadone

- Problems arise from the cumulative effect of risk factors. *Avoid concomitant use of multiple medications, (particularly in high doses):*
  - that can prolong the QTc interval (see *Appendix*)
  - in patients with predisposing QTc prolonging conditions
  - that interact with methadone
    - drugs which undergo CYP450 metabolism
    - CNS depressants

Methadone Rotation Protocol Controversies

- There is no consensus in the literature for the best methadone rotation protocol. Two examples are provided on the next page for general guidance.
- Process differences exist in 4 main areas.
  - Dosage conversion calculations: fixed ratio VERSUS variable
  - Discontinuation of previous opioid: abrupt transition VERSUS tapering over 3-5 days
  - Scheduled dosing intervals: every 6, 8, 12, or 24 hours
  - Breakthrough medication selection: short-acting opioid PRN (morphine, oxycodone, or hydromorphone) VERSUS methadone PRN
- Most clinicians support a ratio of parenteral methadone to oral methadone of 1:2. For example, an oral methadone dose of 20mg is equivalent to an IV or SC dose of 10mg.

Methadone Dosing, Titration, and Monitoring Guidelines

1. Assess patient's appropriateness for methadone
   - Preexisting disease states (e.g., cardiac disease, hypokalemia)
   - Expectations and desire for sedation/euphoria
   - Ability and willingness to comply with instructions
2. Understand the pharmacokinetics of methadone:
   - Long elimination half-live (8-59 hours)
   - Duration of analgesia (4-8 hours – up to 24 hours in some patients with continued use)
   - Dosing guidelines and equianalgesic dosage calculations
3. Maintain an accurate and current medication profile of all medications used by the patients: prescription, over-the-counter, and herbals and dietary supplements.
4. Avoid the use of medications known to interact with methadone. However, adjust methadone doses based on the patient's response rather than the anticipated interactions.
5. Provide education to the patient on the importance of adhering to the prescribed medication regimen.

6. Provide education to the patient and caregiver:
    - Not to take more methadone than prescribed as it can accumulate in the body.
    - Signs of *overdose:* Increased sedation, respiratory depression (respiratory rate < 9 breaths/minute not associated with normal dying process), blurred vision, inability to think, talk or walk normally, and feeling faint, dizzy or confused, and pinpoint pupils.
    - Signs of *opioid withdrawal:* Yawning, sweating, watery eyes, rhinorrhea, anxiety, restlessness, insomnia, dilated pupils, piloerection, chills, tachycardia, hypertension, nausea, vomiting, cramping abdominal pains, diarrhea, and muscle aches and pains.
    - Seek medical attention right away if the patient experiences symptoms suggestive of an arrhythmia such as palpitations, dizziness, lightheadedness, or fainting.
    - Alert all prescribers before starting or stopping other medications due to possible interactions with methadone.

Example 1: AAHPM Methadone Equianalgesic Dosing Ratio[60]	
24 Hour Oral Morphine Equivalent	**Morphine : Methadone Ratio (per 24 hours)**
> 30mg / 24 hrs	2 :1
31-99mg / 24 hrs	4 : 1
100-299mg / 24 hrs	8 : 1
300-499mg / 24 hrs	12 : 1
500-999mg / 24 hrs	15 : 1
>1000 mg / 24 hrs	20 : 1
Divide calculated 24 hour methadone dose by 2 for every 12 hour dosing, or by 3 for every 8 hour dosing.	

Example 2: Methadone Dosing Rotation[61]

1. Calculate 24 hour oral morphine equivalent (OME) dose based on current opioid use.
2. Calculate methadone 24 hour dose equivalent:
    - Use 20% of 24 hour OME (1:5 methadone to morphine ratio).
    - ***Do not exceed starting methadone dose = 60mg PO/24hrs (30mg IV/SC/24hrs).***
3. Assess patient factors necessitating a calculated dose reduction (incomplete cross-tolerance, addition of co-analgesics, non-physical pain component, neurotoxicity, hyperalgesia, etc.).
4. Reduce calculated 24 hour methadone dose by 30% to 50%.
5. Divide calculated 24 hour methadone dose by 2 for every 12 hour dosing, or divide by 3 for every 8 hour dosing.
6. As needed opioids for breakthrough pain:
    - Option 1: use short-acting opioid for breakthrough pain at 10% of the calculated OME dose given every 1-2 hours PRN.
    - Option 2: use methadone for breakthrough pain PRN at 15% of the 24 hour scheduled methadone dose given every 4 hours PRN.
7. Monitor patient daily for the first 5 to 7 days after initiating methadone.
8. If needed due to poor pain control, titrate methadone doses no more frequently than every 3-5 days. When titrating, increase by 25-30% increments.
    - Allow the patient to use breakthrough doses in between dosage titrations.

Note: Patients receiving higher dose (> 300 mg OME) or parenteral opioids may benefit from tapering the previous opioid over 3-5 days rather than an abrupt rotation. Tapering the previous opioid can prevent withdrawal and reduce the potential for psychological methadone failure.

Disposal of Controlled Substances and Other Medication[61-65]

Background
- In recent years, multiple agencies have provided guidance on the disposal of medications, especially controlled substances. *This section addresses the U.S. Drug Enforcement Agency (DEA) rules and the U.S Food and Drug Administration recommendations for disposal of controlled substances and other medications.*
- Unfortunately, existing rules and regulations do not clearly define situations when hospice patients are deceased, or otherwise unable to dispose of medications themselves.
- All clinicians prescribing, dispensing, and administering controlled substances must stay current on local, state, and federal policies, rules and regulations.
- The Drug Enforcement Agency (DEA) published the Final Rule on the Disposal of Controlled Substances (DEA-316). This rule sets requirements for handling controlled substances no longer wanted by patients, or no longer useful to a hospital, health system, or clinic. The effective date of the Final Rule was October 9, 2014.

DEA-316 Disposal of Controlled Substances Summary
- This rule governs the secure disposal of controlled substances by registrants and ultimate users (patients) and implements the Secure and Responsible Drug Disposal Act of 2010 by expanding the options available to collect controlled substances from ultimate users for the purpose of disposal.
- Law enforcement can voluntarily continue to conduct take-back events, administer mail-back programs, and maintain collection receptacles. Additionally, authorized manufacturers, distributors, reverse distributors, narcotic treatment programs (NTPs), hospitals/clinics with an on-site pharmacy, and retail pharmacies can now voluntarily administer mail-back programs and maintain collection receptacles.
- Authorized hospitals, clinics, or pharmacies may voluntarily maintain collection receptacles at long-term care facilities for drug disposal by patients and providers at the facility.
- DEA-316 Final Rule now permits controlled substance disposal via 3 methods:
  - Drug take-back events
  - Mail-back programs
  - Collection receptacles for drug disposal
- DEA-316 Final Rule does NOT require any of the 3 methods listed above, rather it expands the use of those programs to now include disposal of controlled substances.
- Commercial drug disposal kits containing chemicals to adsorb and inactivate medications, including controlled substances, continue to be recommended for *in home* destruction and disposal of unused patient medications.
- To avoid and reduce the risk of diversion and personal safety risks, hospice staff members should NOT remove controlled substances from a patient's home.
- Take-back, mail-back, or collection receptacles can NOT be used for disposal of schedule 1 controlled substances (e.g. marijuana and marijuana products), illicit drugs, or illegally obtained controlled substances.

Flushing Medications
- Flushing controlled substances or mixing with cat litter or coffee grounds does NOT satisfy the requirements for non-retrievable for DEA registrants.
- However, ultimate users (patients) may continue to dispose of controlled substances in accordance with package labeling and local laws which may include sewering (flushing).
- Ultimate users can continue to use the FDA and EPA guidelines for the disposal of medications. Refer to the FDA website, *Medicines Recommended for Disposal by Flushing*, or drug manufacturers' package labeling for updated information on specific disposal processes.

Managing Drug Misuse and Diversion in Hospice[67-80]

Background
- All health care professionals have the responsibility to assess risk for, and identify signs of, drug misuse and addiction.
- Hospice and palliative care programs should have policies in place to manage these situations.
- Many screening tools are available to identify risks. Examples are provided on the following pages.
- Patients may exhibit behaviors which mimic drug abuse but are actually signs of chemical coping or undertreated pain. Involving the entire interdisciplinary team is essential to making these determinations.

Managing Opioid Risk
- Managing opioid risk and chemical coping in patients can be analogous to universal precaution strategies and risk assessment used in other areas of medical practice.
  - Need to protect the health care provider as well as the patient
  - Difficulty in identifying the most "at-risk" patient
  - Incorrect assessment or assumptions about the patient can lead to harm
- Differential diagnosis: identify causes of pain and patient-specific factors influencing an individual's pain perception and expression.
- Risk factor history associated with chemical coping and opioid abuse: tobacco use, depression, history of substance abuse, personality disorder, somatization, sexual abuse.
- Use a risk screening tool at first visit, *for all patients*, to identify those at highest risk.
- Practice informed consent procedures including patient education about addiction, tolerance, opioid side-effects and develop a treatment plan that de-emphasizes opioids as the sole treatment for pain.
- Opioid agreements or other pain and symptom management agreements include an outline of patient and practitioner expectations and obligations (e.g., receive opioids prescriptions from a single provider, no early refills, and random urine drug screening if appropriate).
- Pre-assessment and post-assessment of patient's pain level and function, with routine assessment of 4 As: analgesia, activities of daily living, adverse effects, and aberrant behavior.
- Online Prescription Drug Monitoring Programs are available in nearly all states. These tools can be used to identify "doctor shopping" and problematic prescribing practices.
- Encourage psychological support combined with increased vigilance and structure for those at high risk of opioid misuse (e.g., pill counts, dispensing smaller quantities, lock boxes, and shorter intervals between visits). An interdisciplinary team approach is necessary for those patients at risk of coping in a maladaptive manner. Consider co-management or consultation with a substance abuse specialist as appropriate to patient's prognosis.
- Understand that the source of pain and patient-specific factors related to pain may change over time. For example, patients with stable pain or no evidence of disease should be on a relatively stable opioid dose; whereas patients with progressive, advanced disease will likely require additional breakthrough dose opioids and potentially dose escalations.
- Objectively document all prescriptions, healthcare visits, agreements, and instructions.
- Discharging a patient with a terminal illness and substance misuse can lead to ethical concerns. The interdisciplinary team must have open, non-judgmental, and respectful dialogue with the patient and family about the concerns. Consultation with an ethics advisory board is recommended.
- The safety risks to patient, family, hospice staff and organization, and community must be thoroughly assessed and documented within the scope of the hospice organization's policy and procedures document. The discharge plan should include referral information to community supportive services to avoid a sense of abandonment.

Figure 1. CAGE© and CAGE-AID© Questionnaire[76]

1. In the last three months, have you felt you should cut down or stop drinking or *using drugs?*   **Yes No**
2. In the last three months, has anyone annoyed you or gotten on your nerves by telling you to cut down or stop drinking or *using drugs?*   **Yes No**
3. In the last three months, have you felt guilty or bad about how much you drink *or use drugs?*   **Yes No**
4. In the last three months, have you been waking up wanting to have an alcoholic drink or *use drugs?*   **Yes No**

- *Each affirmative response earns one point.*
- *One point indicates a possible problem.*
- *Two points indicate a probable problem.*

Figure 2. Opioid Risk Tool[77]

		Mark each box that applies	Item Score ☐ Female	Item Score ☐ Male
1. **Family History of Substance Abuse**	Alcohol	[ ]	1	3
	Illegal Drugs	[ ]	2	3
	Prescription Drugs	[ ]	4	4
2. **Personal History of Substance Abuse**	Alcohol	[ ]	3	3
	Illegal Drugs	[ ]	4	4
	Prescription Drugs	[ ]	5	5
3. **Age**	(Mark box if 16-45 yoa)	[ ]	1	1
4. **History of Preadolescent Sexual**		[ ]	3	0
5. **Psychological Disease**	Attention Deficit Disorder Obsessive Compulsive Disorder Bipolar Disorder Schizophrenia	[ ]	2	2
	Depression	[ ]	1	1
	TOTAL		_____	_____

Total Score Risk Category
Low Risk 0 – 3
Moderate Risk 4 – 7
High Risk ≥ 8

Figure 3. Screener and Opioid Assessment for Patients with Pain (SOAPP©)[78]
Please answer the questions below using the following scale:
0 - never; 1 - seldom; 2 - sometimes; 3 - often; 4 - very often

1. How often do you have mood swings?
2. How often do you smoke a cigarette within an hour after you wake up?
3. How often have any of your family members, including parents and grandparents, had a problem with alcohol or drugs?
4. How often have any of your close friends had a problem with alcohol or drugs?
5. How often have others suggested that you have a drug or alcohol problem?
6. How often have you attended an Alcoholics Anonymous or Narcotics Anonymous meeting?
7. How often have you taken medication other than the way that it was prescribed?
8. How often have you been treated for an alcohol or drug problem?
9. How often have your medications been lost or stolen?
10. How often have others expressed concern over your use of medication?
11. How often have you felt a craving for medication?
12. How often have you been asked to give a urine screen for substance abuse?
13. How often have you used illegal drugs (e.g., marijuana, cocaine) in the past 5 years?
14. How often, in your lifetime, have you had legal problems or been arrested?

References

1. IASP Task Force on Taxonomy. Part III: Pain terms, a current list of definitions and notes on usage. In: Merskey H, Bogeuk N, eds. Classification of chronic pain, 2nd ed. Seattle, WA: IASP Press, 1994. Available at: http://www.iasp-pain.org/Education/Content.aspx?ItemNumber=1698. Accessed July 28, 2014.
2. McCaffrey M. *Nursing practice theories related to cognition, bodily pain, and man-environmental interactions.* Los Angeles, CA: UCLA Students' Store; 1968:95.
3. Ferrell B. Ethical perspectives on pain and suffering. *Pain Manag Nurs.* 2005;6(3):83-90.
4. National Comprehesive Cancer Network (NCCN). NCCN clinical practice guidelines in oncology: adult cancer pain. Version 2.2014. Available at http://www.nccn.org/professionals/physician_gls/pdf/pain.pdf. Accessed July 9, 2014.
5. Reynolds J, Drew D, Dunwoody C. American Society for Pain Management Nursing position statement: pain management at the end of life. *Pain Manag Nurs.* 2013;14(3):172-175. Available at http://www.aspmn.org/Pages/positionpapers.aspx. Accessed August 14, 2014.
6. Smith AK, Cenzer IS, Knight SJ, Puntillo KA, Widera E, Williams BA, et al. Epidemiology of pain during the last 2 years of life. *Ann Intern Med.* 2010;153:563-569.
7. McCaffrey M, Pasero C. Assessment: underlying complexities, misconceptions, and practical tools. In: McCaffrey M, Pasero C., eds. *Pain: Clinical Manual.* 2nd ed. St. Louis, MO: Mosby, Inc.; 1999:35-99.
8. Krechel SW, Bildner J. CRIES: A new neonatal postoperative pain measurement score. Initial testing of validity and reliability. *Paediatr Anaesth.* 1995;5:53-61.
9. Merkel SI, Voepel-Lewis T, Shayevitz JR, Malviya S. The FLACC: a behavioral scale for scoring postoperative pain in young children. *Pediatr Nurs.* 1997;23(3):293-7.
10. Malviya S, Voepel-lewis T, Burke C, Merkel S, Tait AR. The revised FLACC observational pain tool: improved reliability and validity for pain assessment in children with cognitive impairment. *Paediatr Anaesth.* 2006;16(3):258-65.
11. Wong D, Baker C. Pain in children: comparison of assessment scales. *Pediatr Nurs.* 14(1):9-17, 1988.
12. Mcconahay T, Bryson M, Bulloch B. Clinically significant changes in acute pain in a pediatric ED using the Color Analog Scale. *Am J Emerg Med.* 2007;25(7):739-42.
13. Warden V, Hurley AC, Volicer L. Development and psychometric evaluation of the pain assessment in advanced dementia (PAINAD) scale. *J Am Med Dir Assoc.* 2003;4:9-15. Available at http://www.amda.com/publications/caring/may2004/painad.cfm. Accessed November 14, 2014.
14. International Association for the Study of Pain (IASP). Faces pain scale – revised. September 11, 2014. Washington, DC; IASP, 2014. Available at http://www.iasp-pain.org/Education/Content.aspx?ItemNumber=1519&&navItemNumber=577. Accessed November 14, 2014.
15. Fuchs-Lacelle S, Hadjistavropoulos T. Development and preliminary validation of the pain assessment checklist for seniors with limited ability to communicate (PACSLAC). Pain Manag Nurs 2004;5(1): 37-49. Available at http://www.geriatricpain.org/Content/Assessment/Impaired/Documents/PACSLAC_Tool.pdf Accessed December 16, 2014.
16. Smith HS. Pathophysiology of pain. In: Smith HS, ed. *Current Therapy in Pain.* Philadelphia, PA: Saunders-Elsevier;2009: 4-8.
17. Fouladbakhsh J, Szczesny S, Jenuwine E, Vallerand A. Nondrug therapies for pain management among rural older adults. *Pain Manag Nurs.* 2011;12(2):70-81.
18. Kwekkeboom K, Bumpus M, Wanta B, Serlin R. Oncology nurses' use of nondrug pain interventions in practice. *J Pain Symptom Manage.* 2008;35(1):83-94.
19. Thorns A, Sykes N. Opioid use in last week of life and implications for end-of-life decision-making. *Lancet.* July 2000; 356(9227): 398–399.
20. Lexi-Comp Online. Lexi-Drugs Online, Hudson, OH: Lexi-Comp, Inc.; Accessed July 15, 2014.
21. Vargas-Schaffer G. Is the WHO analgesic ladder still valid? Twenty-four years of experience. *Can Fam Physician.* 2010;56(6):514-517. Available at http://www.cfp.ca/cgi/pmidlookup?view=long&pmid=20547511.
22. Katz N, Ferrante FM. Nociception. In: Ferrante FM, VadeBoncouer TR eds. *Postoperative Pain Management.* New York, NY: Churchill Livingstone Inc; 1993.
23. Pasero C, Paice J, McCaffrey M. Basic mechanisms underlying the causes and effects of pain. In: McCaffrey M, Pasero C., eds. *Pain: Clinical Manual.* 2nd ed. St. Louis, MO: Mosby, Inc.; 1999:15-34.
24. Mercadante S, Arcuri E. Pharmacological management of cancer pain in the elderly. *Drugs Aging.* 2007;24(9):761-76.
25. Ripamonti C. Pain management. *Ann Oncol.* 2012;23(suppl10):x294-x301.
26. British Pain Society. *Cancer Pain Management: a perspective from the British Pain Society, supported by the Association for Palliative Medicine and the Royal College of General Practitioners.* London: British Pain Society; 2010. Available at https://www.britishpainsociety.org/static/uploads/resources/files/book_cancer_pain.pdf
27. World Health Organization (WHO). *Cancer Pain Relief: with a Guide to Opioid Availability.* 2nd ed. Geneva: WHO; 1996. Available at http://whqlibdoc.who.int/publications/9241544821.pdf
28. Sikandar S, Dickenson A. Visceral pain: the ins and outs, the ups and downs. *Curr Opin Supp Palliat Care.* 2012;6(1):17-26.

29. Baron R, Binder A, Wasner G. Neuropathic pain: diagnosis, pathophysiological mechanisms, and treatment. *Lancet Neurol.* 2010;9(8):807-19.

30. Mercadante S, Arcuri E, Tirelli W, Casuccio A: The analgesic effect of ketamine in cancer patients on opioid therapy: A randomized, controlled, double-blind, cross-over, double dose study. *J Pain Symptom Manage* 2000; 20:246-252.

31. Chaparro LE, Wiffen PJ, Moore RA, Gilron I. Combination pharmacotherapy for the treatment of neuropathic pain in adults. Cochrane Database Syst Rev. 2012;7:CD008943.

32. Caraceni A, Zecca E, Bonezzi C, et al. Gabapentin for neuropathic cancer pain: A randomized controlled trial from the Gabapentin Cancer Pain Study Group. *J Clin Oncol* 2004; 22:2909-2917.

33. Smith HS. Opioids and neuropathic pain. *Pain Physician* 2012; 15(3): 93-110.

34. Mather LE. Trends in the pharmacology of opioids: implications for the pharmacotherapy of pain. *Eur J Pain* 2001;5(suppA):49-57.

35. Rang HP, Dale MM, Ritter JM, Flower RJ, Henderson G. Analgesic drugs. In: *Rang and Dale's Pharmacology*, 7th ed. New York, NY: Elsevier, Inc. 2012;503-524.

36. Trescot AM, Datta S, Lee M, Hansen H. Opioid pharmacology. *Pain Physician* 2008;11:s133-s153. Available at http://www.painphysicianjournal.com/2008/march/2008;11;S133-S153.pdf.

37. Pathan H, Williams J. Basic opioid pharmacology: an update. *Brit J Pain* 2012;6(1):11-16. Available at http://bjp.sagepub.com/content/6/1/11.full.pdf+html.

38. Bosilkovska M, Walder B, Besson M, Daali Y, Desmeules J. Analgesics in patients with hepatic impairment: pharmacology and clinical implications. *Drugs.* 2012;71(12):1645-1669.

39. Rogal S, Winger D, Bielefeldt K, Rollman B, Szigethy E. Healthcare utilization in chronic liver disease: the importance of pain and prescription opioid use. *Liver Int.* 2013;33(10):1497-1503.

40. Carbonara GM. Opioids in patients with renal or hepatic dysfunction. *Pract Pain Manage.* May 1, 2008. Available at http://www.practicalpainmanagement.com/treatments/pharmacological/opioids/opioids-patients-renal-hepatic-dysfunction. Accessed January 30, 2015.

41. Davison S. Prevalence and management of chronic pain in end-stage renal disease. *J Palliat Med.* 2007;10(6):1277-1287.

42. Back IN. *Palliative Medicine Handbook*. 3rd ed. Cardiff, UK: BPM Books; 2001.

43. Cheshire WP, Fealey RD. Drug-induced hyperhidrosis and hypohidrosis: incidence, prevention and management. *Drug Safety* 2008;31(2):109-126.

44. Divvela S, Williams A, Meives C, Gozun E. Opioid analgesics: comparison of pharmacokinetics and equianalgesic doses. *Hospital Pharm.* 2006;42(11):1130-1135.

45. McPherson ML. *Demystifying Opioid Conversion Calculations: A Guide to Effective Dosing*. Bethesda, MD. American Society of Health-System Pharmacists; 2009.

46. Mercadante S, Bruera E. Opioid switching: a systematic and critical review. *Cancer Treat Rev.* 2006;32(4):304-315.

47. Mercadante S, Caraceni A. Conversion ratios for opioid switching in the treatment of cancer pain: a systematic review. *Palliat Med.* 2011 Jul;25(5):504-15.

48. Prommer E. Levorphanol: the forgotten opioid. *Support Care Cancer* 2007;15:259-264.

49. Price LC, Wobeter B, Delate T, Kurz D, Shanahan R. Methadone for pain and the risk of adverse cardiac outcomes. *J Pain Symptom Manage.* 2014;48(3):333-42.e1.

50. Krantz MJ, Martin J, Stimmel B, Mehta D, Haigney MC. QTc Interval Screening in Methadone Treatment. *Ann Intern Med.* 2009;150:387-395.

51. U.S. Food and Drug Administration, Information for Healthcare Professionals Methadone Hydrochloride text version. Available at: http://www.fda.gov/Drugs/DrugSafety/PostmarketDrugSafetyInformationforPatientsandProviders/ucm142841.htm. Accessed October 22, 2014.

52. Davis M: Methadone. In: Davis M, Glare P, Hardy J, ed. *Opioids in Cancer Pain*, Oxford, UK: Oxford University Press; 2005:247-265.

53. Pergolizzi J, Böger RH, Budd K, et al. Opioids and the management of chronic severe pain in the elderly: consensus statement of an International Expert Panel with focus on the six clinically most often used World Health Organization Step III opioids (buprenorphine, fentanyl, hydromorphone, methadone, morphine, oxycodone). *Pain Pract.* 2008;8(4):287-313.

54. Mercadante S, Ferrera P, Villari P, Casuccio A, Intravaia G, Mangione S. Frequency, indications, outcomes, and predictive factors of opioid switching in an acute palliative care unit. *J Pain Symptom Manage.* 2009;37(4):632-41.

55. Ripamonti C, Groff L, Brunelli C, et al: Switching from morphine to oral methadone in treating cancer pain: What is the equianalgesic dose ratio? *J Clin Oncol* 1998; 16:3216-3221.

56. Ayonrinde OT, Bridge DT. The rediscovery of methadone for cancer pain management. *Med J Aust* 2000; 173:536-540.

57. Price LC, Wobeter B, Delate T, Kurz D, Shanahan R. Methadone for pain and the risk of adverse cardiac outcomes. *J Pain Symptom Manage.* 2014;48(3):333-42.e1.

58. Chou R, Cruciani RA, Fiellin DA, et al. Methadone safety: a clinical practice guideline from the American Pain Society and College on Problems of Drug Dependence, in collaboration with the Heart Rhythm Society. *J Pain.* 2014;15(4):321-37.

59. McCance-Katz EF, Sullivan LE, Nallani S. Drug interactions of clinical importance among the opioids, methadone and buprenorphine, and other frequently prescribed medications: a review. *Am J Addict.* 2010;19(1):4-16.

60. Quill TE, Bower KA, Holloway RG, et al. *Primer of Palliative Care.* 6th ed. Chicago, IL: American Academy of Hospice and Palliative Medicine; 2014.

61. Clinical experience Grauer, PA. HospiScript Protocol, Unpublished.

62. Drug Enforcement Agency (DEA). Disposal of controlled substances. Final rule. *Fed Regist.* 2014;79:53520-53570. Codified at 21 CFR Parts 1300, 1301, 1304, 1305, 1307, 1317.

63. American Society of Health-System Pharmacists (ASHP). Frequently asked questions: DEA rule on the disposal of controlled substances (DEA-316). October 10, 2014. Available at http://www.ashp.org/DocLibrary/Advocacy/DEA-Proposed-Rule-on-the-Disposal-of-Controlled-Substances.pdf. Accessed October 13, 2014.

64. National Hospice and Palliative Care Organization (NHPCO). DEA releases new rules for safe and secure prescription drug disposal. October 7, 2014. Available at http://www.nhpco.org/alerts/dea-releases-new-rules-prescription-drug-disposal. Accessed October 10, 2014.

65. Drug Enforcement Agency (DEA). Letter to registrants regarding the disposal of controlled substances; final rule. September 9, 2014. Available at http://www.deadiversion.usdoj.gov/drug_disposal/dear_registrant_disposal.pdf. Accessed October 13, 2014.

66. Food and Drug Administration (FDA) Disposal of Unused Medicines: What You Should Know. Available at http://www.fda.gov/Drugs/ResourcesForYou/Consumers/BuyingUsingMedicineSafely/EnsuringSafeUseofMedicine/SafeDisposalofMedicines/ucm186187.htm#MEDICINES. Accessed November 9, 2014.

67. Gourlay DL, Heit HA, Almahrezi, A. Universal precautions in pain medicine: a rational approach to the treatment of chronic pain. *Pain Med.* 2005;6(2):107-112.

68. Green E. Discharge for cause: a compassionate and ethical response. *NHPCO NewsLine.* 2012;Sept:10-15. Available at http://www.nhpco.org/sites/default/files/public/newsline/2012/NL_September12.pdf

69. Kwon JH, Tanco K, Hui D, Reddy A, Bruera E. Chemical coping versus pseudoaddiction in patients with cancer pain. *Palliat Support Care.* 2014;12(5):413-7.

70. Passik SD, Kirsh KL, Webster L. Pseudoaddiction revisited: a commentary on clinical and historical considerations. *Pain Manag.* 2011; 1:239–248.

71. Meltzer EC, Rybin D, Meshesha LZ, et al. Aberrant drug-related behaviors: unsystematic documentation does not identify prescription drug use disorder. *Pain Med.* 2012;13(11):1436-43.

72. Vadivelu N, Singh-gill H, Kodumudi G, Kaye AJ, Urman RD, Kaye AD. Practical guide to the management of acute and chronic pain in the presence of drug tolerance for the healthcare practitioner. *Ochsner J.* 2014;14(3):426-33.

73. Modesto-Lowe V, Girard L, Chaplin M. Cancer pain in the opioid-addicted patient: can we treat it right? *J Opioid Manag.* 2012; 8:167–175.

74. Del fabbro E. Assessment and management of chemical coping in patients with cancer. *J Clin Oncol.* 2014;32(16):1734-8.

75. Rauenzahn S, Del Fabbro E. Opioid management of pain: the impact of the prescription opioid abuse epidemic. *Curr Opin Support Palliat Care.* 2014;8(3):273-8.

76. Brown RL, Leonard T, Saunders LA, Papasouliotis O. Two-item conjoint screen for alcohol and other drug problems. *J Am Board Fam Pract.* 2001;14:95-106.

77. Webster LR, Webster R. Predicting aberrant behaviors in opioid-treated patients: Preliminary validation of the opioid risk tool. *Pain Med.* 2005; 6(6):432-442.

78. Akbik H, Butler SF, Budman SH, Fernandez K, Katz NP, Jamison RN. Validation and clinical application of the Screener and Opioid Assessment for Patients with Pain (SOAPP). *J Pain Symptom Manage.* 2006;32(3):287-93.

Treatment Algorithm for Nociceptive Pain

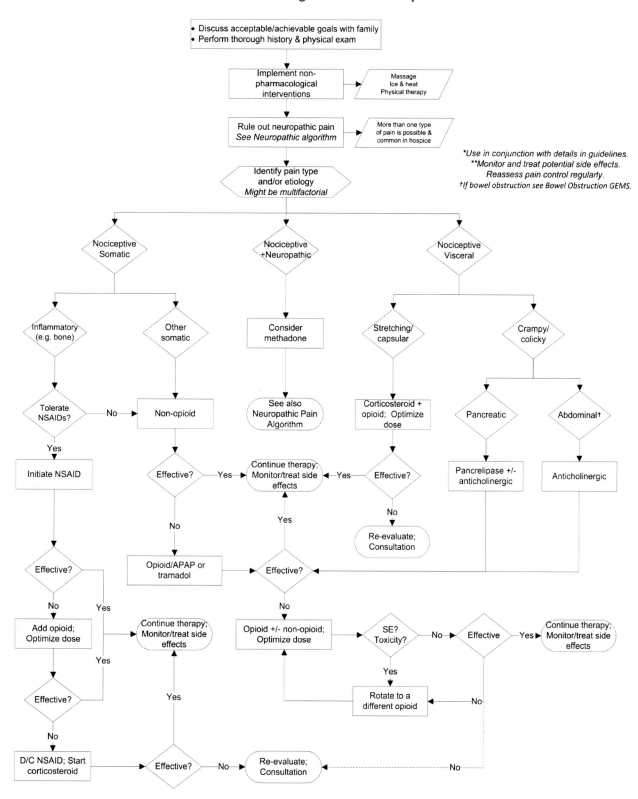

Treatment Algorithm for Neuropathic Pain

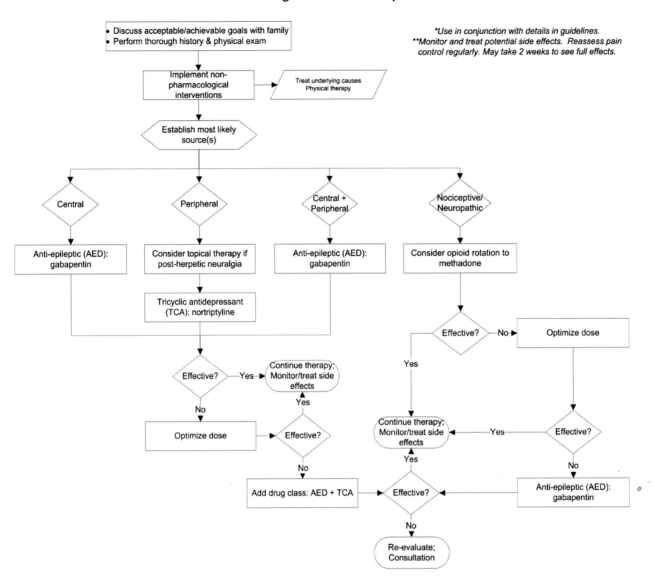

Palliative Sedation

Introduction and Background[1-3]

- Palliative sedation has been defined as the use of specific sedative non-opioid medications to relieve intolerable suffering from refractory symptoms by reducing patient consciousness using appropriate drugs carefully titrated to the cessation of symptoms.
- Palliative sedation may refer to 2 different types of sedation: brief, intermittent, or respite sedation and continuous sedation until death. The level of sedation may vary from light or superficial sedation to deep sedation in which the patient is unconscious with no ability to communicate.
- There is no consensus definition for palliative sedation in the United States.
- Several organizations consider palliative sedation to be an appropriate intervention of last resort to treat otherwise refractory suffering. A few of these organizations do not recommend palliative sedation for primarily existential suffering.
- Proportionality, intent and criteria for success are important principles with regards to palliative sedation. These principles also allow for palliative sedation to be distinguished from euthanasia.
- Proportionality implies that only enough medication will be used to achieve relief from the refractory symptom. The intent of palliative sedation is to relieve suffering from a refractory symptom and the criterion for success is relief of the symptom, not the death of the patient.

Prevalence[3-5]

- Primarily because there is not a consensus definition for palliative sedation, the reported incidence of palliative sedation varies from less than 3% to 64% of terminally ill patients.
- The reported incidence of palliative sedation also likely varies based on cultural differences and differences in clinical settings.

Causes

- Refractory physical symptoms such as delirium, dyspnea and pain are among the most commonly reported symptoms for which palliative sedation is used.
- Many other symptoms have reportedly required palliative sedation including bleeding, nausea & vomiting, fatigue, hiccups and myoclonus.
- The use of palliative sedation for non-physical symptoms of extreme psychological suffering or existential suffering is more controversial.

Clinical Characteristics[6,7]

- A symptom is refractor if any of the following are true:
    o there are no further interventions that are capable of providing relief of the symptom(s)
    o any potential interventions for the symptom(s) are not expected to be tolerated by the patient
    o potential interventions for the symptom(s) will not work in an acceptable timeframe
- Although there is some literature available with regards to palliative sedation in the home setting, this option will depend on the hospice policies and procedures and family and patient preferences.
- The availability of medications and acceptable routes of administration may be impacted by the clinical setting (e.g. home vs. hospice inpatient unit) and the expected timeframe until the patient's death (e.g. hours to days).
- If the patient is receiving artificial nutrition and/or hydration, a discussion covering the potential positive and negative repercussions of continuing these interventions must be held between the hospice team and family. The burden of artificial nutrition and hydration is likely to outweigh any benefits during palliative sedation at end of life.

Non-Pharmacological Treatment[8-10]

- Consideration of palliative sedation should include all members of the interdisciplinary team, the patient's attending physician (if not the hospice medical director), and the patient's family or caregivers.
- An ethics advisory council, or hospice ethics committee, should be involved to review the case prior to initiation of palliative sedation. The ethics committee may be periodically consulted during the course of treatment.

- Palliative sedation for existential suffering is a controversial topic. Palliative sedation for existential suffering should be reserved for rare instances where this suffering does not respond to specific interventions targeted at relief of psychosocial, spiritual, and existential suffering, and all other criteria for appropriate use of palliative sedation are present.

Pharmacotherapy[11,12]

- Opioids are not recommended for initiation or maintenance of palliative sedation. Continue opioids with routine assessment of non-verbal signs of pain; titrate opioids if necessary to control pain.
- If a symptom persists despite use of one class of medication, additive therapy (versus replacement therapy) may be necessary.
- Dosing and initial medication selection depends on several factors:
    - previous and current medications and doses
    - medication intolerances and allergies
    - symptom(s) requiring palliative sedation
    - plans for respite vs continuous sedation
    - clinical setting (home vs inpatient unit)
    - medication availability
    - available routes of administration
    - patient/family/caregiver/clinician preferences
- The specific dose of medication used is less important than the ultimate goal of relieving suffering in a manner proportional to the level of suffering.
- Decision-making about medication doses for palliative sedation must be individualized to patient needs and past medication use. For example, patients who have developed a tolerance to benzodiazepines from long-term use will likely require higher dosing strategies or the addition of alternative sedative medications to induce and maintain sedation.
- Parenteral administration of medications, IV or SC, is preferred for palliative sedation. However, patients under light sedation may be able to accept sublingual medication administration, if necessary.
- Do not combine multiple medications through the same SC port; infuse one medication per site. Consult a pharmacist for stability and compatibility information in available diluents.

Clinical Pearls[13-15]

- Limited data is available with regards to the usefulness of sedation scales in the context of palliative sedation. The Richmond Agitation-Sedation Scale (RASS) or Guideline for Palliative Sedation of the Royal Dutch Medical Association (KNMG) Scale may be among the most useful. Clinician documentation of routine monitoring and evaluation of the sedated patient can be improved using standardized sedation scales.
- Respite sedation is a form of palliative sedation for a specific period of time (often 24-48 hours) with the goal of then reversing the sedation to see if this allows the patient to re-set from the refractory symptoms.
- For respite sedation, especially palliative sedation for existential suffering, medications with shorter half-lives and quicker onset/offset of action (e.g. midazolam) may be drugs of choice.
- Parenteral, oral, sublingual, and rectal doses of the sedative medications commonly used during palliative sedation are approximately equivalent. For example, lorazepam 2mg (oral) is equivalent to lorazepam 2mg (intravenous/subcutaneous).
- Follow standard equianalgesic dosing tables to convert from oral or sublingual opioids to parenteral infusions based on the total daily oral morphine equivalents. See also *Pain GEMS* for additional information.

Pharmacological Management of Palliative Sedation

Generic Name (Trade name)	Adult Dosing Range	Routes	Common Strengths and Formulations	Comments
Benzodiazepines				
Lorazepam (Ativan®)	0.5-2mg Q4-8H	SL PR IV SC IM	**Tablets:** 0.5 mg, 1 mg, 2 mg **Oral solution:** 2 mg/mL **Injection:** 2 mg/mL, 4 mg/mL	• C-IV controlled substance. • May also be given as a continuous IV or SC infusion. • Dilute prior to use. • Consider inline filter for continuous infusion; check frequently for precipitation. • Refrigeration for oral solution and injection is recommended.
Midazolam (Versed®)	0.5-1 mg/hour continuous infusion	SC IV	**Injection:** 1 mg/mL, 5 mg/mL	• C-IV controlled substance. • Drug of choice for respite sedation due to short half-life.
Antipsychotics				
Haloperidol (Haldol®)	0.5-2mg Q4-12H	SL PR IV SC IM	**Tablets:** 0.5 mg, 1 mg, 2 mg, 5 mg, 10 mg, 20 mg **Oral solution:** 2 mg/mL **Injection:** 5 mg/mL	• Drug of choice for patients with delirium/terminal restlessness. • May also be given as a continuous IV or SC infusion.
Chlorpromazine (Thorazine®)	25-100mg Q4-12H	SL PR IV IM	**Tablets:** 10 mg, 25 mg, 50 mg, 100 mg, 200 mg **Injection:** 25 mg/mL	• Drug of choice for patients with delirium/terminal restlessness. • More sedating than haloperidol, but less versatile dosing. • SC use has been reported, irritation and tissue damage may occur. • Oral concentrate (100 mg/mL) can be compounded for sublingual or rectal administration.
Barbiturates				
Pentobarbital (Nembutal®)	1-5 mg/kg/hour continuous infusion	IV	**Injection:** 50 mg/mL	• C-II controlled substance. • Consider loading dose of 50-100mg with initiation of continuous infusion. • May be difficult to obtain; frequently in shortage or at risk of shortage. • Expensive.
Phenobarbital (Luminal®)	60-120mg Q4-12H	SL PR IV SC IM	**Tablets:** 15 mg, 16.2 mg, 30 mg, 32.4 mg, 60 mg, 64.8 mg, 97.2 mg, 100 mg **Injection:** 65 mg/mL, 120 mg/mL	• C-IV controlled substance. • Long half-life may allow for less frequent dosing. • May also give as a continuous IV or SC infusion.
Anesthetic				
Propofol (Diprivan®)	0.3-1 mg/kg/hour continuous infusion	IV	**Injection:** 10 mg/mL	• Consider if other sedative medications are ineffective. • Lower doses are required when used with opioids. • Refer to institutional policies on use.

See Drug Dosing for Liver and Renal Disease for additional drug information.

References

1. De Graeff A, Dean M. Palliative sedation therapy in the last weeks of life: A literature review and recommendations for standards. *J Palliat Med.* 2007;10(1):67-85.

2. National Ethics Committee, Veterans Health Administration. The ethics of palliative sedation as a therapy of last resort. *Am J Hosp Palliat Care.* 2006;23(6):483-91.

3. Van Diejck RH, Hasselaar JG, Verhagen SC, Vissers KC, Koopmans RT. Determinants of the administration of continuous palliative sedation: a systematic review. *J Palliat Med.* 2013;16(12):1624-1632.

4. Vayne-Bossert P, Zulian G. Palliative sedation: from the family perspective. *Am J Hosp Palliat Care.* 2013;30(8):786-790.

5. Miccinesi G, Rietjens JA, Deliens L, Paci E, Bosshard G, et al. Continuous deep sedation: physicians' experience in six European countries. *J Pain Symptom Manage.* 2006;31(2):122-9

6. Mercadante S, Porzio G, Valle A, Fusco F, Aielli F, Costanzo V. Palliative sedation in patients with advanced cancer followed at home: a systematic review. *J Pain Symptom Manage.* 2011;41(4):754-760.

7. Mercadante S, Porzio G, Valle A, Aielli F, Casuccio A. Palliative sedation in patients with advanced cancer followed at home: a prospective study. *J Pain Symptom Manage.* 2014; 47(5):860-866.

8. Koike K, Terui T, Takajashi Y, et al. Effectiveness of multidisciplinary team conference on decision-making surrounding the application of continuous deep sedation for terminally ill cancer patients. *Palliat Support Care.* 2013;4:1-8.

9. Morita T. Palliative sedation to relieve psycho-existential suffering of terminally ill cancer patients. *J Pain Symptom Manage.* 2004;28(5):445-450.

10. Kirk TW, Mahon MM. National Hospice and Palliative Care Organization (NHPCO) position statement and commentary on the use of palliative sedation in imminently dying terminally ill patients. *J Pain Symptom Manage* 2010;39(5):914-923

11. Rousseau P. Palliative sedation in the management of refractory symptoms. *J Support Oncol.* 2004;2(2):181-186.

12. Editorial Board Palliative Care: Practice Guidelines. Palliative sedation. Utrecht, The Netherlands: Association of Comprehensive Cancer Centers (ACCC);2006:33 p.

13. Arevalo JJ, Brinkkemper T, van der Heide A, et al. Palliative sedation: reliability and validity of sedation scales. *J Pain Symptom Manage.* 2012;44(5):704-14.

14. Rousseau P. Palliative sedation. *Am J Hosp Palliat Med.* 2002;19(5):295-297.

15. Lux MR, Protus BM, Kimbrel JM, Grauer PA. Survey of hospice and palliative care physicians regarding palliative sedation practices. Unpublished manuscript; contact druginformation@hospiscript.com for additional information.

16. Richards JH, Protus BM, Grauer PA, Kimbrel JM. Evaluation of subcutaneous phenobarbital administration in hospice patients. *Am J Hosp Palliat Med* 2014 Dec 3; epub ahead of print. DOI: 1049909114555157

Palliative Sedation Algorithm

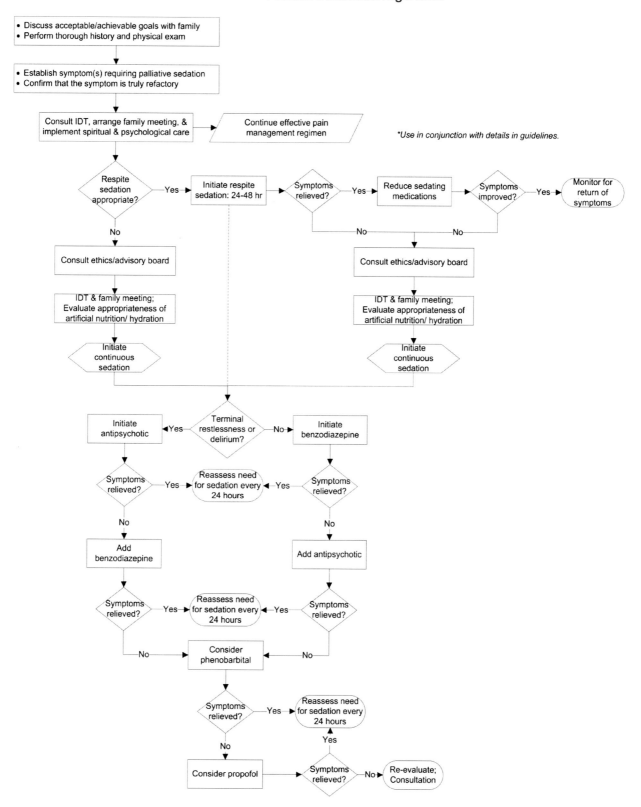

* Discuss acceptable/achievable goals with family
* Perform thorough history and physical exam

* Establish symptom(s) requiring palliative sedation
* Confirm that the symptom is truly refactory

Consult IDT, arrange family meeting, & implement spiritual & psychological care

Continue effective pain management regimen

Use in conjunction with details in guidelines.

Respite sedation appropriate? — Yes → Initiate respite sedation: 24-48 hr → Symptoms relieved? — Yes → Reduce sedating medications → Symptoms improved? — Yes → Monitor for return of symptoms

No

Consult ethics/advisory board

No — No

Consult ethics/advisory board

IDT & family meeting; Evaluate appropriateness of artificial nutrition/ hydration

IDT & family meeting; Evaluate appropriateness of artificial nutrition/ hydration

Initiate continuous sedation

Initiate continuous sedation

Initiate antipsychotic ←Yes— Terminal restlessness or delirium? —No→ Initiate benzodiazepine

Symptoms relieved? — Yes → Reassess need for sedation every 24 hours ← Yes — Symptoms relieved?

No — No

Add benzodiazepine

Add antipsychotic

Symptoms relieved? — Yes → Reassess need for sedation every 24 hours ← Yes — Symptoms relieved?

No — No

Consider phenobarbital

Symptoms relieved? — Yes → Reassess need for sedation every 24 hours

No — Yes

Consider propofol → Symptoms relieved? —No→ Re-evaluate; Consultation

Pruritus

Introduction and Background[1-5]
- Pruritus is a common sensation of itching associated with the urge to scratch. The sensation of itching or the urge to scratch is frequent, generalized in distribution, or severe.
- Scratching associated with pruritus often damages the skin, reducing its function as a protective barrier.
- Patients may describe pruritus as burning, tingling, numbness, or crawling in the skin.
- Many pruritic conditions are a result of underlying systemic abnormalities rather than superficial skin irritation or infection.

Prevalence[3-5]
- Itching is a common symptom, with all persons experiencing acute itch at some point in life; prevalence of pruritus increases with age.
- Dry skin (xerosis) is present in 60-90% of patients with uremic pruritus.
- When pruritus is chronic or severe, sleep, attention, and quality of life are affected.

Causes[1-8]
- Pruritus may be caused by skin disease, skin infection, or systemic causes (Table 1).

Table 1. Causes of Pruritus in Hospice & Palliative Care

Allergens	Soaps, detergents, latex
Endocrine	Hyperthyroidism, hypothyroidism, diabetes
Electrolyte disturbances	Iron deficiency, hypercalcemia, hypermagnesemia, hyperphosphatemia
Hepatic	Biliary cirrhosis, cholestasis, hepatitis
Infections	*Candida spp.*, herpes zoster, cellulitis, folliculitis
Malignancy	Breast, CNS, lung, melanoma, carcinoid syndrome, lymphoma, leukemia
Medication	Opioids, acyclovir, alprazolam, amlodipine, bupropion, SSRIs, donepezil, megestrol, tramadol, antifungals, penicillins, phenytoin
Miscellaneous	Advanced age, neurologic syndromes, AIDS, parasites, insect bites, dry skin, psychogenic
Renal	Chronic renal failure, uremia

Clinical Characteristics[1-8]
- Sensations of pruritus are transmitted by specific itch fibers in peripheral nerves. Itch may be mediated by peripheral histamine, serotonin, and pro-inflammatory cytokines.
- Dryness of the skin causes itch or makes it worse.
- Heat and other causes of peripheral vasodilatation worsen itching.
- Skin that is chronically damp and wet can produce pruritus.
- Though it may give immediate relief, scratching can make pruritus worse, especially if vigorous scratching produces skin injury, excoriation, or inflammation.
- Similar to pain, injury to nerve fibers that transmit itch signals can produce neuropathic pruritus.

Non-Pharmacological Treatment[1-3,5]
- Thorough physical examination focused on the skin for presence of dermatitis or rash; investigate recent exposure to new soaps, detergents, topical products, or medications.
- Treat dry skin regularly with moisturizing, emollient skin lotion such as Aveeno®, Eucerin®, or Aquaphor®. For patients prone to sensitive skin, avoid lotions with lanolin, fragrances, alcohols, or colorants. Look for products with glycerin, niacinamide, or petrolatum to help add and sustain moisture in the skin's surface.
- Gentle, fragrance-free laundry detergent can reduce exposure to potentially irritating chemicals.
- A cool environment, with light clothing, and warm, not hot baths or showers can help reduce itching.
- Cool compresses and oatmeal baths can provide effective, but temporary, relief.

- Avoid vasodilators such as caffeine, alcohol, spicy foods, hot water and excessive sweating.
- Keep nails clean and well-trimmed. Encourage patients to pat or gently rub itchy areas, not scratch.
- Efforts to promote relaxation can also help reduce pruritus.

Pharmacotherapy[1-15]

- Review the patient's medication profile and discontinue potentially pruritogenic medications if possible, prior to adding new medications to treat itching.
- Assessment questions should include:
  - Is the onset of itching related to the initiation of a new medication?
  - Is the patient taking any medications commonly associated with pruritus?
  - Does the patient have a characteristic drug rash, frequently symmetric and truncal, morbilliform (maculopapular) or urticarial?
  - For localized itching, is it near the site of application of a topical medication?
- Treat the underlying cause of pruritus (e.g. infection, anxiety, thyroid problems) as directly as possible.
- In general, manage a localized itch with topical therapies; generalized itch will likely require systemic medication. Pharmacological management tables are not all-inclusive, but will help guide therapy by providing treatment options with best evidence to support use.

Clinical Pearls[1-16]

- If an opioid-induced pruritus is suspected, consider rotating to a different opioid. If opioid rotation or treatment with antihistamines (e.g., diphenhydramine, hydroxyzine) have failed or are not tolerated, ondansetron or mirtazapine may provide relief. Consider naloxone for refractory patients.
- Opioid-induced pruritus is more likely with morphine, codeine, or oxycodone, than with methadone, fentanyl, hydromorphone, or oxymorphone.
- Chronic pruritus has a high treatment failure rate; combinations of topical medicated and non-medicated lotions along with systemic medications may reduce symptoms.
- Fungal skin infections present in areas that likely to retain moisture and warmth: skin folds, mucous membranes, armpits, and underneath breasts.
- Patients treated with systemic antibiotics and corticosteroids for other conditions may increase the risk of fungal skin infections through changes in skin and genitourinary or GI tract flora or immunosuppression.
- *Candida spp.* skin rash is bright red and macular with pustules or papules at the edges of the rash. Peripheral lesions may spread and blend into the larger area of rash. Healing a fungal skin infection requires treating with appropriate anti-fungal medications and keeping skin clean and dry.
- Topical calcineurin inhibitors (tacrolimus, pimecrolimus) may be helpful in atopic dermatitis, though they are expensive and tend to cause burning and stinging at the site of application.
- Neuropathic pruritus may benefit from topical capsaicin products (Zostrix, Capzasin) which deplete substance P from sensory nerves. Initial burning sensation on application and the need for frequent application (3-4 times per day) limit capsaicin use.
- Topical anesthetics such as benzocaine and lidocaine work by interfering with sensory nerve fibers and cutaneous sensory receptors. "Caine"-based topical products may be effective but can cause sensitization. Consider pramoxine +/- menthol lotions (Sarna) as an alternative.
- Rifampin is considered second line therapy for cholestasis-induced pruritus if the patient fails or cannot tolerate a bile acid sequestrant (e.g., cholestyramine). The American Association of Study of Liver Diseases (AASLD) includes the off-label use of rifampin in practice guidelines for primary biliary cirrhosis.
- A small study of patients receiving hemodialysis reported some benefit from ingestion of activated charcoal for dialysis-related uremic pruritus.

Pharmacological Management of Pruritus - TOPICAL

Generic Name (Trade Name)	Adult Starting Dose	Routes	Common Strengths and Formulations	Comments
Skin Products				
Camphor + menthol (Sarna®, Mentholatum®)	Apply as needed	Topical	Cream, Gel, Lotion, Ointment	• For xerosis. • Available OTC with 0.5% camphor, 0.5% menthol. • Avoid application of products containing menthol to excoriated, broken skin. • Avoid contact with mucous membranes, burns, and open wounds.
Calamine (Caladryl®)	Apply as needed	Topical	Lotion	• Astringent, protectant, and soothing properties. • For minor skin irritation, insect bites, poisonous plant exposure. • Avoid contact with mucous membranes, burns, and open wounds.
Corticosteroids				
Hydrocortisone (Cortaid®)	Apply a thin film twice daily	Topical	Cream, Gel, Lotion, Ointment	• For inflammatory rash. • May worsen fungal skin infections. • Excessive use or occlusive dressings can cause systemic absorption. • Prolonged use will cause thinning of skin. • OTC available in 0.5% and 1% strengths. Higher potency products are available by prescription.
Triamcinolone (Kenalog®)	Apply a thin film twice daily	Topical	Cream, Lotion, Ointment	• Rx only. • For inflammatory rash. • May worsen fungal skin infections. • Excessive use or occlusive dressings can cause systemic absorption. • Prolonged use will cause thinning of skin.
Antifungals				
Clotrimazole (Lotrimin AF®)	Apply thin film twice daily	Topical	Cream, Lotion, Ointment	• Available OTC at 1% strength. • Useful for vaginal pruritus and groin infections (*tinea cruris*). • Avoid contact with eyes. • Reassess therapy if no improvement within 7-14 days.
Nystatin (Mycostatin®, Nystop®)	Apply BID to TID	Topical	Cream, Ointment, Powder	• Rx only; 100,000 units/gram • Avoid face and eyes. • Use powder for moist topical lesions.

See Drug Dosing for Liver and Renal Disease for additional drug information.

Pharmacological Management of Pruritus - SYSTEMIC

Generic Name (Trade Name)	Adult Starting Dose	Routes	Common Strengths and Formulations	Comments
Antihistamines				
Diphenhydramine (Benadryl®)	25mg Q8H PRN	PO	**Tablets:** 25 mg, 50 mg **Capsules:** 25 mg, 50 mg **Chewable tablets:** 12.5 mg **Oral liquid:** 12.5 mg/5 mL	• Available OTC. • Anticholinergic side effects: sedation, dry mouth, constipation, urinary retention, confusion. • Use cautiously in geriatrics. • Tablets may be split or crushed; additional dosage forms available.
Hydroxyzine (Atarax®, Vistaril®)	25mg Q8H PRN	PO	**Tablets:** 10 mg, 25 mg, 50 mg **Capsules:** 25 mg, 50 mg, 100 mg **Oral liquid:** 10 mg/5 mL	• Antihistamine with some anxiolytic properties. • Anticholinergic side effects: sedation, dry mouth, constipation, urinary retention, confusion. • Use cautiously in geriatrics. • Tablets may be split or crushed.
Antidepressants				
Doxepin (Sinequan®, Zonalon®)	10mg at bedtime	PO, Topical	**Capsules:** 10 mg, 25 mg, 50 mg, 75 mg, 100 mg, 150 mg **Oral liquid:** 10 mg/mL **Cream:** 5%	• Tricyclic antidepressant (TCA) with potent antihistamine activity; pruritus dosing is well below antidepressant dose. • Anticholinergic side effects: sedation, dry mouth, constipation, urinary retention, confusion. • Use cautiously in geriatrics. • Cream is expensive and provides no benefit over oral products. • Cream is well absorbed and reaches systemic levels similar to oral for efficacy and side effects.
Mirtazapine (Remeron®)	7.5mg at bedtime	PO	**Tablets:** 7.5 mg, 15 mg, 30 mg, 45 mg **Oral disintegrating tablets:** 15 mg, 30 mg, 45 mg	• Non-TCA, non-SSRI antidepressant with antihistamine, alpha-adrenergic blocking, 5HT$_3$-blocking properties. • Consider for patients with comorbid insomnia and depression.
Paroxetine (Paxil®)	10mg daily	PO	**Tablets:** 10 mg, 20 mg, 30 mg, 40 mg **Oral liquid:** 10 mg/5 mL	• SSRI antidepressant studied in chronic pruritus associated with advanced cancer. • Antipruritic effects begin in 2-3 days but may wear off within 4-6 weeks. • Taper slowly when discontinuing.
Sertraline (Zoloft®)	25mg daily	PO	**Tablets:** 25 mg, 50 mg, 100 mg **Oral liquid:** 20 mg/mL	• Studied in patients with chronic liver disease and cholestatic pruritus. • Titrate to 75-100mg daily. • Consider for patients with comorbid insomnia and depression.

Continued

Generic Name (Trade Name)	Adult Starting Dose	Routes	Common Strengths and Formulations	Comments
Corticosteroids				
Dexamethasone (Decadron®)	4mg daily	PO	**Tablets:** 0.25 mg, 0.5 mg, 0.75 mg, 1 mg, 1.5 mg, 2 mg, 4 mg, 6 mg **Solution:** 0.5 mg/5 mL, 1mg,mL **Injection:** 4 mg/mL, 10 mg/mL	• Has less mineralocorticoid effect than prednisone. • Anti-inflammatory and immunosuppressant effects. • Use for short courses, "steroid bursts" for inflammatory causes of pruritus. • Studied in Hodgkin's lymphoma.
Prednisone (Deltasone®)	20mg daily	PO	**Tablets:** 1 mg, 2.5 mg, 5 mg, 10 mg, 20 mg, 25 mg, 50 mg **Solution:** 5 mg/5 mL, 5 mg/mL	• Anti-inflammatory and immunosuppressant effects. • Use for short courses, "steroid bursts" for inflammatory causes of pruritus. • Studied in Hodgkin's lymphoma.
Miscellaneous				
Cholestyramine (Questran®)	2g BID	PO	**Powder:** 4 g	• Bile acid sequestrant; may provide benefit in refractory cases of cholestatic pruritus. • Very constipating; recommend use of a stimulant laxative during therapy. • May decrease absorption of other medications. Separate from other medications by 2 hours.
Gabapentin (Neurontin®)	300mg at bedtime	PO	**Tablets:** 600 mg, 800 mg **Capsules:** 100 mg, 300 mg, 400 mg **Solution:** 250 mg/5 mL	• May be useful for neuropathic pruritus. • Consider in chronic itch unresponsive to other treatments. • Studied in hemodialysis for CKD-associated pruritus, give 100mg after each dialysis session.
Naloxone (Narcan®)	0.25 mcg/kg/hour	IV	**Injection:** 0.4 mg/mL, 1 mg/mL	• May be beneficial in severe cases of uremic or cholestatic pruritus. • Will reverse opioid analgesia; trial very low doses to avoid pain crisis.
Ondansetron (Zofran®)	4mg BID	PO	**Tablets:** 4 mg, 8 mg **Oral disintegrating tablets:** 4 mg, 8 mg	• May provide benefit in refractory cases of uremic or cholestatic pruritus. • Consider after failure of topical products, oral antihistamines and oral antidepressants list above.
Rifampin (Rifadin®)	150mg daily	PO	**Capsules:** 150 mg, 300 mg	• Risk of drug interactions; review medication profile with pharmacist prior to initiating. • Consider for patients with cholestatic pruritus unable to tolerate cholestyramine. • Monitor liver function tests, CBC.

See Drug Dosing for Liver and Renal Disease for additional drug information.

References

1. Twycross R, Greaves MW, et al. Itch: scratching more than the surface. *Q J Med* 2003; 96: 7-26.
2. Lovell P, Vender B. Management and treatment of pruritus. *Skin Therapy Letter* 2007; 12(1): 1-10.
3. Moses S. Pruritus. *Am Fam Physician*. 2003;68:1135-1146.
4. Patel T, Yosipovitch G. Therapy of pruritus. *Expert Opin Pharmacother* 2010 July; 11(10): 1673–1682.
5. Krajnik M, Zylicz Z. Understanding pruritus in systemic disease. *J Pain Symptom Manage*. 2001;21(2):151-168.
6. Manenti L, Tansinda P, Vaglio A. Uraemic pruritus: clinical characteristics, pathophysiology and treatment. *Drugs* 2009; 69(3): 251-63.
7. Keczkes K, Lyell A. Intractable pruritus due to hepatic cirrhosis relieved by cholestyramine. *Postgrad Med J* 1965; 41: 155-157.
8. Khandelwal M, Malet PF. Pruritus associated with cholestasis: a review of pathogenesis and management. *Dig Dis Sci* 1994; 39(1): 1-8.
9. Mayo MJ, Handem I, Saldana S, et al. Sertraline as a first-line treatment for cholestatic pruritus. *Hepatology* 2007; 45: 666-674.
10. Bergasa NV, et. al. A controlled trial of naloxone infusions for the pruritus of chronic cholestasis. *Gastroenterology*. 1992 Feb; 102(2): 544-9.
11. O'Donohue JW, Pereira SP, Ashdown AC, et al. A controlled trial of ondansetron in the pruritus of cholestasis. *Aliment Pharmacol Therap* 2005;21:1041-45.
12. Siddik-Sayyid SM, Yazbeck-Karam VG, Zahreddine BW et al. Ondansetron is as effective as diphenhydramine for treatment of morphine-induced pruritus after cesarean delivery. *Acta Anaesth Scand* 2010;54:764-69.
13. Generali JA, Cada DJ. Off-label drug uses: ondansetron (oral): uremic pruritus (adults). *Hosp Pharm* 2010;45(7):534-7.
14. Pederson, JA, Matter BJ, Czerwinski AW, et al. Relief of idiopathic generalized pruritus in dialysis patients treated with activated oral charcoal. *Ann Intern Med* 1980; 93: 446-8
15. LexiComp Online. LexiDrugs Online. Hudson, OH:LexiComp, Inc. Accessed November 12, 2012.
16. Lindor KD, Gershwin ME, Poupon R, et al. AASLD practice guidelines: primary biliary cirrhosis. *Hepatol*. 2009; 50(1):291-308.

Treatment Algorithm for Pruritus

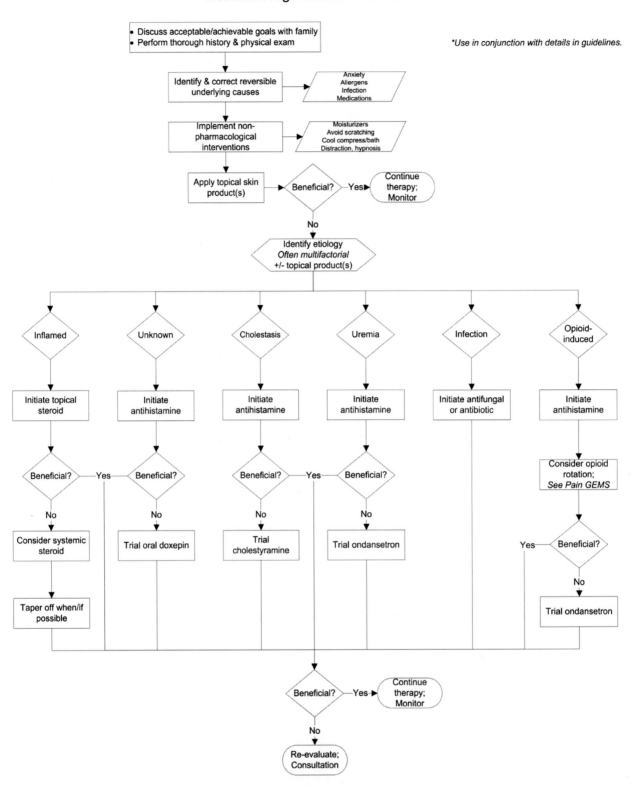

*Use in conjunction with details in guidelines.

Secretions

Introduction and Background[1-3,9]
- Thick and excessive respiratory secretions can be problematic in end-of-life care.
- Thick pulmonary secretions
  - Abnormally thick pulmonary secretions (mucus plugs) can partially obstruct the airway, lead to increased airway resistance, and increase breathing exertion.
  - The goal of treatment for thick secretions is to decrease morbidities such as dyspnea, fatigue, insomnia, infection, and improve quality of life.
  - Dehydration produces adhesion of mucus to the airway surface, leading to a failure to clear mucus from the airways both by normal ciliary and cough-dependent mechanisms.
- Sialorrhea
  - Also known as drooling or excessive secretions.
  - Sialorrhea is seen as leakage of saliva from the mouth as a result of diminished swallowing ability or neurodegenerative disorders making control of saliva difficult.
- Terminal respiratory secretions (TRS)
  - Terminal respiratory secretions, commonly known as "death rattle," are the accumulation of fluid in the lungs or oropharynx which can occur if a patient unconscious and dying or if the patient is too weak to clear secretions and cannot swallow. TRS generally occurs within the last 48 hours of life.
  - The wet, noisy, rattling and gurgling sound occurs as air passes over the accumulated secretions during inhalations and exhalations.
  - Palliative care professionals should advise families and caregivers that the sound does not represent any discomfort for the patient. TRS does not require treatment unless the sound is very distressing for the family.

Prevalence[3,4]
- Death rattle caused by tracheal secretion in the absence of a functioning cough reflex is a common symptom reported in 23% to 92% of dying patients and witnessed by 41% to 44% of family members.
- In a quantitative study, 78% of family members who witnessed this symptom reported high distress levels.

Causes[1,2,4-6]
- Sialorrhea can be caused by three different factors:
  - Excessive production of saliva
  - Inability to retain saliva in the mouth
  - Difficulty swallowing
- Excessive saliva production alone is generally not a problem, unless accompanied by one or both of the other two factors.
- Both sialorrhea and thick secretions often have reversible causes that should be identified and treated if possible (Table 1).

Table 1. Causes of Problematic Secretions

Causes of Sialorrhea	Causes of Thick Secretions
Abnormalities of the mouth, jaw, or nasopharynx	Cigarette smoke
Cancer affecting the mouth	Dehydration
Dysphagia	Fluid overload and edema
Fluid overload and edema	Inability to clear secretions/cough
Neurodegenerative disorders	Infection - purulent sputum
Psychological	Tube feedings
Medications: benzodiazepines, clozapine, pilocarpine, carbidopa-levodopa, donepezil, rivastigmine, galantamine, pyridostigmine, bethanechol, carbachol, cevimeline, ropinirole	*Medications:* anticholinergics, decongestants, antihistamines, oxybutynin, tolterodine, tricyclic antidepressants (TCAs), opioids, aclidinium, ipratropium, tiotropium, dicyclomine, benztropine

Clinical Characteristics[1,2]

- The noise of terminal secretions is produced by the oscillatory movements of secretions in the upper airways; it is typically seen only in patients who are obtunded or are too weak to expectorate.
- Drugs that decrease secretions are best initiated at the first sign of noisy breathing, as they do not affect existing respiratory secretions.
- These agents have limited or no impact when the secretions are secondary to pneumonia or pulmonary edema.

Symptoms of Sialorrhea

Aspiration pneumonia	Coughing
Breathing difficulties	Dermatitis around mouth, lips, chin
Choking	Dysphagia
Constant need to change bibs or clothing	Social stigma

Non-Pharmacological Treatment[1,2,4,6-8,10]

- Inform and educate the family about what to expect.
- Management of thick pulmonary secretions:
  - Water is the best way to thin secretions; increase fluid intake.
  - Nebulized normal saline or hypertonic saline can break up secretions.
  - Encourage the patient to cough.
  - If possible, place the patient in Trendelenburg's position (lowering the head of the bed), this allows fluids to move into the oropharnyx, facilitating an easy removal. Do not maintain this position for long, as there is a risk of aspiration.
  - Oropharyngeal suctioning is another option but may be disturbing to both the patient and visitors.
- Management of "death rattle":
  - Repositioning the patient with the head slightly elevated can help alleviate some of the concerns.
  - Aggressive suctioning can cause localized tracheal edema and pulmonary congestion.
  - Continuing oral fluids, parenteral hydration, or tube feedings may increase secretions at the end of life; discontinue lessening excess fluid accumulation and overhydration.
  - Position the patient on his/her side or in a semi-prone position to help facilitate drainage of secretions.
  - Gentle swabbing of the mouth and lips with a moist oral swab (Toothette®) can help reduce pooling of saliva in the mouth.

Pharmacotherapy[5-12]

- Evaluate the patient's medication profile for medications that may be contributing to problematic secretions (Table 1). If possible, taper and discontinue the offending medication(s) rather than add another medication to treat these medication side effects.
- Anticholinergic drugs remain standard therapy for preventing excessive terminal secretions.
- All anticholinergic drugs are similar pharmacologically and one can be selected by anticholinergic potency, onset of action, route of administration, alertness of patient, and cost.
- Anticholinergic side effects are common and similar in this class including blurred vision, constipation, urinary retention, confusion, delirium, restlessness, hallucinations, dry mouth, and heart palpitations.
- Differences among agents exist, for example, glycopyrrolate does not cross the blood brain barrier and is associated with fewer central nervous system side effects.
- If the patient is alert and secretions are thick but the patient is able to expectorate, then focus pharmacotherapy on thinning mucus.
- If patient is unable to expectorate, cough, or swallow, the emphasis of pharmacotherapy is to dry secretions.

Clinical Pearls[1,6-8,10]

- Fluid, particularly water, administered oral or parenteral remains the best approach to thin secretions.
- Avoid anticholinergic agents if patients are still able to expectorate secretions.
- Preventing the accumulation of large amounts of secretions is easier than treating the condition. However, premature use of anticholinergic medications in a patient who is still alert may lead to unacceptable drying of oral and pharyngeal mucosa or CNS side effects (sedation, confusion).
- All anticholinergic drugs have similar actions and side effects; do not use these agents in combination.
- Anticipate and prepare for possible anticholinergic side effects, especially urinary retention and constipation. Consider having a catheter available in case needed acutely. Prevent constipation with laxatives.

Pharmacological Management of Secretions: Focus on DRYING

Generic Name (Trade Name)	Adult Starting Dose	Routes	Common Strengths and Formulations	Comments
Anticholinergics				
atropine 1% (Isopto® Atropine)	2 drops SL Q4H PRN	SL	**Ophth. solution:** 1%	• 1% ophthalmic solution is given *sublingually;* educate caregivers about non-standard route. • 1 drop of 1% atropine solution delivers approximately 0.5mg atropine. • Easiest dosage form for caregivers to administer.
glycopyrrolate (Robinul®, Cuvposa®)	0.2mg SC Q6H PRN 1mg PO Q6H PRN	PO SC IM IV	**Tablets:** 1 mg, 2 mg **Oral solution:** 1 mg/ 5mL **Injection:** 0.2 mg/mL	• Fewer CNS effects (sedation, confusion) but more xerostomia than other anticholinergics. • Bioavailability of oral formulations is low (< 15%). • Oral tablets not appropriate for terminal secretions, but may be used for chronic sialorrhea. • Oral solution (Cuvposa®) is expensive.
hyoscyamine (Levsin®, Hyomax-SL®)	0.125mg SL Q4H PRN	PO SL	**Oral solution:** 0.125 mg/mL, 0.125 mg/5 mL **Oral disintegrating tablets** : 0.125 mg **Tablets:** 0.125 mg **ER tablets:** 0.375 mg	• May give SL tablet with a few drops of water to help dissolve tablets. • SL tablets may leave chalky residue. • ER tablets not appropriate for terminal secretions, but may be used for chronic sialorrhea.
scopolamine (Transderm Scōp®)	1 patch Q72H 0.4mg SC Q6H PRN	TD SC IM IV	**Transdermal patch:** 1.5 mg **Injection:** 0.4 mg/mL	• Apply patch to hairless area behind ear. • If using for chronic sialorrhea, rotate patch site to avoid skin irritation. • Do not cut transdermal patches. • Non-ideal for terminal secretions due to slow onset of action and difficult titration. • Dilute 1:1 with sterile water for injection prior to IV administration.

See Drug Dosing for Liver and Renal Disease for additional drug information.

Pharmacological Management of Secretions: Focus on THINNING

Generic Name (Trade Name)	Adult Starting Dose	Routes	Common Strengths and Formulations	Comments
Mucolytics				
acetylcysteine (Mucomyst®)	5mL of 10% solution via nebulizer Q8H PRN	Inh	**Solution, nebulization:** 10%, 20%	• Administer bronchodilator 15 minutes prior to use. • Dilute 20% solution with equal parts normal saline or sterile water prior to use. • Acute flushing and redness may occur, but usually resolves spontaneously. • May require postural drainage or suctioning after inhalation. Prepare patient for increased bronchial secretions. • Solution has unpleasant, sulfurous odor.
saline, nebulized	3-5mL via nebulizer Q2H PRN	Inh	**Solution, nebulization:** 0.9%, 3%	• Cost effective. • May also use in between nebulized bronchodilators to prevent overuse. • Moisturizes airways and loosens secretions.
Expectorants				
guaiFENesin (Robitussin®, Mucinex®)	200mg PO Q4H PRN ER tablets: 600mg PO BID	PO	**Oral solution:** 100 mg/5 mL **Tablets:** 200 mg, 400 mg **ER tablets:** 600 mg, 1200 mg **Granules:** 50 mg, 100 mg	• Drug of choice, but patient must have good fluid intake for best effect. • Do not crush ER tablets. • Acts as irritant to gastric mucosa to stimulate respiratory tract secretions and decrease mucus viscosity.

See Drug Dosing for Liver and Renal Disease for additional drug information.

References

1. Müller-Busch HC, Jehser T. Death rattle. In Walsh TD, Caraceni AT, Fainsinger R, eds. *Palliative Medicine.* Philadelphia, PA: Saunders, an imprint of Elsevier Inc, 2009. http://www.expertconsultbook.com. Accessed July 1, 2014.

2. Borasio GD. Amyotrophic lateral sclerosis. In Walsh TD, Caraceni AT, Fainsinger R, eds. *Palliative Medicine.* Philadelphia, PA: Saunders, an imprint of Elsevier Inc, 2009. http://www.expertconsultbook.com. Accessed July 1, 2014.

3. Shimizu Y, Miyashita M, Morita Y, et al. Strategy for death rattle in cancer patients: recommendations from a cross-sectional nationwide survey of bereaved family members' perceptions. *J Pain Symptom Manage.* 2014;48(1)2-12.

4. Hirsch CA, Marriott JF, Faull CM, Influences on the decision to prescribe or administer anticholinergic drugs to treat death rattle: a focus group study. *Palliat Med* 2013;27:732-738.

5. Kintzel PE, Chase SL, Thomas W, et al. Anticholinergic medications for managing noisy respirations in adult hospice patients. *Am J Health-Syst Pharm* 2009;66(1):458–464.

6. Protus BM, Grauer PA, Kimbrel JM. Evaluation of atropine 1% ophthalmic solution administered sublingually for the management of terminal respiratory secretions. *Am J Hosp Palliat Care.* 2013;30(4):388-92.

7. Kintzel PE, Chase SL, Thomas W, et al. Anticholinergic medications for managing noisy respirations in adult hospice patients. *Am J Health-Syst Pharm* 2009; 66(1):458–464.

8. Prommer E. Anticholinergics in palliative medicine: an update. *Am J Hosp Palliat Care*. 2013;30(5):490-498.

9. Seagrave J, Albrecht H, Park Y S, Rubin B, Solomon G, Kim KC. Effect of guaifenesin on mucin production, rheology, and mucociliary transport in differentiated human airway epithelial cells. *Experiment Lung Res.* 2011; 37(10) 606-614.

10. Eng PA, Morton JA, Riedler DJ, Wilson J Robertson CF. Short-term efficacy of ultrasonically nebulized hypertonic saline in cystic fibrosis." *Pediatr Pulmonol.* 1996; 21(2): 77-83.

11. Davies L, Calverley P. The evidence for the use of oral mucolytic agents in chronic obstructive pulmonary disease (COPD). *Brit Med Bull.* 2010; 93: 217-27.

12. Seckel, MA. Normal saline and mucous plugging. *Crit Care Nurse* 2012;32(5): 66-8

13. Rubin, BK. The role of mucus in cough research. *Lung* 2010;188: 69-72.

Treatment Algorithm for Secretions

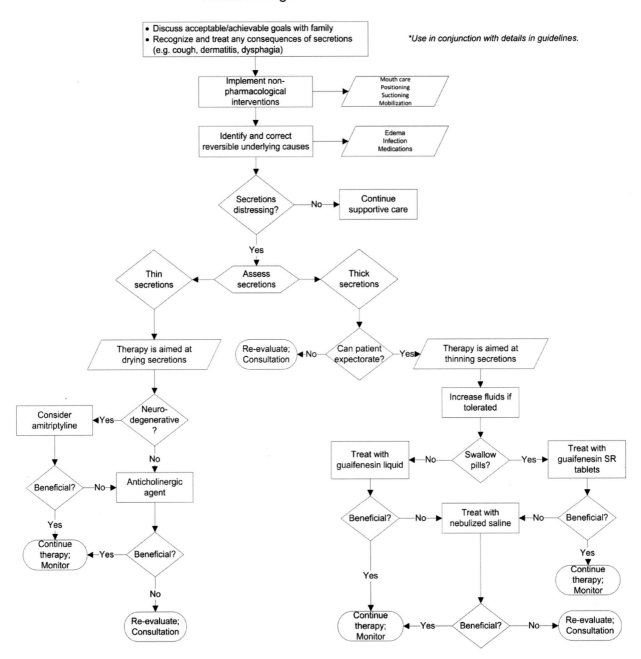

Seizures

Introduction and Background[1]

- Seizures are caused by a brief, excessive surge of electrical activity in the brain. This surge causes changes in sensations, perceptions, and/or behaviors and is typically brief (lasting < 5 minutes).
- The brain phenomenon called a seizure can be manifest in a number of ways, not just convulsions.
- Patients may report odd physical sensations, describe strange smells (usually unpleasant ones like burning rubber or burning hair), or demonstrate brief episodes of staring into space, or loss of attention or awareness.
- Patients with recurrent, unprovoked seizures are diagnosed with epilepsy.
- Seizures can be sorted into two general groups: focal (partial) seizures and generalized seizures.
  - Focal seizures, also called partial or localized seizures, result from an abnormal electrical discharge restricted to one part of the brain (or a localized region of the brain). Focal seizures are further divided into simple (consciousness or memory is preserved) and complex (consciousness or memory before, during and immediately after the seizure is compromised).
  - Generalized seizures are the result of a widespread, excessive electrical discharge simultaneously involving both sides of the brain.
  - The focal vs generalized distinction is not absolute. The electrical activity surge of a focal seizure may spread throughout the brain and the seizure then becomes generalized.

Prevalence[2-5]

- The prevalence of emergent seizures in the hospice setting is not well documented.
- Seizure prevalence in patients with primary CNS tumors or CNS metastases is reported at > 57%.
- Epilepsy and isolated seizure events occur more commonly in patients over 65 years of age than any other age group, including pediatrics. Seizures were reported in 10% to 17% of patients with Alzheimer's disease.
- Otherwise, new-onset seizures are relatively unusual overall and rare in the absence of one of the causes listed below.

Causes[3-7]

- In the hospice and palliative care setting, the following are the most common causes of new onset seizures.

Disease Related Causes of Seizures	Medication Related Causes of Seizures

• Alzheimer's disease and other dementias
• CNS infection (meningitis)
• CNS malignancy – primary and metastatic
• Head injury or trauma
• Hypoglycemia
• Hypoxia
• Metabolic disturbances
  o uremia
  o hypocalcemia
  o hyponatremia
  o hypomagnesemia
• Stroke – both hemorrhagic and thrombotic
	• Drug toxicities
	  o especially in renal or hepatic failure
	  o some antibiotics
	  o bupropion
	  o meperidine
	  o tramadol
	  o tricyclic antidepressants
	• Drug withdrawal
	  o alcohol
	  o benzodiazepines
	  o anticonvulsants
	  o opioids

- Conditions often confused with seizures include:
  - Anxiety (especially panic attacks)
  - Delirium (confusion and agitation)
  - Migraines
  - Myoclonus (from opioid toxicity)
  - Syncope
  - Transient ischemic attacks (TIAs)
  - Unexpected falls

- Laboratory studies may be required to detect the cause of a new onset seizure in hospice, since infectious or metabolic causes are possible.
- In patients without known CNS tumors, a brain imaging study may be considered within the context of the patient's goals of care.
- Electroencephalography (EEG) is the standard diagnostic test for seizures and epilepsy. In many cases, the EEG shows a widespread increase in brain electrical activity.
- In partial seizures, brain waves may show a localized increase in electrical activity. EEG tracings may be normal in between seizure episodes, however, or even apparently abnormal in patients who have never had a seizure.
- An EEG tracing must be interpreted by an neurologist experienced in the diagnosis of seizures.

Clinical Characteristics[7-9]

- In a generalized, tonic-clonic seizure, the patient's body becomes rigid, followed by convulsions and loss of consciousness. If standing, the patient will fall.
  - o Noises or cries made by the patient result from air being forced through contracted vocal cords.
  - o After this initial period of muscle stiffness, the patient's arms and legs jerk rhythmically.
  - o Patients may drool, bite their tongues, or lose bowel or bladder control during the seizure.
- The entire process (the "ictal" stage of a seizure) usually lasts from 1 to 3 minutes.
- In the post-ictal stage of a seizure, the person may appears drowsy, confused, or may even fall asleep.
- Not every seizure manifests with convulsions. Sensory disturbances including visual and auditory hallucinations can occur, or a patient may simply loose awareness and stare blankly for 1-2 minutes.
- Partial complex seizures can mimic psychiatric syndromes.
- Partial or complex partial seizures can produce treatment refractory problems such as episodic focal pain, paresthesias, confusion, or gastrointestinal symptoms.
- Hospice programs can benefit from a working relationship with a neurologist experienced in epilepsy to assist the interdisciplinary team with complex patients.

Non-Pharmacological Treatment[2, 10]

- When a patient is having a seizure, quickly prepare surroundings to avoid falls or injury.
- Gently move the patient to a stable, prone position; place the patient on one side to minimize the risk of aspiration.
- Do not insert anything into patient's mouth. Do not attempt to restrain the patient.
- Assess the patient's airway, breathing, and circulation during recovery from the seizure. At the peak of seizure activity there may be a brief period of apnea or asystole.
- Observe the patient until the seizure resolves to the post-ictal phase; occurring in a matter of seconds to a few minutes.
- For patients with known history of diabetes or hypoglycemia, administer glucose (orally or parenterally), if available.
- Teach the patient and family seizure precautions, what to expect during a seizure, and how to manage them if they recur.

Pharmacotherapy[2-4, 9-15]

- Medications for Alzheimer's disease, especially donepezil (Aricept®) and galantamine (Razadyne®) can interact with metabolism of AEDs (e.g., phenytoin, carbamazepine, phenobarbital, oxcarbazepine) causing both increased risk of adverse effects and reduced clinical benefit.
- AEDs are not usually initiated in patients presenting with a single, idiopathic seizure.
- Patients over the age of 65 years are at higher risk of drug side effects and risk from drug interactions. If AED therapy is required, initiate with a single medication and titrate slowly to improve safety and medication tolerability. When testing serum levels, target the lower end of the therapeutic range.
- Not all oral AEDs are effective and well-absorbed when given per rectum. If the patient can no longer swallow whole tablets or capsules, consider switching to a crushable or sprinkle capsule formulation. Simplify the AED regimen to monotherapy if possible. Refer to Table 1 for rectal administration information on commonly used AEDs. All benzodiazepines and phenobarbital may be given rectally.

Table 1. Routes of Administration for Anti-Epileptic Drugs (AEDs)

Medication	ROA	Dosage Forms	Comments
Carbamazepine (Tegretol®)	PO, PR	Tabs, oral suspension, chewables, caps	• PR dose same as PO dose • Use immediate release forms for PR administration • Partial (simple and complex), generalized seizures
Divalproex (Depakote®)	PO, PR	EC tabs, sprinkle caps, ER tabs	• EC/ER forms NOT recommended for PR use • Convert to Depakene® solution; give BID – TID • Partial seizures (simple and complex)
Ethosuximide (Zarontin®)	PO, PR?	Caps, oral solution	• Insufficient data to recommend PR administration, but well absorbed in GI tract • Absence (petit mal) seizures
Gabapentin (Neurontin®)	PO	Caps, oral solution, tabs	• Poorly absorbed rectally, not recommended • Partial seizures (simple and complex)
Fosphenytoin (Cerebyx®)	IV, IM	Injectable	• Used only for control of status epilepticus when other forms of phenytoin are not available • Status epilepticus, emergency treatment
Lacosamide (Vimpat®)	PO, IV	Injectable, oral solution, tabs	• Insufficient data for PR administration • Partial onset seizures
Lamotrigine (Lamictal®)	PO, PR	Tabs, chewables, ER tabs, ODT	• PR absorption acceptable • PR dose is 2x PO dose • Partial (simple and complex), generalized seizures
Levetiracetam (Keppra®)	PO, PR?	Tabs, oral solution, injectable, ER tabs	• Insufficient data for PR administration • Suggest continue IR tabs given PR only if patient not tolerant of lorazepam or phenobarbital • Partial onset, generalized, & myoclonic seizures
Methsuximide (Celontin®)	PO	Caps	• Insufficient data for PR administration • Absence (petit mal) seizures
Oxcarbazepine (Trileptal®)	PO	Tabs, oral suspension	• Poorly absorbed rectally, not recommended for PR administration • Partial (simple and complex) and generalized seizures
Phenytoin (Dilantin®)	PO, IV	ER caps, injectable, chewables, oral suspension	• Poorly absorbed rectally, not recommended for PR administration • Oral suspension is 125mg/5mL; dosed TID • Partial (complex) and generalized seizures
Pregabalin (Lyrica®)	PO	Caps	• Insufficient data for PR administration • Partial onset seizures
Tiagabine (Gabitril®)	PO	Tabs	• Insufficient data for PR administration • Partial seizures (simple and complex)
Topiramate (Topamax®)	PO, PR	Tabs, sprinkle caps, ER caps	• PR dose same as PO dose • Use tabs rectally; do not use sprinkle caps • Partial (simple and complex) and generalized seizures
Vigabatrin (Sabril®)	PO	Tabs, oral suspension	• Insufficient data for PR administration • Refractory partial seizures (complex)
Valproic acid (Depakene®)	PO, IV, PR	Injectable, caps, syrup, oral solution	• PR dose same as PO dose • Instill liquid form rectally; do not use coated tabs or caps • Partial (simple and complex) and absence (petit mal) seizures
Zonisamide (Zonegran®)	PO	Caps	• Insufficient data for PR administration • Animal study (rats) shows good PR absorption • Adjunctive treatment partial seizures

ODT=oral dissolving tablet   ER=extended release   EC=enteric coated

Clinical Pearls[7,9-15]

- Assessing patients for seizure risk on admission to hospice can help both the interdisciplinary team plan for the patient's care. The team can then prepare the patient and family with instructions to follow in the event of a seizure. Baldwin, et al have outlined an approach to proactive screening for seizure risk in hospice, risk assessment templates, and suggested contents of a hospice "seizure cessation kit."
- Do not wait to administer a benzodiazepine to stop a seizure until after a blood glucose test can be given. Prepare patient surroundings to safety, administer the acute benzodiazepine seizure dose, and then consider a finger-stick blood glucose test for hypoglycemia.
- If AED toxicity is suspected check AED serum levels (e.g., phenobarbital, phenytoin, valproic acid); check AED serum levels if breakthrough seizures occur despite apparent adherence to AED regimen.
- For acute seizures, IV access is preferred since it allows more rapid control of seizures. However, if access is unavailable, often the case in the hospice setting, rectal administration of benzodiazepines is effective in controlling acute seizures.
- When discontinuing a maintenance dose of an AED, slow taper to discontinuation minimizes the risk of withdrawal seizures. Advise patients and families against stopping AEDs abruptly.
- Severe or frequent seizures are rare as death approaches, but may require sedation to control.
- *Status epilepticus* is a special condition of prolonged seizure activity and is generally considered a medical emergency. Traditionally, status epilepticus is defined as a seizure lasting longer than 30 minutes or seizures recur without return of consciousness between seizures. Seizures lasting longer than 5 minutes are unlikely to self-terminate and may cause neuronal injury.

Pharmacological Management of Seizures

Generic Name (Trade Name)	Adult Starting Dose	Routes	Common Strengths and Formulations	Comments
Acute Management of Seizures				
Lorazepam (Ativan®)	2mg, may repeat every 15 minutes, up to 8 mg total.	PO SL IM IV PR SC	**Tablets:** 0.5 mg, 1 mg, 2 mg **Oral solution:** 2 mg/mL **Injection:** 2 mg/mL, 4 mg/mL	• C-IV controlled substance. • No ceiling dose to control acute seizures, though control may come at the cost of prolonged sedation. • Repeat dose every 15 minutes until seizure subsides.
Diazepam (Valium®)	10mg, may repeat every 15 minutes, up to 40mg total	PO SL IM IV PR	**Tablets:** 2 mg, 5 mg, 10 mg **Oral solution:** 5mg/mL **Injection:** 5 mg/mL **Rectal gel:** 2.5 mg, 10 mg, 20 mg	• C-IV controlled substance. • No ceiling dose to control acute seizures, though control may come at the cost of prolonged sedation. • Repeat dose every 15 minutes until seizure subsides. • Rectal gel is expensive.
Maintenance Management of Seizures				
Clonazepam (Klonopin®)	2mg daily	PO PR	**Tablets:** 0.5 mg, 1 mg, 2 mg	• C-IV controlled substance. • Long acting benzodiazepine. • Useful in absence seizures and myoclonus.
Phenobarbital	100mg daily	PO PR IV SC	**Tablets:** 7.5 mg, 15 mg, 30 mg, 60 mg, 90 mg, 100 mg **Injection:** 30 mg/mL, 60 mg/mL, 130 mg/mL	• C-IV controlled substance. • Long half-life allows once daily maintenance dose (ideally at bedtime). • Signs of toxicity: drowsiness, nystagmus, ataxia. • Therapeutic range: 20-40 mcg/mL

Continued

Generic Name (Trade Name)	Adult Starting Dose	Routes	Common Strengths and Formulations	Comments
Maintenance Management of Seizures				
Phenytoin (Dilantin®)*	IR caps: 100mg TID ER caps: 300mg daily	PO IV	**Chewable tablets:** 50 mg **Capsules**: 30 mg, 100 mg **ER Capsules:** 100 mg, 200 mg, 300 mg **Injection:** 50 mg/mL	• Maintenance AED of choice in hospice. • Long half-life allows once daily maintenance dose (ideally at bedtime). • Signs of toxicity: drowsiness, diplopia, ataxia. • Therapeutic range: 10-20 mcg/mL; 5-10 mcg/mL may also be effective.
Valproic acid, Divalproex sodium (Depakene®, Depakote® ER, Stavzor®)*	15 mg/kg/day in 2-4 divided doses	PO PR IV	*Valproic acid* **Capsules:** 250mg **DR capsules:** 125 mg, 250 mg, 500 mg **Syrup:** 250 mg/5 mL **Injection**: 100 mg/mL *Divalproex sodium* **Sprinkle capsules:** 125 mg **DR tablets:** 125 mg, 250 mg, 500 mg **ER tablets:** 250 mg, 500 mg	• Regular release and delayed release formulations are usually given in 2-4 divided doses/day. • Extended release formulation (Depakote® ER) is given once daily. • Conversion to ER tablets from a stable IR dose may require an increase in total daily dose between 8% and 20% to maintain similar serum concentrations. • Divalproex sodium is a compound of sodium valproate and valproic acid; converts to valproate in the GI tract. • Therapeutic range: 50-100 mcg/mL
Management of Seizures due to Brain Tumor or Metastases				
Dexamethasone (Decadron®)	16mg daily or 8mg BID	PO IV PR	**Tablets:** 0.25 mg, 0.5 mg, 0.75 mg, 1 mg, 1.5 mg, 2 mg, 4 mg, 6 mg **Oral solution:** 1 mg/mL **Injection:** 4 mg/mL, 8 mg/mL, 10 mg/mL, 16 mg/mL, 24 mg/mL	• To reduce risk of seizures related to CNS malignancy or increased intracranial pressure (ICP) from other causes. • May give dose once daily or BID (morning and noon) to prevent insomnia. • Give with food to reduce stomach upset. • Consider monitor blood glucose levels periodically during corticosteroid use.

See Drug Dosing for Liver and Renal Disease for additional drug information.

References

1. Ropper AH, Brown RH. *Adams and Victor's Principles of Neurology*, 8th ed. New York: McGraw-Hill; 2005.
2. Krouwer HGJ, Pallagi JL, Graves NM. Management of seizures in brain tumor patients at the end of life. *J Palliative Med* 2000;3(4):465-475.
3. Jenssen S, Schere D. Treatment and management of epilepsy in the elderly demented patient. *Am J Alzheimer's Dis Oth Dement*. 2010;25(1):18-26.
4. Van Cott A, Pugh MJ. Epilepsy and the elderly. *Ann Long Term Care* 2008;16(1):28-32.
5. Gofton TE, Graber J. Identifying palliative care needs of patients living with cerebral tumors and metastases: a retrospective analysis. *J Neurooncol*. 2012;108:527-534.

6. Paramanandam G, Prommer E, Schwenke D. Adverse effects in hospice patients with chronic kidney disease receiving hydromorphone. *J Palliat Med.* 2011; 14(9):1029-1033.

7. Baldwin K, Miller L, Scott JB. Proactive identification of seizure risk improves terminal care. *Am J Hosp Palliat Care.* 2002; 19:251-258.

8. Eisenschenk S, Gilmore R. Strategies for successful management of older patients with seizures. *Geriatrics.* 1999; 54:31-40.

9. American College of Emergency Physicians (ACEP) Clinical Policies Committee; Clinical Policies Subcommittee on Seizures. Clinical policy: Critical issues in the evaluation and management of adult patients presenting to the emergency department with seizures. *Ann Emerg Med.* 2014; 63(4):437-447.

10. Beskind D, Rhodes S, Stolz U, et al. When should you test for and treat hypoglycemia in pre-hospital seizure patients? *Prehospital Emerg Care* 2014;18(3):433-441.

11. LaRoche SM, Helmers SL. The new antiepileptic drugs: scientific review. *JAMA.* 2004; 291:605-614.

12. Sirven JI, Waterhouse E. Management of status epilepticus. *Am Fam Physician.* 2003; 68:469-476, 2003.

13. Droney J, Hall E. Status epilepticus in a hospice inpatient setting. *J Pain Symptom Manage.* 2008;36:97-105.

14. Warren DE. Practical use of rectal medications in palliative care. *J Pain Symptom Manage.* 1996; 11:378-387.

15. Rey E, Treluyer JM, Pons G. Pharmacokinetic optimization of benzodiazepine therapy for acute seizures: focus on delivery routes. *Clin Pharmacokinet.* 1999;3: 409-424.

16. Richards JH, Protus BM, Grauer PA, Kimbrel JM. Evaluation of subcutaneous phenobarbital administration in hospice patients. *Am J Hosp Palliat Med.* 2014 Dec 3; epub ahead of print. DOI 1049909114555157

Treatment Algorithm for Seizures

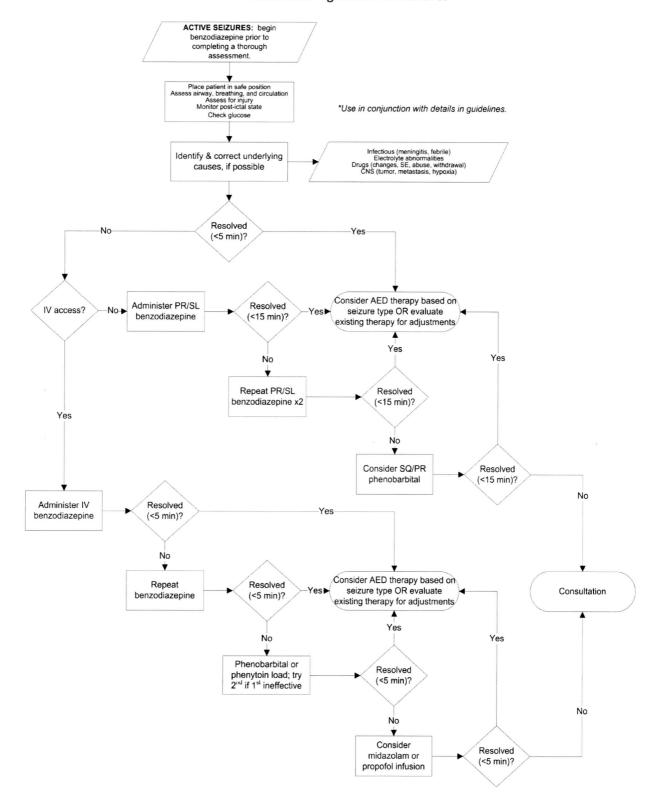

Xerostomia

Introduction and Background[1-6]

- Saliva is produced by the parotid, submandibular and sublingual glands as well as by the hundreds of smaller salivary glands that are located throughout the oral cavity. These glands are innervated by both the parasympathetic and sympathetic nervous system.
- Parasympathetic stimulation produces thin, watery secretions while the sympathetic stimulation leads to less volume and more viscous saliva.
- Approximately one liter of saliva is produced daily. Flow rates fluctuate due to diurnal rhythms.
- Xerostomia is a subjective, uncomfortable feeling of dry mouth related to either a decrease in the production and flow of saliva or a change in the composition of saliva.
- Saliva consists of water, electrolytes and glycoproteins.
- The major functions of saliva are to lubricate food and enhance taste, swallowing, and speech.
- The antimicrobial components and buffering activity of saliva also protect the teeth from dental caries and the upper digestive tract from oral candidiasis.

Prevalence[3,4,6]

- The prevalence of xerostomia in the general population is about 6-13% of males and 20-40% of females. For patients over the age of 65, the prevalence is up to 60%.
- In patients with advanced cancer, up to 77% report xerostomia. Nearly all patients who have received radiotherapy to the head and neck experience xerostomia.
- A recent study of terminally ill patients cancer and a very short life expectancy (2-3 weeks) reported symptoms of salivary hypofunction (98%), mucosal erythema (50%) and ulceration (20%) along with other oral problems such as mouth pain, oral fungal infections, and taste changes.

Causes[1-5]

- Xerostomia is most commonly caused by:
  - Connective tissue disorders
  - Immunological disorders
  - Destruction of salivary glands by radiation therapy or surgery
  - Medications (Table 1)

Table 1. Medication Causes of Xerostomia

Categories	Examples
Analgesics	Opioids, NSAIDs (celecoxib, diclofenac, felbamate, meloxicam, oxaprozin, piroxicam)
Anticholinergics	Atropine, glycopyrrolate, benztropine, oxybutynin, scopolamine, tolterodine, solifenacin, darifenacin, trospium
Antidepressants	Paroxetine, amitriptyline, desipramine, nortriptyline, imipramine, venlafaxine, mirtazapine, trazodone, sertraline, fluoxetine
Anti-emetics	Prochlorperazine, promethazine
Antihistamines	Diphenhydramine, dimenhydrinate, loratadine, meclizine
Antihypertensives	ACE inhibitors (e.g., lisinopril, enalopril, ramipril), clonidine, amlodipine
Antipsychotics	Chlorpromazine, haloperidol, olanzapine, quetiapine, risperidone, ziprasidone
Anxiolytics	Benzodiazepines (e.g., alprazolam, lorazepam, diazepam, clonazepam)
Bronchodilators	Aclidinium, albuterol, ipratropium, tiotropium, umeclidinium
Chemotherapy	Anastrozole, erlotinib, everolimus, letrozole, sunitinib, sorafenib
Diuretics	Chlorothiazide, furosemide, hydrochlorothiazide, bumetanide, torsemide
Muscle relaxants	Baclofen, cyclobenzaprine, tizanidine
Other	Anticonvulsants, anti-arrhythmics, carbidopa/levodopa, nicotine

- Sjögren's syndrome, (pronounced "show-grens") is a condition that presents with both xerostomia and xerophthalmia (dry eyes). Sjögren's syndrome is a chronic autoimmune disease, occurring primarily in women in their late 40s. Secondary Sjögren's syndrome is associated when another autoimmune or

- connective tissue diseases (e.g., rheumatoid arthritis, systemic lupus erythematosus, systemic sclerosis) is present.
- Other conditions associated with xerostomia include renal dialysis, diabetes (hyperglycemia), primary biliary cirrhosis, vasculitis, chronic hepatitis, HIV/AIDS, bone marrow transplantation, and graft-versus-host disease (GVHD).
- Xerostomia is commonly seen in patients with fibromyalgia, chronic fatigue syndrome, and Raynaud's phenomenon.
- Patients who are anxious or depressed often complain of dry mouth.
- Mouth breathing, dehydration, non-humidified oxygen therapy, and hypercalcemia can worsen the symptom of xerostomia.

Clinical Characteristics[1,4-6]
- Patients with xerostomia or hyposalivation complain of dry mouth, a burning sensation, soreness of the mouth, altered taste and loss of appetite.
  - The flavor of foods is strongly associated with the aroma of the food. Patients with chronic sinus problems or other disorders of the nasal passages will report lack of flavor in food and drink, leading to loss of appetite.
- Caregivers may notice increased requests for water (especially when speaking or swallowing), difficulty swallowing, or avoidance of dry or hard foods.
- As xerostomia progresses, the mouth may manifest erythematous pebbled, cobblestoned, or fissured tongue. Mucosal surfaces may become sticky to the touch.

Non-Pharmacological Treatment[5,7-13]
- Saliva substitutes: over the counter formulations are available as solutions, gels, sprays, lozenges
  - May contain sorbitol, sodium carboxymethylcellulose, methylparaben or porcine and bovine mucin.
- Water or ice chips; frequent sips of water.
- Milk may be effective in moistening and lubricating, and may also buffer oral acids
- Frozen grapes, popsicles, lemon sugar-free candy, vitamin C tablets, frozen tonic water
- Lubricate lips; use water-based lubricants if patient is using oxygen therapy.
- Stimulate salivary glands: sour or acidic candy
- Diet: encourage foods that are soft, moist, and cool or at room temperature.
- Olive oil or olive oil containing products can serve as mucosal lubricants.
- Masticatory stimulants: sugar-free chewing gum or hard candies
  - Usually contain sugar alcohols (e.g., sorbitol) which can lead to bloating and diarrhea if overused.

Pharmacotherapy[7-13]
- Identifiable, underlying causes of xerostomia should be corrected if possible. Alternate drugs should be considered, hydration corrected if possible, and psychological factors addressed.
- Data regarding superiority of any treatment is lacking; treatment selection should take into consideration of patient preference, cost, availability, and dosage form.
- Treatment is primarily palliative, with emphasis on the use of saliva substitutes.
- Cholinergic agonists may be considered if saliva substitutes are inadequate, but salivary glands must be at least partially functional for clinical benefit.

Clinical Pearls[3,8,9]
- Advise the patient to avoid use of caffeine, alcohol, and tobacco products.
- Patients with xerostomia have an increased risk for dental caries and oral thrush. Oral hygiene is thus very important; fluoride (alcohol-free) or chlorhexidine rinses may be used.
- Sublingual tablets may be inappropriate in patients with xerostomia since the lack of saliva will decrease the ability to dissolve the tablet.
- Saliva substitutes with porcine or bovine mucin-based derivatives may not be acceptable to vegetarians, Jews, or Muslims. Animal mucin-based saliva substitutes are not available in the United States.
- Always check ingredient lists of saliva substitutes; ingredients vary by dosage form even within the same brand line.

Pharmacological Management of Xerostomia

Generic Name (Trade Name)	Adult Starting Dose	Routes	Common Strengths and Formulations	Comments
Saliva Substitutes & Oral Lubricants				
Aquoral®	2 sprays 3-4 times daily	PO	**Oral spray**; citrus flavor	• Oxidized glycerol triesters, silicon dioxide, aspartame. • Rx only.
Biotène®	Use as directed for each product form	PO	**Mouthwash, spray, toothpaste**; mint flavor	• Polyglycitol, propylene glycol, sunflower oil, xylitol, milk protein extract, acesulfame K, enzymes • Available OTC.
Caphasol®	Use as directed	PO	**Mouthwash**	• Use immediately after mixing. • Do not refrigerate. • Rx only.
Moi-Stir®	Use as needed	PO	**Oral spray**; mint flavor	• Sorbitol, carboxymethylcellulose, methylparaben, glycerin. • Available OTC.
Mouth Kote®	Spray 3-5 times, swirl for 8-10 seconds, then swallow or spit	PO	**Oral spray**, lemon-lime flavor	• Xylitol, sorbitol, yerba santa, citric acid, ascorbic acid, saccharin. • Available OTC.
Numoisyn®	1 lozenge PRN 2 mL, rinse and swallow PRN	PO	**Lozenge, oral liquid**	• Lozenges contain sorbitol, polyethylene glycol, malic acid, citric acid, cottonseed oil. • Liquid contains sorbitol, linseed extract, parabens, citric acid. • Do not refrigerate Numoisyn® liquid. • Rx only.
Oasis®	Use as directed for each product form	PO	**Mouthwash, spray**; mint flavor	• Glycerin, sorbitol, poloxamer 338, castor oil, copovidone, sodium benzoate, carboxymethylcellulose. • Available OTC.
Sialogogues (Cholinergic Agonists)				
Pilocarpine (Salagen®)	5 mg TID 5 drops TID (5 drops of 2% ophth solution = 5mg)	PO	**Tablets:** 5 mg, 7.5 mg **Ophth. solution:** 2%	• Avoid taking with dairy products. • May take up to 2 months for full effect. • Use of ophthalmic solution may be easier and more cost effective than tablets. • Avoid oral pilocarpine in patients with glaucoma. Oral pilocarpine can antagonize the effects of anti-cholinergic agents and produce cardiac conduction abnormalities in patients taking beta-blockers.
Cevimeline (Evoxac®)	30 mg TID	PO	**Capsules:** 30 mg	• Similar side effects as pilocarpine. • Avoid in poorly controlled asthma, narrow angle glaucoma. • Use caution in patients with gallstones or kidney stones. • Expensive.

See Drug Dosing for Liver and Renal Disease for additional drug information.

References

1. Plemons J, Al-Hashimi I, Marek C. Managing xerostomia and salivary gland hypofunction: executive summary of a report from the American Dental Association Council on Scientific Affairs. *JADA*. 2014;145:867-873

2. Davies AN, Broadley K, Beighton D. Xerostomia in patients with advanced cancer. *J Pain Sym Manage*. 2001:22;820-825.

3. Guggenheimer J, Moore PA. Xerostomia: etiology, recognition and treatment. *JADA*. 2003;134: 61-69.

4. Porter SR. Xerostomia: prevalence, assessment, differential diagnosis and implications for quality of life. *Oral Dis* 2010;16:501-502

5. Narhi TO, Meurman JH, Ainamo A. Xerostomia and hyposalivation: causes, consequences, and treatment in the elderly. *Drugs Aging.* 1999;15:103-116.

6. Fischer DJ, Epstein JB, Yao Y, Wilkie DJ. Oral health conditions affect functional and social activities of terminally ill cancer patients. *Support Care Cancer* 2014;22:803-810.

7. Hoegh-Guldberg N. Treatment of Drug-Induced Xerostomia. Drymouth.info [Internet] http://www.drymouth.info/practitioner/treatment.asp. Accessed September 25, 2014.

8. Neiuw Amerongen AV, Veerman ACI. Current therapies for xerostomia and salivary gland hypofunction associated with cancer therapies. *Support Care Cancer.* 2003;11: 226-231.

9. Scully C, Felix DH: Oral medicine – update for the dental practitioner: dry mouth and disorders of salivation. *Br Dental J.* 2005;199:423-427.

10. Dost F, Farah CS. Stimulating the discussion on saliva substitutes: a clinical perspective. *Austral Dent J* 2013;58:11-17

11. Radvansky LJ, Pace MB, Siddiqui A. Prevention and management of radiation-induced dermatitis, mucositis, and xerostomia. *Am J Health-Syst Pharm* 2013;70:1025-1032

12. Yasuda H, Niki H: Review of the pharmacological properties and clinical usefulness of muscarinic agonists for xerostomia in patients with Sjögren's syndrome. *Clin Drug Invest.* 2002;22:67-73.

13. Ship JA, McCutcheon JA, Spivakovsky S, Kerr AR. Safety and effectiveness of topical dry mouth products containing olive oil, betaine, and xylitol in reducing xerostomia for polypharmacy-induced dry mouth. *J Oral Rehabil* 2007;34:724-732

Treatment Algorithm for Xerostomia

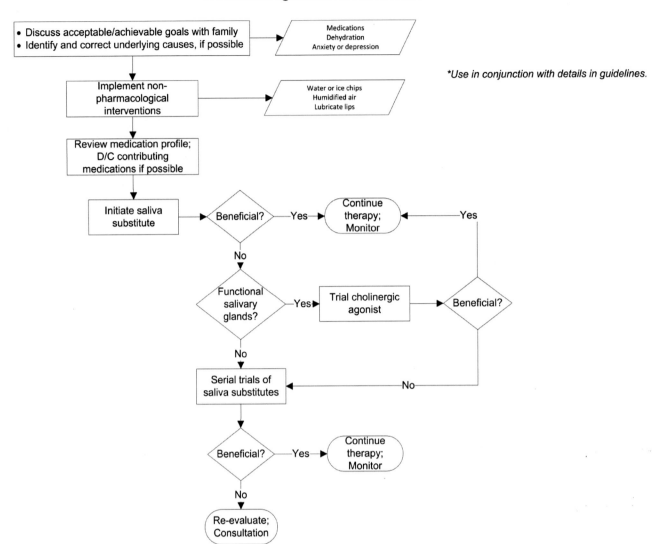

*Use in conjunction with details in guidelines.

Section III:

Disease State Management

- Acquired Immune Deficiency Syndrome (AIDS)
- Amyotrophic Lateral Sclerosis (ALS)
- Cancer
- Cardiac Disease
- Chronic Obstructive Pulmonary Disease (COPD)
- Dementia
- End Stage Liver Disease
- End Stage Renal Disease
- Parkinson's Disease
- Stroke

Human Immunodeficiency Virus (HIV) &
Acquired Immune Deficiency Syndrome (AIDS)

Introduction[1-5]

Compared to other primary hospice diagnoses, admissions for persons with HIV-AIDS comprise only about 0.2% of the total annual hospice admissions. With the introduction of protease inhibitors in the mid-late 1990s, highly active anti-retroviral therapies (HAART) have transformed HIV-AIDS from a terminal diagnosis to a chronic disease. Up to 50% of the 15,000 deaths per year in patients with HIV/AIDS in the United States are attributed to non-AIDS defining comorbidities, such as liver disease, malignancies, cardiovascular disease, and complications of substance abuse. However, due to the chronic nature of HIV-AIDS, disease related illness and cumulative effects of HAART treatment-related adverse effects and toxicity, integration of palliative care is crucial to provide comprehensive patient-centered medical and psychosocial support to patients and families. Additionally, patients with HIV are less likely to openly discuss advanced care planning and are at high risk of underlying psychiatric disorders.

Prognosis[4-9]

Life expectancy for patients with HIV-AIDS is affected by age, availability of HAART treatment options, drug resistant opportunistic infections, functional status, nutritional status, CD4 and viral load counts, and development of difficult to treat complications. Patients may choose to discontinue HAART due to side effects, multidrug resistance, lack of access, or belief that burden of medications outweighs the benefit (e.g., at end of life). When antiretroviral therapies are discontinued, the CD4 count drops and the viral load rises, increasing susceptibility to opportunistic infections and increasing AIDS-related symptom burden. CD4 and viral load correlates with prognosis, but must be considered along with the presence of AIDS-related syndromes and non-AIDS related comorbidities before deciding on hospice eligibility. Consultation with an infectious disease physician specializing in HIV-AIDS is recommended.

Guidance for Determination of Hospice Eligibility: HIV-AIDS[8,9]
Patient with HIV-AIDS meets the following criteria:
- Palliative performance status (PPS) < 50%
- CD4 (T Cell) count ≤ 25 cells/mL
  OR
- Viral load ≥ 100,000 copies/mL

At least one of the following AIDS-related conditions:
- Wasting, defined as a loss of > 33% of lean body mass
- *Mycobacterium avium* complex (MAC) bacteremia (untreated or unresponsive to treatment)
- Progressive multifocal leukoencephalopathy (PML)
- Renal failure in the absence of dialysis
- CNS lymphoma or poorly responsive systemic lymphoma
- Refractory cryptosporidium infection
- Refractory toxoplasmosis
- Refractory Kaposi's sarcoma

Supporting documentation includes:
- Chronic diarrhea (≥ 1 year)
- Persistent serum albumin < 2.5 g/dL
- Active substance abuse
- Age > 50 years
- Advanced AIDS dementia
- Symptomatic CHF (at rest)
- Lack of antiretroviral, chemotherapeutic, and prophylactic medications directly related to HIV treatment.

In the absence of one or more of the above criteria, rapid decline or comorbidities may also support the physician's determination of a life expectancy of < 6 months and hospice eligibility. Certification or recertification is based upon a physician's clinical judgment. According to the Benefits Improvement and Protection Act of 2000 (BIPA), hospice certification of terminal illness "shall be based on the physician's or medical director's clinical judgment regarding the normal course of the individual's illness."[9]

Prevalent Symptoms[3,10]

Symptoms reported to be the most bothersome by patients with HIV-AIDS include pain, anxiety and depression, anorexia and weight loss, insomnia and daytime fatigue, nausea, and diarrhea. The prevalence of symptoms reported by patients with HIV increases as the CD4 count decreases and viral load increases, with about 50% of patients reporting between 2 and 7 undesirable symptoms. Younger patients, those with a history of injection drug use, and those with less formal education are more bothered by symptoms attributed to HIV. For symptoms that do not respond well to pharmacotherapy, support from psychosocial and spiritual staff is critical to help the patient cope with expected decline.

- Anorexia, see *Anorexia GEMS*
- Anxiety, see *Anxiety GEMS*
- Constipation, see *Constipation GEMS*
- Depression, see *Depression GEMS*
- Diarrhea, see *Diarrhea GEMS*
- Fatigue, see *Fatigue GEMS*
- Insomnia, see *Insomnia GEMS*
- Nausea, see *Nausea & Vomiting GEMS*
- Pain, see *Pain GEMS*

HAART[2,3,11-14]

HAART suppresses viral replication, resulting in improved immune function and higher levels of CD4 cells. Some patients cannot tolerate HAART adverse effects (e.g., fatigue, headache, nausea, diarrhea, neuropathy, anemia, hepatotoxicity, rash, and hyperglycemia). Even incomplete suppression of viral load is associated with immunologic benefits, which may make continuation of HAART appropriate near the end of life. Similar to patients with cancer making the decision to forgo or stop chemotherapy, discontinuing HAART may feel as though the patient is "giving up." Patients should be actively involved in discussions regarding changes to medications prescribed to manage HIV or sequelae. Assess benefits and burdens of HAART with the patient to assist in decision-making (Table 1) about treatment goals.

- If HAART is discontinued, viral load will rise and CD4 count will decrease resulting in increased incidence of viral symptoms: fatigue, anorexia, fevers or sweats, depression, dementia, pain, myopathy, and neuropathy. The decreased immunologic response following HAART discontinuation increases a patient's risk for opportunistic infections.
- HAART regimens contain at least 3 drugs. Many antiretroviral medications have extensive drug interactions with commonly used symptom management medications (Table 2).
- Continued HAART therapy may result in prolonged survival complicating prognostication.

Opportunistic Infections[2,5,7,13,15]

- Patients with HIV-AIDS are at higher risk for opportunistic infections with atypical organisms. As with other medications, always discuss the risk vs benefits of anti-infective therapy.
- As CD4 counts decrease, most patients will benefit from primary prophylaxis with trimethoprim-sulfamethoxazole (Bactrim®) and azithromycin (Zithromax®) to prevent *Pneumocystis* pneumonia (PCP), *Toxoplasma gondii* encephalitis (TE), and *Mycobacterium avium* complex (MAC).
- Oropharyngeal and esophageal candidiasis is common in patients with HIV-AIDS. Systemic antifungals (fluconazole, itraconazole) are needed for effective treatment of esophageal candidiasis. Reserve itraconazole for fluconazole-resistant infections. Chronic suppressive therapy may be needed if infections are recurrent or severe. Consult with an HIV physician for advice in treatment refractory patients.
- *Clostridium difficile* infection (CDI) is common in patients with HIV-AIDS; CD4 <50 cells/mL is an independent risk factor in addition to the patient's traditional risk factors (e.g., exposure to antibiotics or hospitals and nursing facilities). Treatment of CDI in patients with HIV-AIDS is the same as for those not HIV-infected.

Table 1. Benefit vs Burden of HAART[11-13]

Potential Benefits	Comments
Prevention of retroviral syndrome	• Not all patients experience symptoms with discontinuation of HAART; if presenting, onset of symptoms may be within 1-2 months of discontinuation. • Recommend discontinue if life expectancy is < 1 month.
Managing syndromes associated with viral load	• HIV-related neuropathy severity, fatigue, and weight loss correlates with higher viral load. • Suppressing the viral load may lessen symptom severity.
Prevention of opportunistic infections	• HAART reduces the incidence and risk of opportunistic infections by decreasing viral load; protease inhibitors can reduce virulence of some infectious organisms.
Delay progression of AIDS dementia complex (ADC)	• ADC may be triggered by viral replication. • Zidovudine may provide benefit in slowing progression of ADC.
Potential Burdens	**Comments**
Adverse effects and drug interactions	• Common side effects include nausea, headache, diarrhea, fatigue; more significant adverse effects pancreatitis, myopathy, arthralgias, depression, and neuropathy are associated with many antiretrovirals. • Many of the HAART medications affect drug metabolism via liver enzymes (CYP450 3A4); dose adjustments may be required – consult with pharmacist for medication review.
Pill burden and treatment complexity	• Complexity of medication regimens and number of pills taken each day is associated with decreased quality of life • Risk of non-adherence to complex regimens increases problems with multidrug resistance limiting the patient's effective antiretroviral options.
Cost of therapy	• Typical regimens such as efavirenz (Sustiva®) + tenofovir (Viread®)+ emtricitabine (Emtriva®) average about $2,700 /month when taken individually. • To reduce pill burden the triple combination above is available in a single tablet (Atripla®) average cost about $2,500/month. • Hospices struggle to decide if continuing HAART therapy is appropriate based on patient goals, benefits, burdens, and therapy costs. • Few patients can afford to cover the out-of-pocket cost of HAART and may decline hospice enrollment if hospice declines payment for the medications.

Table 2. Drug Interactions with HAART and Symptom Management Medications[2,5,12-14]

Palliative Medication	HAART Medication	Comment & Recommendation
Antidepressants (trazodone, bupropion, mirtazapine, duloxetine)	Ritonavir, indinavir, nelfinavir, saquinavir, amprenavir, delaviridine	HAART medication (protease inhibitors) can inhibit the metabolism of these antidepressants leading to increased risk of adverse effects or treatment failure. Monitor patient closely with HAART discontinuation or dosage changes. Avoid use of trazodone with saquinavir.
Benzodiazepines (clonazepam, diazepam, midazolam, triazolam)	Ritonavir, indinavir	Avoid use of clonazepam, midazolam, and triazolam with HAART medication (protease inhibitors). Recommend lorazepam as benzodiazepine of choice due to no CYP450 metabolism and no interactions with any HAART medication.
Carbamazepine	Efavirenz, nevirapine	Avoid combination; risk of treatment failure. HAART medication decreases the serum concentration of carbamazepine.
Chlorpromazine	Saquinavir	Avoid concomitant use; increased exposure of drug leading to excess side effects and QT interval prolongation risk.
Haloperidol	Saquinavir	Avoid concomitant use; increased exposure of drug leading to excess side effects and QT interval prolongation risk.
Methadone	Ritonavir, indinavir, nelfinavir, saquinavir, amprenavir, delaviridine	HAART medication (protease inhibitors) can inhibit the metabolism of methadone leading to increased sedation and risk of toxicity. Monitor patient closely with HAART discontinuation or dosage changes.
	Efavirenz, nevirapine	Monitor for decreased serum concentration of methadone associated with withdrawal symptoms, poor pain control if nevirapine or efavirenz dose is increased. Methadone dose may need to be lowered if nevirapine or efavirenz is discontinued.
Fentanyl, hydrocodone, oxycodone, tramadol (opioids metabolized by CYP3A4)	Ritonavir, indinavir, nelfinavir, saquinavir, amprenavir, delaviridine	HAART medication (protease inhibitors) can inhibit the metabolism of opioids leading to increased sedation and risk of toxicity. Monitor patient closely with HAART discontinuation or dosage changes.
	Efavirenz, nevirapine	Monitor for decreased pain control with opioids if nevirapine or efavirenz dose is increased. Opioid dose may need to be lowered if nevirapine or efavirenz is discontinued.
Phenobarbital	Efavirenz, nevirapine	Phenobarbital can decrease serum concentration of HAART medication potentially causing treatment failure.
Phenytoin	Efavirenz, nevirapine	Phenytoin can decrease serum concentration of HAART medication potentially causing treatment failure.
Prochlorperazine	Saquinavir	Avoid concomitant use; increased exposure of drug leading to excess side effects and QT interval prolongation risk.
SSRI antidepressants	Saquinavir	Use paroxetine and sertraline cautiously; dose adjustments may be needed to avoid adverse effects or treatment failure.
Tricyclic antidepressants	Saquinavir	Avoid use of amitriptyline, doxepin, nortriptyline with saquinavir; excess side effects and QT interval prolongation risk.
Zolpidem	Ritonavir, indinavir, nelfinavir, saquinavir, amprenavir, delaviridine	Use zolpidem cautiously; dose adjustments may be needed to avoid adverse effects or treatment failure.

Note: chart information not comprehensive. Consultation with a pharmacist to review patient's complete medication profile is strongly recommended. Additional information available at **www.hiv-druginteractions.org***.*

References

1. National Hospice & Palliative Care Organization (NHPCO). NHPCO's facts and figures: hospice care in America. 2014 edition. Alexandria, VA; NHPCO, October 2014. Available at http://www.nhpco.org/sites/default/files/public/Statistics_Research/2014_Facts_Figures.pdf.
2. Selwyn PA. Palliative care for patient with human immunodeficiency virus/acquired immune deficiency syndrome. *J Palliat Med.* 2005;8(6):12481268.
3. Matthews W C, McCutchan JA, Asch S, et al. National estimates of HIV-related symptom prevalent from the HIV cost and services utilization study. *Med Care.* 2000;38(7):750-762.
4. Stewart A, Carusone SC, To K, Schaefer-McDaniel N, Halman M, Grimes R. Causes of death in HIV patients and the evolution of an AIDS hospice: 1988-2008. *AIDS Res Treat.* 2012;390406. Available at http://www.hindawi.com/journals/art/2012/390406/
5. Selwyn PA, Forstein M. Overcoming the false dichotomy of curative vs palliative care for late-stage HIV/AIDS: "Let me live the way I want to live, until I can't." *JAMA.* 2003;290:806-814.
6. Oppenheim S. Prognosis in HIV and AIDS. *J Palliat Med.* 2009;12(9):833-835. Available at https://www.capc.org/fast-facts/213-prognosis-hiv-and-aids/
7. Fausto JA, Selwyn PA. Palliative care in the management of advanced HIV-AIDS. *Prim Care Clin Office Pract.* 2011;38:311-326.
8. Centers for Medicare & Medicaid Services (CMS). Local coverage determination (LCD): hospice determining terminal status. Available at http://www.cms.gov/medicare-coverage- database/details/lcd-details.aspx. Accessed December 18, 2014.
9. Centers for Medicare & Medicaid Services (CMS). Medicare program; hospice care amendments. *Fed Register* 2005;70:FR70532-70548. Available at https://federalregister.gov/a/05-23078.
10. Whalen CC, Antani M, Carey J, and Landefeld CS. An index of symptoms for infection with human immunodeficiency virus: reliability and validity. *J Clin Epidemiol* 1994;47(5):537-546.
11. Vandekieft G, Cohen M. Highly active antiretroviral therapy and hospice. March 2009. Fast Facts 102. Available at https://www.capc.org/fast-facts/102-highly-active-antiretroviral-therapy-and-hospice/
12. Lexi-Comp Online, Lexi-Drugs Online, Hudson, OH: Lexi-Comp, Inc. Accessed December 28, 2014.
13. Aberg JA, Gallant JE, Ghanem KG, et al. Primary care guidelines for the management of persons infected with HIV: 2013 update by the HIV Medicine Association of the Infectious Disease Society of America. Clin Infect Dis. 2014;58(1):e1-e34. Available at http://cid.oxfordjournals.org/content/58/1/e1.full.pdf+html
14. Gourevitch MN and Friedland GH. Interactions between methadone and medications used to treat HIV infection: a review. *Mt Sinai J Med.* 2000;67(5&6):429-436.
15. Panel on Opportunistic Infections in HIV-Infected Adults and Adolescents. Guidelines for the prevention and treatment of opportunistic infections in HIV-infected adults and adolescents: recommendations from the CDC, the NIH, and the HIV Medicine Association of ISDA. 2014. Available at http://aidsinfo.nih.gov/contentfiles/lvguidelines/adult_oi.pdf.

Amyotrophic Lateral Sclerosis (ALS)

Introduction[1-2]

Amyotrophic lateral sclerosis (ALS) is a progressive neurodegenerative disorder causing muscle weakness, disability, and death. About 0.5% of annual hospice admissions are for patients with a primary diagnosis of ALS. Because there is no cure or effective treatment, palliative care for patients with ALS should begin at the time of diagnosis. As the disease progresses, hospice referral is appropriate when patient and family treatment goals change from maximizing function to symptom control and psychosocial support for the patient, family and caregivers.

Prognosis[3-6]

The median survival for patients with ALS is about 3 to 5 years, however about 10-20% of patients may survive up to 10 years. Longer term survival may be associated with younger age, male gender, and limb type rather than bulbar. ALS tends to progress in a linear pattern with the overall rate of decline fairly constant. Some patients decline rapidly while others progress much more slowly; history of rate of progression can assist in estimating prognosis. Mechanical ventilation and artificial nutrition and hydration can prolong survival and make prognostication more difficult.

Guidance for Determination of Hospice Eligibility: ALS

Rapid disease progression with ALL of the following in the preceding 12 months:
- o Progression from independent ambulation to wheelchair or bed-bound status
- o Progression from normal to barely intelligible or unintelligible speech
- o Progression from normal to pureed diet
- o Progression from independence in most or all activities of daily living (ADLs) to needing major assistance for all ADLs

And at least one of the following:

Critically impaired breathing capacity with ALL of the following in the preceding 12 months:
- o Significant dyspnea at rest
- o Vital capacity less than 30%
- o Requirement for supplemental oxygen at rest
- o Patient declines mechanical ventilation [external, noninvasive ventilation (NIV) such as BiPAP may be used for comfort]

Critical nutritional impairment with ALL of the following in the preceding 12 months:
- o Oral intake of nutrients and fluids insufficient to sustain life
- o Continued weight loss
- o Dehydration or hypovolemia
- o Absence of artificial feeding methods (tube feedings or parenteral nutrition)

Life-threatening complications with 1 or more of the following in the preceding 12 months:
- o Recurrent aspiration pneumonia (with or without tube feedings)
- o Upper urinary tract infection
- o Sepsis
- o Recurrent fever after antibiotic therapy
- o Pressure ulcers (stage 3 or 4)

In the absence of one or more of the above criteria, rapid decline or comorbidities may also support the physician's determination of a life expectancy of < 6 months and hospice eligibility. Certification or recertification is based upon a physician's clinical judgment. According to the Benefits Improvement and Protection Act of 2000 (BIPA), hospice certification of terminal illness "shall be based on the physician's or medical director's clinical judgment regarding the normal course of the individual's illness."

Prevalent Symptoms

In addition to the symptoms listed below, developing a plan of care with the patient and family regarding nutrition and dysphagia, and breathing support and dyspnea or respiratory failure.

- Constipation, see *Constipation GEMS*
- Depression, see *Depression GEMS*
- Dyspnea, see *Dyspnea GEMS*
- Fatigue, see *Fatigue GEMS*
- Insomnia, see *Insomnia GEMS*
- Muscle spasms, see *Muscle Spasms GEMS*
- Pain, see *Pain GEMS*
- Sialorrhea, see *Secretions GEMS*

Medication Management in ALS[5-12]

- Riluzole (Rilutek®) is the only FDA-approved medication to treat ALS. Riluzole may slow progression of ALS and prolongs survival an average of 2 – 3 months. The exact mechanism of action is unknown, but riluzole has an inhibitory effect on glutamate release; inactivates voltage-depended sodium channels; and interferes with transmitter binding at excitatory amino acid receptors.
- Riluzole use may be appropriate to continue in some patients while under hospice care. Those patients tend to meet the following criteria: higher functional level of patient (e.g., some level of ambulation or ability to propel self in wheelchair and/or provide some self-care); history of riluzole use is less than 12 months and ALS symptoms less than 5 years; If known, forced vital capacity > 60%; age less than 75 years.
- Clinical trials comparing use of lithium with riluzole vs placebo and riluzole demonstrated no benefit to the use of lithium to prolong survival.
- Amitriptyline (Elavil®), a TCA antidepressant, is usually avoided at end of life due to anticholinergic side effects. Amitriptyline may be appropriate for patients with ALS to reduce sialorrhea and insomnia, and may be effective for pseudobulbar affect. Titrate doses cautiously to lessen the risk of overly thick secretions or mucus plugs.
- Pseudobulbar affect (PSA), a disorder of involuntary emotional outbursts, usually uncontrollable laughing or crying can be difficult to manager. A combination of dextromethorphan and quinidine (Nuedexta®) may alleviate the PSA syptoms in patients with insufficient response to other antidepressants (SSRIs or tricyclic antidepressants).

Clinical Pearls[5-9]

- Clinical trials studying the use vitamin E and creatinine have failed to demonstrate improvements in symptoms or survival time.
- Degeneration of the nervous system can lead to decreased sensation of the need to defecate; despite stool softeners and laxatives patients will often need manual stimulation usually in the form a suppository or enema to move their bowels.
- As patients become weaker they are more likely to have dysphagia. Initial management of dysphagia should be with done with modifications to the diet to increase the food and fluid consistency. The use of a percutaneous gastrostomy tube (PEG) can be advantageous for some patients with ALS.
  - Marked weight loss not associated with dysphagia. Nutritional supplementation is often recommended for these individuals to supplement their ability to continue enteral nutrition since dysphagia is not present.
  - Patients who have dysphagia and weight loss that still have a pulmonary vital capacity that has not fallen below 50 of predicted and are not in the beginning stages of the terminal phase.

References

1. National Hospice & Palliative Care Organization (NHPCO). NHPCO's facts and figures: hospice care in America. 2014 edition. Alexandria, VA; NHPCO, October 2014. Available at http://www.nhpco.org/sites/default/files/public/Statistics_Research/2014_Facts_Figures.pdf.
2. Amyotrophic Lateral Sclerosis Society of Canada. A guide to ALS patient care for primary care physicians. Markham, Ontario: ALS Society of Canada, 2009. Available at

http://www.als.ca/sites/default/files/files/Physicians%20CD/A%20Guide%20to%20ALS%20Patient%20Care%20For%20Primary%20Care%20Physicians%20English.pdf

3. Centers for Medicare & Medicaid Services (CMS). Local coverage determination (LCD): hospice determining terminal status. Available at http://www.cms.gov/medicare-coverage- database/details/lcd-details.aspx. Accessed December 18, 2014.

4. Centers for Medicare & Medicaid Services (CMS). Medicare program; hospice care amendments. *Fed Register* 2005;70:FR70532-70548. Available at https://federalregister.gov/a/05-23078.

5. Mitsumoto H, Rabkin JG. Palliative care for people with amyotrophic lateral sclerosis: prepare for the worst and hope for the best. *JAMA.* 2007;298(2):207-216.

6. Borasio GD, Voltz R, Miller RG. Palliative care in amyotrophic lateral sclerosis. *Neurol Clin.* 2001;19(4):829-847.

7. Miller RG, Jackson CE, Kasarkis EJ, et al. Practice parameter update: the care of the patient with amyotrophic lateral sclerosis: multidisciplinary care, symptom management, and cognitive/behavioral impairment (an evidence-based review). *Neurology.* 2009;73:1227-1233.

8. Miller RG, Jackson CE, Kasarkis EJ, et al. Practice parameter update: the care of the patient with amyotrophic lateral sclerosis: drug, nutritional, and respiratory therapies (an evidence-based review). *Neurology.* 2009;73:1218-1226.

9. Lexi-Comp Online, Lexi-Drugs Online, Hudson, Ohio: Lexi-Comp, Inc; January 15, 2015.

10. Miller RG, Mitchell JD, Lyon MD, Moore DH. Riluzole for amyotrophic lateral sclerosis (ALS)/motor neuron disease (MND) review. *The Cochrane Library.* 2008;2:1-25.

11. Zoccolella S, Beghi E, Palagano G, et al. Riluzole and amyotrophic lateral sclerosis survival: a population-based study in southern Italy. *European Journal of Neurology.* 2007;14:262-68.

12. Morrison KE, Dhariwal S, Hornabrook R, et al. Lithium in patients with amyotrophic lateral sclerosis (LiCALS): a phase 3 multicenter, randomized, double-blind, placebo controlled trial. *Lancet Neurol.* 2013;12(4):338-345. Available at http://www.ncbi.nlm.nih.gov/pmc/articles/PMC3610091/.

Cancer

Introduction[1-4]

Patients with a terminal diagnosis of cancer compose nearly 40% of hospice admissions annually, making cancer the most common reason for hospice admission.[1] Of those patients, lung, colorectal, blood and lymphatic, breast, pancreas, and prostate are the most common primary cancer site diagnoses.[2] Home hospice care for patients with cancer provides improved symptom control (pain and anxiety) and increased likelihood of dying at the place of choice (home). More patients in home hospice care also have advanced directives in place than those who die of cancer without home hospice.[3] Additionally, the American Society of Clinical Oncology (ASCO) expert consensus states that palliative care should be combined with standard oncology care at the time of diagnosis for any patient with metastatic cancer or high symptom burden to improve quality of life, increase patient satisfaction with care, and reduce caregiver burden.[4]

Metastatic Cancer[5,6]

Nearly all types of cancer have the ability to metastasize. Metastases can occur in 3 ways:

- Direct growth into tissue surrounding the tumor
- Cancer cells migrate through blood vessels to other areas of body
- Cancer cells migrate through the lymph system to nearby or distant nodes

Common Sites of Metastasis[5,6]

The brain, bones, lungs, and liver are the most common sites for cancers to metastases. Metastatic disease may be discovered without a known primary cancer (cancer of unknown primary) even after extensive diagnostic testing. Table 1 shows primary sites of metastasis by cancer type.

Table 1. Common Sites of Metastasis

Cancer Type	Metastatic sites *(alphabetical order)*
Bladder	Bone, liver, lung
Breast	Bone, brain, liver, lung
Colorectal	Liver, lung, peritoneum
Kidney	Adrenal gland, bone, brain, liver, lung
Lung	Adrenal gland, bone, liver, contralateral lung
Melanoma	Bone, brain, liver, lung, skin, muscle
Ovarian	Liver, lung, peritoneum
Pancreas	Liver, lung, peritoneum
Prostate	Adrenal gland, bone, liver, lung
Stomach	Liver, lung, peritoneum
Thyroid	Bone, liver, lung
Uterine	Bone, liver, lung, peritoneum, vagina

Prognosis[7-11]

Clinicians tend to overestimate survival in patients with advanced cancer. Prognostication can be improved and individualized to the patient when population-based statistics (e.g., scoring tools and indexes) are used in combination with clinician's assessment of the patient's functional ability, comorbidities, and pertinent symptoms. The Eastern Cooperative Oncology Group Performance Status is a commonly used scale to assess how the patient's disease is progressing as well as effects on activities of daily living. ECOG scores tend to correlate with life expectancy and may be used to assist in determining appropriateness of treatment.

Table 2. Eastern Cooperative Oncology Group (ECOG) Performance Status[11]

Grade	ECOG Description
0	Fully active, able to carry on all pre-disease performance without restriction
1	Restricted in physically strenuous activity but ambulatory and able to carry out work of a light or sedentary nature, e.g., light house work, office work
2	Ambulatory and capable of all selfcare but unable to carry out any work activities. Up and about more than 50% of waking hours
3	Capable of only limited selfcare, confined to bed or chair more than 50% of waking hours
4	Completely disabled. Cannot carry on any selfcare. Totally confined to bed or chair.
5	Dead

Guidance for Determination of Hospice Eligibility: Cancer[9,10]
Patient with cancer that meets the following criteria:
- Metastatic cancer with increasing symptoms and/or worsening lab values
- Impaired performance status with a PPS ≤ 70%
- Patient refuses further life-prolonging therapy *or* continues to decline despite disease directed therapy

Supporting documentation includes:
- Hypercalcemia (serum calcium ≥ 12 mg/dL)
  - Corrected calcium = Total calcium (mg/dL) + [4 - serum albumin(g/dL)]*0.8
- Cachexia or weight loss of 5% in the preceding 3 months
- Recurrent disease after surgery/radiation/chemotherapy
- Signs and symptoms of advanced disease (e.g., refractory nausea, requirement for transfusions, malignant ascites, pleural effusion, etc.)

In the absence of one or more of the above criteria, rapid decline or comorbidities may also support the physician's determination of a life expectancy of < 6 months and hospice eligibility. Certification or recertification is based upon a physician's clinical judgment. According to the Benefits Improvement and Protection Act of 2000 (BIPA), hospice certification of terminal illness "shall be based on the physician's or medical director's clinical judgment regarding the normal course of the individual's illness."[10]

Prevalent Symptoms
Patients with cancer experience a complex set of symptoms related to both the physical and psychological impact of the disease. Symptom severity and presentation may be linked to location of primary site of tumor and metastatic disease, history of cancer interventions (surgery, chemotherapy, radiation), and psycho-social situations. For example, bowel obstruction is especially problematic in patients with gastrointestinal or genitourinary cancers while all patients experience pain, dyspnea, fatigue, and anxiety.
- Agitation, see *Agitation & Delirium GEMS*
- Anorexia, see *Anorexia GEMS*
- Anxiety, see *Anxiety GEMS*
- Ascites, see *Ascites & Edema GEMS*
- Bowel obstruction, see *Bowel Obstruction GEMS*
- Constipation, see *Constipation GEMS*
- Depression, see *Depression GEMS*
- Dyspnea, see *Dyspnea GEMS*
- Edema, see *Ascites & Edema GEMS*
- Fatigue, see *Fatigue GEMS*
- Insomnia, see *Insomnia GEMS*
- Nausea, see *Nausea & Vomiting GEMS*
- Pain, see *Pain GEMS*
- Xerostomia, see *Xerostomia GEMS*

Palliative Radiotherapy[12-15]

Palliative radiotherapy can help patients manage symptoms of advanced cancer including pain, neurologic symptoms, and obstructive symptoms. About 50% of patients with cancer receive palliative radiotherapy at some point during the course of illness, with painful bone metastases being the most common symptom treated. See Table 3 for symptoms which may respond to palliative radiotherapy. Always review the options for palliative radiotherapy in the context of patient performance status, expected tolerability of treatment, possible improvement in quality of life, and patient goals of care.

Avoid use of palliative radiotherapy in patients with very poor prognosis due to the delay between delivery of radiotherapy treatment and onset of symptom relief. Standard fractionation can require weeks of daily irradiation appointments which may cause an unreasonable burden on the patient and family. Single fraction radiotherapy may be preferred for many patients to limit the amount of travel and appointments for consultation and treatment applications needed.

Table 3. Palliative Radiotherapy for Symptom Management[13,14]

Symptom	Comment
Bone metastases	Useful for painful bone metastases; not for patients with asymptomatic bone metastases. May reduce need for opioids for pain control. Elderly and younger patients tolerate treatment well.
Spinal cord compression	May be useful for patients who are not good candidates for surgical decompression. Not for patients without pain, with related paralysis > 2 days, compression caused by vertebral body collapse, or if spine is structurally unstable. Elderly and younger patients tolerate treatment well.
Brain metastases	May be useful for patients with higher performance status or life expectancy of at least 2-3 months to provide modest survival benefit or delay in further neurological symptoms.
Dysphagia with esophageal cancer	May be useful if patient can tolerate several weeks of therapy required for meaningful treatment.
Bleeding in various primary malignancy sites	May be useful bleeding and pain and possibly obstructive symptoms in head and neck, genitourinary, and gastrointestinal tumors.

Palliative Chemotherapy[16-20]

According to recent studies, up to 43% of patients are treated with palliative chemotherapy in the last months of their lives. Even the term "palliative chemotherapy" can create misunderstanding among patients, families, and clinicians. An offer of palliative chemotherapy may be with life-prolonging intent, to provide specific symptom management, or to reduce tumor burden and stabilize disease. Treatment may or may not provide palliative symptom management benefit for the patient but often causes undesirable side effects such as nausea, vomiting, weakness, and pain. Patients with advanced cancer receiving aggressive treatment of the disease in the last week of life experienced more physical distress, a lower quality of death, and were less likely to die in their preferred place. ASCO strongly suggests that treatments should not be recommended to patients unless there is evidence that the patient will benefit.

Patients, families, and health care providers must communicate openly about goals of care, risks of toxicity, side effects, and costs associated with palliative chemotherapy. Open communication between the hospice team, patient, caregivers, and the patient's family physician or oncologist is crucial to aid in decision making and maintain focus on patient-centered care. Sample assessment questions (Figure 1) are provided below that can be used to determine whether or not continued chemotherapy use is appropriate and beneficial for the patient.

Figure 1. Palliative Chemotherapy Assessment Questions

1. What is the patient's current status?
    a. ECOG performance status ≤ 3
    b. Primary cancer diagnosis
    c. Sites of metastases
2. What symptom(s) is being palliated?
3. Has the target symptom(s) improved as a result of therapy?
4. What are the potential adverse effects of the therapy?
5. Is the patient able to tolerate these adverse effects, if experienced?
6. How is palliative chemotherapy impacting the patient's quality of life?
7. Will the treatment prolong life beyond 6 months?
8. What clinical indications/symptoms will determine appropriateness to discontinue therapy?
    a. What tests are necessary to evaluate response?
    b. How frequently will testing be required?
    c. What is the expected effectiveness of this medication to palliate the patient's symptom? (including response rate and duration of therapy required)

References

1. National Hospice & Palliative Care Organization (NHPCO). NHPCO's facts and figures: hospice care in America. 2014 edition. Alexandria, VA; NHPCO, October 2014. Available at http://www.nhpco.org/sites/default/files/public/Statistics_Research/2014_Facts_Figures.pdf.
2. Centers for Medicare & Medicaid Services (CMS). Medicare hospice data: Medicare hospice data trends, 1998-2009. April 12, 2013. Available at http://www.cms.gov/Medicare/Medicare-Fee-for-Service-Payment/Hospice/Medicare_Hospice_Data.html. Accessed December 31, 2014.
3. Bentur N, Resnizky S, Balicer R, Eilat-Tsanani T. Quality end-of-life care for cancer patients: dose home hospice care matter? *Am J Manag Care.* 2014;20(12):988-992. Available at http://www.ajmc.com/publications/issue/2014/2014-vol20-n12/quality-of-end-of-life-care-for-cancer-patients-does-home-hospice-care-matter.
4. Smith TJ, Temin S, Alesi ER, Abernethy AP, et al. ASCO provisional clinical opinion: the integration of palliative care into standard oncology care. *J Clin Oncol.* 2012;30(8):880-887. Available at http://www.instituteforquality.org/asco-provisional-clinical-opinion-integration-palliative-care-standard-oncology-care.
5. National Cancer Institute (NCI). Metastatic cancer. March 28, 2013. Available at http://www.cancer.gov/cancertopics/factsheet/Sites-Types/metastatic. Accessed December 31, 2014.
6. Cleveland Clinic. Diseases & Conditions: Metastatic Cancer. Available at http://my.clevelandclinic.org/health/diseases_conditions/metastatic-cancer-can-overview. Accessed December 31, 2014.
7. Glare PA, Sinclair CT. Palliative medicine review: prognostication. *J Palliat Med.* 2008;11(1):84-103.
8. Hui D, Bansal S, Morgado M, Dev R, et al. Phase angle for prognostication of survival in patients with advanced cancer: preliminary findings. *Cancer.* 2014;120(14):2207-2214.
9. Centers for Medicare & Medicaid Services (CMS). Local coverage determination (LCD): hospice determining terminal status. Available at http://www.cms.gov/medicare-coverage- database/details/lcd-details.aspx. Accessed December 18, 2014.
10. Centers for Medicare & Medicaid Services (CMS). Medicare program; hospice care amendments. *Fed Register* 2005;70:FR70532-70548. Available at https://federalregister.gov/a/05-23078.
11. Oken MM, Creech RH, Tormey DC, Horton J, Davis TE, McFadden ET, et al. Toxicity and response criteria of the Eastern Cooperative Oncology Group. *Am J Clin Oncol.* 1982;5:649-55.
12. American Cancer Society (ACS). Radiation therapy principles. October 27, 2014. Available at http://www.cancer.org/treatment/treatmentsandsideeffects/treatmenttypes/radiation/radiationtherapyprinciples/index. Accessed December 31, 2014.
13. Jones JA, Lutz ST, Chow E, Johnstone PA. Palliative radiotherapy at the end of life: a critical review. *CA Cancer J Clin.* 2014;64:295-310.
14. Lutz ST, Korytko T, Nguyen J, et al. Palliative radiotherapy: when is it worth it and when is it not? *Cancer J.* 2010;16:473-482.

15. Gripp S, Mjartan S, Boelke E, Willers R. Palliative radiotherapy tailored to life expectancy in end-stage cancer patients: reality or myth? *Cancer.* 2010;116(13):3251-3256.

16. Nappa U, Linqvist O, Axelsson B. Avoiding harmful palliative chemotherapy treatment in the end of life: Development of a brief patient-completed questionnaire for routine assessment of performance status. *J Support Oncol.* 2012; 20(10):1-8

17. Earle C, Landrum M, Souza M, Neville B, Weeks J, Ayanian J. Aggressiveness of cancer near the end of life: Is it a quality of care issue? *J Clin Oncol.* 2008 Aug 10;26(23):3860-6

18. Silverman GK. Do aggressive treatments in the last week of life harm quality of death? Program and abstracts of the American Geriatrics Society 2007 Annual Scientific Meeting; May 2-6, 2007; Seattle, Washington. Abstract P4.

19. Kadakia KC, Moynihan TJ, Smith TJ, Loprinzi CL. Palliative communications: addressing chemotherapy in patients with advanced cancer. *Ann Oncol.* 2012;23(suppl3):s29-s32.

20. Gonsalves WI, Abuzetun J, Silberstein PT. Palliative chemotherapy: an outdated term for life-prolonging systemic therapies for incurable malignancies. *J Palliat Med.* 2010;13(6):641.

End Stage Heart Disease

Introduction[1-3]
Advanced heart failure, New York Heart Association (NYHA) Class IV or American Heart Association/American College of Cardiology (AHA/ACC) Stage D, is defined as persistent symptoms that limit daily living despite optimal therapy with medications known to provide benefit. About 14% of patients are admitted to hospice with end stage heart disease as a primary diagnosis. Patients have significant cardiac dysfunction with marked symptoms of dyspnea, fatigue, or symptoms relating to end organ hypoperfusion at rest or with minimal exertion despite optimal medical therapy. Advanced care planning should begin at the time of heart failure diagnosis. As with severe pulmonary disease because of the uncertainty of the disease course, discussions about quality of life and prognosis should be an ongoing part of disease management. Once the patient has made the decision for comfort care, discussions and planning for deactivation of implantable defibrillators (IACD) are needed.

Prognosis[4-10]
Expected 1-year mortality of patients with advanced heart failure is 30-50%. Despite optimizing medication and device therapy (IACD and pacemakers), patients with heart failure continue to have a difficult to predict disease trajectory and a relatively high rate of sudden death. Survival at 5 years was only 20% for patients with ACC/AHA stage D heart failure. Elderly patients with stage D heart failure along with other burdensome comorbidities should be offered hospice services.

ACC/AHA Stages of Heart Failure[5-7]
A: Patient at high risk for HF but without structural heart disease or symptoms of HF.
B: Patient with structural heart disease but without signs or symptoms of HF.
C: Patient with structural heart disease with prior or current symptoms of HF.
D: Patient with refractory HF requiring specialized interventions.

NYHA Functional Classification of Heart Failure[5-8]
I: Patient with no limitation of physical activity. Ordinary activity does not cause symptoms of HF.
II: Patient with slight impairment of physical activity. Comfortable at rest, but ordinary activity results in symptoms of HF.
III: Patient with marked limitation of physical activity. Comfortable at rest, but less than ordinary activity causes symptoms of HF.
IV: Patient is unable to carry on any physical activity without symptoms of HF or symptoms (e.g., fatigue, dyspnea, angina) of HF are present at rest.

B-type Natriuretic Peptide (BNP)[9,10]
Serum BNP may be a useful prognostic indicator for patients with HF at all stages of the disease, however BNP has not been directly studied as a component in hospice or palliative care decision-making. BNP levels may correlate with symptoms and possibly with functional capacity. The relative risk of death from HF increases by approximately 35% for each 100 pg/mL rise in BNP. A BNP level greater than 700 pg/mL prior to hospital discharge has been correlated with a risk of death of 31% in 1 month and 93% in 6 months.

Guidance for Determination of Hospice Eligibility: Cardiovascular Disease[11,12]
Patient with severe cardiovascular disease that meets the following criteria:
- Poor response to optimal guideline-directed medical therapy (e.g. diuretics, vasodilators, angiotensin converting enzyme (ACE) inhibitors, hydralazine, nitrates)
- Patient is not a candidate for surgical procedure or has declined offered procedures
- NYHA Class IV HF with significant symptoms of recurrent congestive heart failure (CHF) and/or angina at rest and inability to carry on minimal physical activity or exertion without discomfort, symptoms of heart failure (dyspnea) or angina.

Supporting documentation includes:
- Ejection fraction ≤ 20%
- Treatment resistant symptomatic supraventricular or ventricular arrhythmias
- History of unexplained or cardiac-related syncope

- o   CVA secondary to cardiac embolism
- o   History of cardiac arrest or resuscitation
- o   Concomitant HIV disease

In the absence of one or more of the above criteria, rapid decline or comorbidities may also support the physician's determination of a life expectancy of < 6 months and hospice eligibility. Certification or recertification is based upon a physician's clinical judgment. According to the Benefits Improvement and Protection Act of 2000 (BIPA), hospice certification of terminal illness "shall be based on the physician's or medical director's clinical judgment regarding the normal course of the individual's illness."[12]

Prevalent Symptoms[5,10,13-16]

Patients with end stage cardiac disease and heart failure commonly experience dyspnea, fatigue, anxiety, pain, and edema. Additionally, many symptoms experienced are similar to patients with cancer, including nausea, anorexia, constipation, insomnia, and depression. Dyspnea and pain become the most significant symptoms reported in the last week of life in patients dying from heart failure.

- Anorexia, see *Anorexia GEMS*
- Anxiety, see *Anxiety GEMS*
- Constipation, see *Constipation GEMS*
- Depression, see *Depression GEMS*
- Dyspnea, see *Dyspnea GEMS*
- Fatigue, see *Fatigue GEMS*
- Insomnia, see *Insomnia GEMS*
- Nausea, see *Nausea & Vomiting GEMS*
- Pain, see *Pain GEMS*

Clinical Pearls[6,10,15-19]

- Goals of therapy for patients with stage D (refractory HF) include control of symptoms, improving quality of life, reducing hospital admissions, and establishing patient's end-of-life goals.
- Assess for pulmonary congestion associated with volume overload. Long term use of loop diuretics can lead to enhanced sodium reabsorption from the proximal and distal tubules leading to diuretic resistance.
- Changing route of administration from oral to parenteral, increasing dosing from daily to twice daily, or changing to a different loop diuretic may help overcome resistance. Use of 2 loop diuretics concurrently is not recommended.
- Short term addition of an intermittent thiazide diuretic (metolazone) may enhance diuresis, especially if the patient is requiring oral doses of furosemide exceeding 120mg.
- Consider morphine for patients who fail maximized diuretic or vasodilator therapy and continue to report dyspnea.
- Nebulized furosemide for refractory dyspnea may be effective in patients with HF with a mechanism unrelated to diuresis.
- In hospitalized patients with heart failure, 41% experienced moderate to severe pain in the last 3 days of life. This is comparable to patients with lung or colon cancer.
- Severe pain is second to dyspnea in last 3 days of life. Etiology of pain in heart failure is not entirely understood but may be due to angina and edema, or common comorbid conditions such as arthritis or diabetic neuropathy.
- Due to the risk of worsening peripheral edema, avoid NSAIDs (ibuprofen, naproxen) and COX2 inhibitors (celecoxib). If a corticosteroid is needed, dexamethasone has less mineralocorticoid effect and less risk of associated edema.

Table 1. Medication Considerations in End Stage HF[2,18,19]

Medication Class & Examples	Symptomatic HF Benefit?	Comments
Angiotensin converting enzyme inhibitors (ACE): captopril, lisinopril, enalapril, ramipril	Likely	• Reduced mortality and hospitalizations, equivalent to ARB • Consider discontinuing or dose reduction if symptomatic hypotension is present • Risk of irritating cough, hyperkalemia, angioedema
Angiotensin receptor blockers (ARB): valsartan, candesartan, losartan	Likely	• Reduced mortality and hospitalizations, equivalent to ACE • Consider discontinuing or dose reduction if symptomatic hypotension is present • For patients with ACE intolerance
Beta blockers: bisoprolol, carvedilol, metoprolol	Likely	• Usually not initiated in hospice, but may reduce mortality • Consider dose reduction if bradycardia present • Consider discontinuing or dose reduction if hypotension still present after ACE or ARB stopped
Loop diuretics: furosemide, bumetanide, torsemide	Likely	• Continue for symptom management • Monitor for hypovolemia, dehydration, hypokalemia • Dose adjustments may be necessary to overcome resistance
Thiazide diuretics: metolazone, hydrochlorothiazide	Possibly	• Risk of hypovolemia and electrolyte disturbance • May be helpful to overcome loop diuretic resistance
Vasodilators: hydralazine, nitrates, nitroglycerin	Possibly	• Reduced mortality and hospitalizations • Hydralazine may be more effective in African Americans • Nitrates provide benefit for ischemic chest pain, angina
Aldosterone antagonists: spironolactone, eplerenone	Possibly	• Consider discontinuation • Monitor potassium level; discontinue potassium supplements • Risk of hyperkalemia, especially with renal insufficiency
Cardiac glycoside: digoxin	Limited	• Risk often outweighs benefit; consider discontinuing if any renal insufficiency present • May exacerbate anorexia, confusion, and nausea
Calcium channel blockers: amlodipine, felodipine, verapamil, diltiazem	Limited	• Consider for patients with angina despite treatment with beta-blockers and nitrates (amlodipine, felodipine) • May exacerbate peripheral edema • May help with rate control in patients who cannot tolerate beta-blockers (diltiazem, verapamil)
Antianginal agents: ranolazine	Limited	• Only for chronic, stable angina refractory to optimized beta-blockers, calcium channel blockers, and nitrates • May be discontinued abruptly if patient can no longer swallow or if patient continues to have angina symptoms
Anti-arrhythmics: amiodarone	No benefit	• No clear indication for HF at end of life • Very long half-life, effects may persist for weeks after discontinuation • Avoid in patients with bradycardia • High risk of drug interactions

Managing Pacemakers or Implantable Cardiac Defibrillators (ICDs)[3,10,20-23]

Patients who have pacemakers or implantable cardiac defibrillators (ICDs) to prevent sudden arrhythmic death may ask about deactivation of these devices on hospice admission. Consider the patient's goals of care and life expectancy when discussing options. Some patients with a terminal illness but a life expectancy of weeks to months of acceptable quality of life may choose to accept the risk of a painful ICD shock; other patients may request deactivation at hospice admission or only as their illness progresses. Actively dying patients may develop arrhythmias triggered by electrolyte imbalance or hypoxia. Unless the ICD has been deactivated, the patient will continue to receive painful shocks as the device attempts to restore normal heart rhythm. Pacemakers do not need to be deactivated and will continue to support quality of life by helping to prevent worsening of HF, AV-node block, and syncope. A sample ICD deactivation policy statement is provided in the supplementary materials of reference 23.

Important information patients and families should know includes:

- Deactivating the ICD means that the device will no longer provide life-saving therapy if a fatal heart rhythm occurs. Turning off the ICD means that the device will not prevent sudden death in the event of a dangerous rapid heart rhythm.
- Deactivation of the ICD will not cause death. Although ICDs may prevent sudden death, they do not always prolong life and may worsen symptoms.
- ICD shocks are painful for most people. Deactivating the ICD will not be painful; the patient's death will not be more painful if the ICD is deactivated.
- Some clinicians may be reluctant or simply refuse to deactivate an ICD on the basis of personal beliefs. If the patient and family desire ICD deactivation, they may request a referral to another physician to fulfill this request.

References

1. National Hospice & Palliative Care Organization (NHPCO). NHPCO's facts and figures: hospice care in America. 2014 edition. Alexandria, VA; NHPCO, October 2014. Available at http://www.nhpco.org/sites/default/files/public/Statistics_Research/2014_Facts_Figures.pdf.
2. Caccamo MA, Eckman PM. Pharmacologic therapy for New York Heart Association class IV heart failure. *Congest Heart Fail.* 2011;17(5):213-219.
3. Lewis WR, Luebke DL, Johnson NJ, et al. Withdrawing implantable defibrillator shock therapy in terminally ill patients. *Am J Med* 2006;119:892-896.
4. Stevenson L. Design of therapy for advanced heart failure. *Eur J Heart Fail* 2005;7:323-331.
5. Jessup M, Abraham WT, Casey DE, Feldman AM, et al. 2009 focused update: ACCF/AHA Guidelines for the Diagnosis and Management of Heart Failure in Adults: a report of the American College of Cardiology Foundation/American Heart Association Task Force on Practice Guidelines: developed in collaboration with the International Society for Heart and Lung Transplantation. Circulation 2009;119(14):1977-2016 Available at http://circ.ahajournals.org/content/119/14/1977.long.
6. Yancey CW, Jessup M, Bozkurt B, Butler J, et al. 2013 ACCF/AHA guideline for the management of heart failure. *J Am Coll Cardiol (JACC).* 2013;62(16):147-239. Available at http://linkinghub.elsevier.com/retrieve/pii/S0735-1097(13)02114-1.
7. Ammar KA, Jacobsen SJ, Mahoney DW, Kors JA, et al. Prevalence and prognostic significance of heart failure stages: application of American College of Cardiology/American Heart Association heart failure staging criteria in the community. *Circulation.* 2007;115:1563-1570. Available at http://circ.ahajournals.org/content/115/12/1563.long.
8. Criteria Committee of the New York Heart Association. Nomenclature and criteria for diagnosis of diseases of the heart and great vessels. 9th ed. Boston, MA: Little & Brown; 1994.
9. Doust JA, Pietrzak E, Dobson A, Glasziou P. How well does B-type natriuretic peptide predict death and cardiac events In patients with heart failure: systematic review. BMJ 2005;330:625 Available at http://www.bmj.com/content/330/7492/625.full.pdf+html.
10. Stuart B. Palliative care and hospice in advanced heart failure. *J Palliat Med.* 2007;10(1):210-228.

11. Centers for Medicare & Medicaid Services (CMS). Local coverage determination (LCD): hospice determining terminal status. Available at http://www.cms.gov/medicare-coverage- database/details/lcd-details.aspx. Accessed December 18, 2014.

12. Centers for Medicare & Medicaid Services (CMS). Medicare program; hospice care amendments. *Fed Register* 2005;70:FR70532-70548. Available at https://federalregister.gov/a/05-23078.

13. Zambroski C, Moser D, Roser L. Patients with heart failure who die in hospice. *Am Heart J* 2005;149:558-564.

14. Levenson J, McCarthy E, Lynn J. The last six months of life for patients with congestive heart failure. *J Am Ger Soc* 2000;48 (5 suppl): S101-109.

15. Nordgren L, Sorensen S. Symptoms experienced in the last six months of life in patients with end-stage heart failure. *Eur J Card N* 2003;2:213-217.

16. Zambroski C, Moser D, Bhat G. Impact of symptom prevalence and symptom burden on quality of live in patients with heart failure. *Eur J Card N* 2005;4:198-206.

17. Kohara H, Ueoka H, Aoe K, et al. Effect of nebulized furosemide in terminally ill cancer patients with dyspnea. *J Pain Symptom Manage* 2003;26:962-967.

18. Foley P. Heart failure. First Consult, ClinicalKey [Internet]. Available at https://www.clinicalkey.com/#!/content/medical_topic/21-s2.0-1014218. January 30, 2014. Accessed January 12, 2015.

19. Lexi-Comp Online, Lexi-Drugs Online, Hudson, OH: Lexi-Comp, Inc. Accessed December 28, 2014.

20. Lampert, R, Hayes DL., Annas, GJ, et. al. HRS Expert Consensus Statement on the Management of Cardiovascular Implantable Electronic Devices (CIEDs) in patients nearing end of life or requesting withdrawal of therapy. *Heart Rhythm*; 2010; 7(7):1008-1026.

21. Morrison LJ, Calvin AO, Nora H, Storey CP. Managing cardiac devices near end of life: a survey of hospice and palliative care providers. *Am J Hosp Palliat Med* 2010;27(8):545-551.

22. Russo JE. Deactivation of ICDs at end of life: a systematic review of clinical practices and provider and patient attitudes. *Am J Nurs.* 2011;111(10):26-35.

23. Goldstein N, Carlson M, Livote E, Kutner JS. Management of implantable defibrillators in hospice. *Ann Intern Med.* 2010;152(5):296-299. Available http://annals.org/article.aspx?articleid=745635.

Chronic Obstructive Pulmonary Disease

Introduction[1,2]

Patients with end stage lung disease comprise about 10% of hospice admissions annually.[1] Most of those patients have chronic obstructive pulmonary disease (COPD) with a slow decline, punctuated by periods of exacerbation or crisis. After each symptom crisis, patients generally return to a lower baseline of function compared to before the exacerbation. Accurate prognostication of life expectancy in very severe COPD is challenging. When COPD progression can no longer be slowed and bronchodilators have limited effectiveness, the focus changes to management of symptoms and quality of life.

Prognosis[2-9]

Reported statistics for patient death after hospitalization for a COPD exacerbation ranges between 23% and 80%.[2] Assessment of patients with COPD should include symptom impact on quality of life, degree of airflow limitation with spirometry, risk of exacerbations, and comorbidities. Validated assessment questionnaires that measure the impact of COPD symptoms on quality of life, such as the COPD Assessment Test (CAT), the British Medical Research Council (mMRC) breathlessness have been developed.[2] The body-mass index, airflow obstruction, dyspnea, and exercise capacity (BODE) index correlates scores with longer term (12 - 52 month) mortality, but doesn't predict shorter term mortality risk as is needed for hospice eligibility prognostication. Severity staging from these tests contribute supportive evidence for appropriateness of patients for hospice care.

Global Initiative for Chronic Obstructive Lung Disease (GOLD)[2]
- Classifies airflow limitation based on FEV1 following bronchodilator use
- GOLD1 (mild disease) – GOLD4 (very severe disease)
- GOLD4 3-year mortality is 24%

mMRC Questionnaire for Assessing the Severity of Breathlessness[4,5]
- Assesses the severity of breathlessness as reported by the patient
- Can predict future mortality risk
- Scale: 0 ("I only get breathless with strenuous exercise") - 4 ("I am too breathless to leave the house or I am breathless while dressing or undressing") scale

BODE Index[6]
- Scores severity of 4 components to predict mortality at 12, 24, 52 months
- Clinician scores based on FEV1, BMI, mMRC, and 6 minute walking test
- Higher scores correlate to higher mortality risk

COPD Assessment Test (CAT) [8,9]
- 8 item test to measure the impact of COPD on the patient's daily life
- Patient self-administers
- Developed by GlaxoSmithKline

Table 1. GOLD Combined Assessment of COPD[2]

Patient	Characteristic	Spirometric Classification	Exacerbations per Year	mMRC Score	CAT Score
A	Low Risk Less Symptoms	GOLD 1-2	≤ 1	0-1	<10
B	Low Risk More Symptoms	GOLD 1-2	≤ 1	≥ 2	≥ 10
C*	High Risk Less Symptoms	GOLD 3-4	≥ 2	0-1	< 10
D*	High Risk More Symptoms	GOLD 3-4	≥ 2	≥ 2	≥ 10

Highest risk of hospitalization and/or mortality

Guidance for Determination of Hospice Eligibility: COPD[10,11]
Patient with severe COPD that meets the following criteria:
- o Disabling dyspnea at rest or with minimal exertion
- o Little or no response to bronchodilator medications
- o Decreased functional capacity (e.g. bed to chair existence, fatigue and cough)
- o Progression of disease (e.g., recent history of increasing physician office or emergency visits and/or hospitalizations for pulmonary infection and/or respiratory failure)

Documentation within the past 3 months of one or more of the following:
- o Hypoxemia at rest on room air (p02 ≤ 55 mmHg by ABG) or oxygen saturation ≤ 88%
- o Hypercapnia evidenced by pCO2 ≥ 50 mmHg

Supporting documentation includes:
- o Cor pulmonale and right heart failure secondary to pulmonary disease
- o Unintentional weight loss > 10% of body weight over the preceding 6 months
- o Resting tachycardia > 100 bpm

In the absence of one or more of the above criteria, rapid decline or comorbidities may also support the physician's determination of a life expectancy of < 6 months and hospice eligibility. Certification or recertification is based upon a physician's clinical judgment. According to the Benefits Improvement and Protection Act of 2000 (BIPA), hospice certification of terminal illness "shall be based on the physician's or medical director's clinical judgment regarding the normal course of the individual's illness."[11]

Prevalent Symptoms
Patients with COPD experience a complex set of symptoms related to the physical and psychological impact of the disease.
- Agitation, see *Agitation & Delirium GEMS*
- Anxiety, see *Anxiety GEMS*
- Cough, see *Cough GEMS*
- Depression, see *Depression GEMS*
- Dyspnea, see *Dyspnea GEMS*
- Fatigue, see *Fatigue GEMS*
- Infection, see *Infection GEMS*
- Insomnia, see *Insomnia GEMS*
- Pain, see *Pain GEMS*

Non-Pharmacological Management
- Providing an over the bed table will help allow patients to position themselves more comfortably in bed. Patients can physically expand the chest cavity by tripod positioning (head up with support on elbows and arms).
- Circulation of cool air, avoidance of closed-in spaces, minimizing odors, and providing visual signs of air movement such as ribbons tied to fans can help reduce the patient's sense of suffocation.
- Psychosocial, emotional, and spiritual support from members of the interdisciplinary team is helpful in reducing fear, anxiety, and depression.
- Consider oxygen therapy for any patient with chronic hypoxemia and during periods of exacerbation.

Medications for Management of COPD[12, 13]
Optimizing medication use, especially inhalers, is challenging in severe and end stage COPD. As a patient's disease progresses, the ability to effectively use inhalers decreases. Additionally, patients with poor dexterity or cognitive impairment have an added layer of difficulty with inhaler use. Patients must be able to understand the difference between their controller medications and their rescue inhalers and be able to decide when to use each medication (Table 2). Nebulized medications and oral corticosteroids can help reduce symptoms and do not rely on patient inhaler technique for delivery of medication. Patients with functional or cognitive impairments will still require assistance in preparation, use, and maintenance of the nebulizer device.

Table 3 lists inhaler devices currently available in the U.S. market. Each manufacturer tends to develop a specialized device for delivery of their proprietary medications. As medications become available as generics, the inhaler device used to deliver the medication may be different than in the former proprietary inhaler. Table 4 provides general guidance for assessing a patient's inhaler technique for dry powder inhalers (DPI) and metered dose inhalers (MDI). Each type of device, DPI or MDI, follows different preparation and use instructions; patients frequently have both types of devices. Valved chambers, or spacers, are recommended for use with all MDIs for most efficient use, especially if timing the spray with inhalation is difficult. Patients using valved chambers with MDIs still need to breathe correctly and be able to follow use instructions for each device they are prescribed.

Table 2. Controller vs Rescue Medications

Controller Medications	Rescue Medications
Goal: To reduce COPD-related inflammation and bronchoconstriction • Used on a scheduled basis • Usually longer-acting medications • Risk of adverse effects with overuse • Inhalers and nebulizers (inhaled corticosteroids, long-acting beta agonists, long-acting anti-cholinergics) • Oral medications (theophylline, prednisone, dexamethasone)	*Goal:* To quickly provide bronchodilation and reduce dyspnea and wheezing • Commonly used "as needed" (PRN) • May be used ATC • Risk of adverse effects with overuse • Usually shorter-acting medications • Inhalers and nebulizers (albuterol, ipratropium)

Table 3. DPI and MDI Inhaler Devices[13]

Device Name	Type	Medications
Aerolizer®	DPI	Formoterol (Foradil®)
Diskus®	DPI	Fluticasone (Flovent®), salmeterol (Serevent®), salmeterol-fluticasone (Advair®),
Ellipta®	DPI	Fluticasone-vilanterol (Breo®), umeclidinium (Incruse®), umeclidinium-vilanterol (Anoro®)
Flexhaler®	DPI	Budesonide (Pulmicort®)
Handihaler®	DPI	Tiotropium (Spiriva®)
Neohaler®	DPI	Indacaterol (Arcapta®)
Pressair®	DPI	Aclidinium (Tudorza®)
Respimat®	MDI	Ipratropium-albuterol (Combivent®), olodaterol (Striverdi®), tiotropium (Spiriva®)
Twisthaler®	DPI	Mometasone (Asmanex®)
Traditional inhalers (CFC-free, HFA)	MDI	Ipratropium (Atrovent®), levalbuterol (Xopenex®), albuterol (Ventolin®, Proventil®, Proair®), beclomethasone (QVAR®), budesonide-formoterol (Symbicort®), ciclesonide (Alvesco®), flunisolide (Aerospan®), fluticasone (Flovent®), mometasone (Asmanex®), mometasone-formoterol (Dulera®), salmeterol-fluticasone (Advair®)

Table 4. Assessing the Patient's Ability to Use Inhalers

Dry Powder Inhaler (DPI)	Metered Dose Inhaler (MDI)
For efficient use, patient must be able to:	*For efficient use, patient must be able to:*
1. **Follow instructions to prepare specific DPI device for use**	1. **Follow instructions to prepare specific MDI device for use**
2. Turn head away from device to exhale completely	2. Shake inhaler, if appropriate, and hold properly
3. Close mouth around mouthpiece	3. Position for open airway inhalation
4. Inhale forcefully, steadily, and deeply to propel medicated powder into lungs	4. Exhale completely
5. Hold breath for 10 seconds	5. Close mouth around device mouthpiece
6. Remove DPI from mouth and exhale slowly	6. Activate inhaler device timed to start of inspiration
7. Repeat steps 1-6 if more than 1 inhalation is prescribed	7. Slowly and deeply inhale medication over 5-7 seconds
	8. Hold breath for 10 seconds
	9. Wait 1 minute and repeat steps 2-8 if more than 1 inhalation is ordered

Always review device specific instructions prior to assessing or teaching the patient

Clinical Pearls

- In general, patients with end stage COPD no longer have the ability to use inhalers correctly due to lack of breath control. Administering medications using a nebulizer does not require additional breathing effort from the patient. Also, nebulized medications do not require patients to coordinate activation of device and inspiratory breath, or to hold breath while waiting for the inhaled medication to deposit in the lungs.
- Oral corticosteroids, such as prednisone or dexamethasone, may be more effective than inhaled corticosteroids. Oral corticosteroids can also palliate associated symptoms by increasing appetite and helping with fatigue and inflammatory pain.
- Low, non-sedating doses of benzodiazepines, such as lorazepam, scheduled around-the-clock (ATC) and on an as needed (PRN) basis will help reduce the anxiety component which can exacerbate the sensation of dyspnea.
- Normal saline via nebulizer, offered as frequently as the patient would like, provides moisture to the airways and gives the individual the feeling that they are "doing something" to help with breathing.
- Patients with end stage pulmonary disease should receive the seasonal influenza vaccine.

References

1. National Hospice & Palliative Care Organization (NHPCO). NHPCO's facts and figures: hospice care in America. 2014 edition. Alexandria, VA; NHPCO, October 2014. Available at http://www.nhpco.org/sites/default/files/public/Statistics_Research/2014_Facts_Figures.pdf.
2. Global Initiative for Chronic Obstructive Lung Disease (GOLD). Global strategy for the diagnosis, management, and prevention of chronic obstructive pulmonary disease (updated 2014). GOLD, Inc. 2014. Available from http://www.goldcopd.org. Accessed December 31, 2014.
3. Abrahm J, Hansen-Flaschen J. Hospice care for patients with advanced lung disease. Chest 2002;121:220-229. Available from http://publications.chestnet.org/data/Journals/CHEST/21972/220.pdf
4. Bestall J, Paul E, Garrod R, Garnham R, Jones P, Wedzicha J. Usefulness of the Medical Research Council (MRC) dsypnoea scale as a measure of disability in patients with chronic obstructive pulmonary disease. *Thorax* 1999;54:581-586.
5. Stenton C. the MRC breathlessness scale. Occup Med 2008;58(3):226-227. Available from http://occmed.oxfordjournals.org/content/58/3/226.full#F1
6. Celli B, Cote C, Marin J, Casanova C, Montes de Oca M, et al. The body mass index, airflow obstruction, dyspnea, and exercise capacity index (BODE Index) in chronic obstructive pulmonary disease. *N Engl J Med* 2004;350(10):1005-1012. Available from http://www.nejm.org/doi/full/10.1056/NEJMoa021322
7. Nishmura K, Izumi T, Tsukino M, Oga T. Dyspnea is a better predictor of 5-year survival than airway obstruction in patients with COPD. *Chest* 2002; 121:1434-40.

8. COPD Assessment Test (CAT). Healthcare professional user guide. GlaxoSmithKline, Inc. 2012. Available from http://www.catestonline.org/images/pdfs/CATest.pdf

9. Jones PW, Harding G, Berry P, Wiklund I, et al. Development and first validation of the COPD assessment test (CAT). *Eur Respir J* 2009;34:648-54

10. Centers for Medicare & Medicaid Services (CMS). Local coverage determination (LCD): hospice determining terminal status. Available at http://www.cms.gov/medicare-coverage- database/details/lcd-details.aspx. Accessed December 18, 2014.

11. Centers for Medicare & Medicaid Services (CMS). Medicare program; hospice care amendments. *Fed Register* 2005;70:FR70532-70548. Available at https://federalregister.gov/a/05-23078.

12. Barrons R, Pegram A, Borries A. Inhaler device selection: special considerations in elderly patient with chronic obstructive pulmonary disease. *Am J Health-Syst Pharm.* 2011;68:1221-1232.

13. Lexi-Comp Online, Lexi-Drugs Online, Hudson, OH: Lexi-Comp, Inc. Accessed December 28, 2014.

Dementia

Introduction[1-3]

Dementia is a term for diseases that cause progressive loss of memory, cognitive function impairment, and changes in behavior. Dementia is caused by damage to the neurons, eventually leading to loss of function and cell death. Alzheimer's disease (AD) is the most common type of dementia. According to NHPCO, patients with a terminal diagnosis of dementia make up about 15% of hospice admissions, the highest percentage of all non-cancer admitting diagnoses. Approximately two-thirds of patients with dementia die in nursing homes. Table 1 provides characteristics of AD and other types of dementia.

Table 1. Types of Dementia[1,4]

Type	Characteristics
Alzheimer's disease (AD)	Most common type: 60-80% of patients with dementia have AD; often other types of dementia are also present; slowly progressive brain disease caused by accumulation of amyloid plaques and neurofibrillary tangles (NFT); average life expectancy of 4-8 years after diagnosis
Creutzfeldt-Jakob disease (CJD)	Rare and rapidly fatal; caused by an abnormal protein like substance (prion); may be hereditary or resulting from prion infection (variant CJD)
Frontotemporal lobe dementia	Includes Pick's disease, corticobasal degeneration, and progressive supranuclear palsy; initial symptoms are often distinct personality and behavioral changes with less effect on memory than in AD; develop in patients < 60 years of age
Lewy body dementia (LBD)	Patients may experience symptoms common to AD but also with some Parkinsonian features (gait imbalance, rigidity); patients often have visual hallucinations and sleep disturbances; development of cognitive impairment tends to happen before motor impairment
Mixed dementia	Symptoms of multiple types of dementia may be present, frequently vascular dementia or LBD combined with AD; about 50% of patients with dementia have a mixed etiology
Normal pressure hydrocephalus (NPH)	Symptoms include difficulty walking and gait disturbances, memory loss, and bladder incontinence; caused by impaired reabsorption of cerebrospinal fluid leading to increased fluid accumulation in the brain; NPH may be corrected with placement of a ventricular-peritoneal shunt
Parkinson's disease dementia (PDD)	Motor disorders of Parkinson's disease present first caused by degeneration of dopamine-producing are of the brain (substantia nigra); as Parkinson's progresses Lewy bodies, amyloid plaques, and NFTs may develop and accumulate causing progressive dementia.
Vascular dementia	Also called post-stroke or multi-infarct dementia; about 10% of patients with dementia; caused by brain injury following hemorrhage or thrombosis in the brain; commonly coexists with AD
Wernicke-Korsakoff syndrome	Chronic memory disorder (Korsakoff syndrome) caused by severe thiamine deficiency usually related to heavy alcohol use; this syndrome may follow an episode of encephalopathy (Wernicke's encephalopathy); also associated with AIDS, chronic infections, and poor nutrition

Prognosis[5-10]

Predicting 6-month survival in patients with advanced dementia seems to be more difficult than other terminal diagnoses. Although the various types of dementia present with clinical differences in earlier stages, the end result is loss of cognition, complete functional dependency, frailty, cachexia, and recurrent infections. The most commonly used predictor of 6-month mortality is the eligibility guidance criteria from NHPCO which is based on the Functional Assessment Staging (FAST) score and comorbidities. Other tools may provide additional supportive assessments of mortality risk for patients in nursing homes by including information from the Minimum Data Set (MDS) – the Mortality Risk Index (MRI) and its successor, the Advanced Dementia Prognostic Tool (ADEPT). Regardless of the prognostication method used, the need for quality palliative care for patients with dementia is great. Care must be provided based on patient and family goals for comfort rather than mortality risk estimates.

Functional Assessment Staging (FAST)[6]

Stage	Description
1	No difficulties
2	Forgetting location of objects; work difficulties
3	Decreased work functioning; noticeable to coworkers
4	Decreased ability to perform complex tasks (planning dinner, handling finances)
5	Requires assistance to choose proper clothing for season/weather
6a	Difficulty putting clothing on properly
6b	Unable to bathe properly; may develop fear of bathing
6c	Inability to handle mechanics of toileting (forgetting to flush, clean up properly)
6d	Urinary incontinence
6e	Fecal incontinence
7a	Ability to speak limited to 1 – 5 words per day
7b	All intelligible vocabulary lost
7c	Nonambulatory
7d	Unable to sit up independently
7e	Unable to smile
7f	Unable to hold head up

Note: the FAST score was developed for patients with Alzheimer's dementia and has not been validated for use in other types of dementia.

Mortality Risk Index (MRI)[5] & Advanced Dementia Prognostic Tool (ADEPT)[7]

The MRI and ADEPT composite scoring tools predicting risk of death in nursing home residents based on the MDS. In the study describing the development and validation of the MRI, 70% of patients with an MRI score of 12 or greater died within 6 months. Components of the MRI include an Activities of Daily Living (ADL) score, history of cancer or heart failure, bowel incontinence, poor nutritional intake, age greater than 83 years, bedbound status, and limited time awake during the day. The ADEPT study modified the MRI with additional components of recent nursing home admission, stratified age of resident in 5-year increments, presence of pressure ulcers, and body mass index (BMI) less than 18.5. The complete studies and scoring tools are available online; see References 5 and 7.

Guidance for Determination of Hospice Eligibility: Dementia[11,12]
End stage dementia demonstrated by:
- o FAST score of 7 or beyond
- o Unable to ambulate without assistance
- o Unable to dress without assistance
- o Unable to bathe without assistance
- o Urinary and fecal incontinence, intermittent or constant
- o No consistently meaningful verbal communication (stereotypical phrases only or speech is limited to 6 or fewer intelligible words)

End stage dementia is present; patient has 1 of the following within the past 12 months:
- o Aspiration pneumonia
- o Pyelonephritis or other upper urinary tract infection
- o Septicemia
- o Pressure ulcers, multiple, stage 3-4
- o Fever, recurrent after antibiotics
- o Inability to maintain sufficient fluid and calorie intake; 10% weight loss during the previous 6 months or serum albumin <2.5 g/dL

These criteria, particularly FAST scoring, are specific for Alzheimer's disease and may not fit other types of dementia, such as vascular dementia. In the absence of one or more of the above criteria, rapid decline or comorbidities may also support the physician's determination of a life expectancy of < 6 months and hospice eligibility. Certification or recertification is based upon a physician's clinical judgment. According to the Benefits Improvement and Protection Act of 2000 (BIPA), hospice certification of terminal illness "shall be based on the physician's or medical director's clinical judgment regarding the normal course of the individual's illness."[12]

Prevalent Symptoms

- Agitation, see *Agitation & Delirium GEMS*
- Anorexia, see *Anorexia GEMS*
- Dysphagia, see *Dysphagia GEMS*
- Dyspnea, see *Dyspnea GEMS*
- Infections, see *Infections GEMS*
- Insomnia, see *Insomnia GEMS*
- Pain, see *Pain GEMS*
- Seizures, see *Seizures GEMS*

Clinical Pearls[13-15]

- Because of the limited effectiveness of drug treatments for dementia and related behavioral and psychological symptoms of dementia (BPSD), management must focus on non-pharmacological interventions.
  - Limited evidence supports aromatherapy and music therapy for agitation in patients with dementia.
  - Multisensory stimulation therapy (Snoezelen®) study results are mixed with no apparent long-term effect on mood or behaviors, but immediate and short-term improvement may be seen.
  - Teach caregivers problem solving strategies, communication techniques, and activities and task engagement to improve patient-caregiver interactions.
- Currently, no medications are FDA-approved to treat BPSD. Fully assess patient and address unmet needs (e.g., pain, hunger, thirst, toileting, injury, illness) prior to implementing medications to control behaviors.
- A combination medication, memantine-donepezil (Namzaric®), was FDA-approved in late 2014. There are no studies demonstrating improved efficacy over administration of the individual medications, but adherence may be improved with simpler daily dosing.
- Antipsychotic medications, both conventional and atypical, have FDA black box warnings for increased risk of mortality in elderly patients with dementia-related psychosis.
- When selecting medications for patients with dementia, avoid anti-cholinergic medications if possible. For patients with mild-moderate dementia, anti-cholinergic medications can counteract the benefit of cholinesterase inhibitors for cognition. See Table 3 for medications to avoid and their alternatives for patients with dementia.
- Anti-cholinergic medications can worsen cognitive impairment, and contribute to dry mouth, constipation, urinary retention, and sedation.

Table 2. Medication for Management of Dementia[14]

Medication (Brand)	Dosage Forms	Usual Dose Range	FDA Indications
Acetylcholinesterase Inhibitors: inhibits hydrolysis of acetylcholine to increase acetylcholine available for synaptic transmission in the central nervous system.			
Donepezil (Aricept®)	Tablets; oral disintegrating tablets	10-23mg daily	Treatment of mild, moderate, or severe Alzheimer's dementia
Galantamine (Razadyne®)	24-hour ER capsule; oral solution; tablets	IR tabs, solution: 8-12mg BID ER capsules: 16-24mg daily	Treatment of mild to moderate Alzheimer's dementia
Rivastigmine (Exelon®)	Capsules; oral solution; transdermal patch	Oral: 3-6mg BID Patch: 9.5mg daily	Treatment of mild, moderate, or severe Alzheimer's dementia; mild to moderate Parkinson's dementia
NMDA Receptor Antagonists: blocks excessive NMDA receptor stimulation thought to occur as part of pathogenesis of Alzheimer's disease. Only effects receptor under excessive stimulation, will not affect normal neuronal transmission.			
Memantine (Namenda®)	24-hour ER capsule; oral solution; tablets	IR tabs and solution: 10mg BID ER capsules: 14-28mg daily	Treatment of moderate to severe Alzheimer's dementia

Table 3. Medication Selection for Patients with Dementia[15]

Medication to Avoid	Alternative to Consider
Antidepressants	
Amitriptyline, doxepin, amoxapine, clomipramine	• Avoid tricyclic antidepressants with the most AC activity. • Sertraline is preferred SSRI for depression or generalized anxiety. • Trazodone or mirtazapine for sleep or anxiety. • Desipramine, nortriptyline may be used for neuropathic pain.
Anti-emetics	
Dimenhydrinate, promethazine, meclizine, trimethobenzamide	• Avoid anti-emetics with AC activity, if possible. • Metoclopramide, haloperidol, prochlorperazine may be used in lower doses. • Ondansetron may be useful for post-op or chemo-induced nausea.
Anti-parkinsonism agents	
Benztropine, trihexyphenidyl	• For antipsychotic side effects decrease antipsychotic dose and change to an atypical antipsychotic.
Antipsychotics	
Chlorpromazine, clozapine	• Many, if not all, behaviors associated with dementia result from an unmet patient need; fully assess patient for pain, hunger, fear, toileting need, loneliness and manage appropriately prior to use of antipsychotic medications. • All antipsychotics increase risk of mortality in elderly patients with dementia and none are FDA-approved to manage BPSD. • Always use non-pharmacological approaches prior to initiating antipsychotic medications; continue non-pharmacological approach during antipsychotic medication use. • Haloperidol, risperidone, quetiapine are most well studied, if needed.
Anxiolytics	
Long-acting benzodiazepines	• SSRIs or buspirone will treat generalized anxiety. • If buspirone is chosen to help manage generalized anxiety, schedule the dose twice daily; PRN use is not effective. • If benzodiazepine is needed, consider shorter-acting (lorazepam preferred).

AC = anti-cholinergic

References

1. Alzheimer's Association. 2014 Alzheimer's disease facts and figures: includes a special report on women and Alzheimer's disease. Chicago, IL; Alzheimer's Association, 2014. Available at http://www.alz.org/alzheimers_disease_facts_and_figures.asp.
2. National Hospice & Palliative Care Organization (NHPCO). NHPCO's facts and figures: hospice care in America. 2014 edition. Alexandria, VA; NHPCO, October 2014. Available at http://www.nhpco.org/sites/default/files/public/Statistics_Research/2014_Facts_Figures.pdf.
3. Mitchell SL, Teno JM, Miller SC, Mor V. National study of the location of death for older persons with dementia. *J Am Geriatr Soc.* 2005;53:299-305.
4. National Institute of Neurological Disorders and Stroke (NINDS). Disorders A-Z. Bethesda, MD; National Institutes of Health. Available http://www.ninds.nih.gov/disorders/disorder_index.htm.
5. Mitchell SL, Kiely DK, Hamel MB, Park PS, et al. Estimating prognosis for nursing home residents with advanced dementia. *JAMA.* 2004;291;2734-2740. Available at http://jama.jamanetwork.com/article.aspx?articleid=198894.
6. Reisberg B. Functional assessment staging (FAST). *Psychopharmacol Bull.* 1988;24(4):653-659.
7. Mitchell SL, Miller SC, Teno JM, Kiely DK, et al. Prediction of 6-month survival of nursing home residents with advanced dementia using ADEPT and hospice eligibility guidelines. *JAMA.* 2010;304(17):1929-1935. Available at http://jama.jamanetwork.com/article.aspx?articleid=186837.

8. Aminoff BZ, Adunsky A. Their last 6 months: suffering and survival of end-stage dementia patients. *Age Aging* 2006;35:597-601.

9. Olson E. Dementia and neurodegenerative disorders. In: Morrison RS, Meier DE, eds. *Geriatric Palliative Care*. New York, NY: Oxford University Press; 2003.

10. Sekerak RJ, Stewart JT. Caring for patients with end stage dementia. Ann Long Term Care. 2014;22(12): 36-42. Available at http://www.annalsoflongtermcare.com/article/caring-patient-end-stage-dementia.

11. Centers for Medicare & Medicaid Services (CMS). Local coverage determination (LCD): hospice determining terminal status. Available at http://www.cms.gov/medicare-coverage- database/details/lcd-details.aspx. Accessed December 18, 2014.

12. Centers for Medicare & Medicaid Services (CMS). Medicare program; hospice care amendments. *Fed Register* 2005;70:FR70532-70548. Available at https://federalregister.gov/a/05-23078.

13. O'Neill ME, Freeman M, Christensen V, Telerant R, et al. Systematic evidence review of non-pharmacological interventions for behavioral symptoms of dementia. Evidence-based synthesis program. VA-ESP Project 05-225; 2011. Available at http://www.ncbi.nlm.nih.gov/books/NBK54971/.

14. Lexi-Drugs Online. Hudson, OH; Lexi-Comp, Inc. Accessed December 18, 2014.

15. Pharmacotherapy choices for patients with dementia. *Pharmacist's Letter/Prescriber's Letter* 2008;24(5):240510.

End Stage Liver Disease

Introduction[1,2]

According to NHPCO statistics, patients with a terminal diagnosis of end stage liver disease (ESLD) compose just over 2% of hospice admissions annually. Patients with ESLD gradually experience an increase in disability, fatigue, changes in mental status, and protein-wasting. The gradual progression is often interspersed with periods of exacerbations of hepatic encephalopathy, variceal bleeding, or severe infection.

Prognosis[3-6]

The Model for End Stage Liver Disease (MELD) and the Child-Turcotte-Pugh scoring systems may be used independently and as a combined risk assessment process for mortality in patients with liver disease. MELD was initially designed to assess short-term mortality in patients with cirrhosis undergoing a transjugular intrahepatic portosystemic shunts (TIPS) procedure. It has since been validated to predict survival in patients with varying levels of liver disease in both inpatient and ambulatory care settings and has become the basis for allocating and prioritizing organs for liver transplantation. Child-Turcotte-Pugh (CTP) can predict survival outcomes in patients with portal hypertension and cirrhosis. CTP calculation is based on a simple point summary of 5 liver disease related parameters and estimates risk of death at 3-month, 1 year, and 2 year intervals.

Estimated 3-month Mortality by MELD Score					
MELD score	≤9	10-19	20-29	30-39	≥40
Hospitalized	4%	27%	76%	83%	100%
Outpatient	2%	6%	50%	No data	No data

MELD Score = $[9.57 \times \log_e(creatinine)] + [3.78 \times \log_e(total\ bilirubin)] + [11.2 \times \log_e (INR) + 6.43]$

A MELD score calculator is available at:

http://www.mayoclinic.org/medical-professionals/model-end-stage-liver-disease/

Child-Turcotte-Pugh (CTP) Classification for Severity of Cirrhosis			
Criteria	**Points***		
	1	**2**	**3**
Encephalopathy	None	Mild-moderate (grade 1 or 2)	Severe (grade 3 or 4)
Ascites	None	Mild-moderate (diuretic responsive)	Severe (diuretic refractory)
Bilirubin (mg/dL)	< 2	2-3	>3
Albumin (g/dL)	>3.5	2.8-3.5	<2.8
Prothombin Time/ International Normalized Ratio (PT/INR)	<4 seconds prolonged <1.7 INR	4-6 seconds prolonged 1.7-2.3 INR	>6 seconds prolonged >2.3 INR
Class A	5 – 6 points (least severe disease)		
Class B	7 – 9 points (moderately severe disease)		
Class C	10 – 15 points (severe disease): *score > 13 predict 3-month mortality of 40%*		

Point scores from each of the 5 criteria are added to determine severity classification (A, B, or C)

Guidance for Determination of Hospice Eligibility: Liver Disease[7,8]
End stage liver disease as demonstrated by:
- Prothrombin time (PT) prolonged more than 5 seconds over International Normalized Ratio (INR) >1.5
- Serum albumin <2.5 g/dL

End-stage liver disease is present; the patient has 1 or more of the following conditions:
- Ascites, refractory to treatment or patient is non-compliant
- History of spontaneous bacterial peritonitis
- Hepatorenal syndrome (elevated creatinine and BUN; oliguria <400 mL/day) and urine sodium concentration <10 mEq/L
- Hepatic encephalopathy, refractory to treatment or patient is non-compliant
- Recurrent variceal bleeding despite therapy or patient declines sclerosing therapy

Supporting documentation includes:
- Progressive malnutrition
- Muscle wasting with reduced strength
- Ongoing alcoholism (> 5-6 drinks/day)
- Hepatocellular carcinoma
- Hepatitis B surface antigen positive
- Hepatitis C refractory to interferon treatment

Patients eligible and waiting for liver transplant may be admitted to hospice but should be discharged in the event that a donor organ is procured. In the absence of one or more of the above criteria, rapid decline or comorbidities may also support the physician's determination of a life expectancy of < 6 months and hospice eligibility. Certification or recertification is based upon a physician's clinical judgment. According to the Benefits Improvement and Protection Act of 2000 (BIPA), hospice certification of terminal illness "shall be based on the physician's or medical director's clinical judgment regarding the normal course of the individual's illness."[8]

Prevalent Symptoms[9-11]
Patients with ESLD report a high symptom burden. Advanced cirrhosis is complicated with ascites, hepatic encephalopathy (HE), and bleeding. Grading of HE is provided in Table 1; medications to manage ammonia levels in HE are in Table 2. Most common symptoms reported were pain, nausea, depression, anxiety, dyspnea, fatigue, pruritus, and anorexia. According to patient reports, lack of energy, nausea, and pain are the most distressing symptoms with the most impact on quality of life. See chapters below for additional information on symptom management.
- Anorexia, see *Anorexia GEMS*
- Anxiety, see *Anxiety GEMS*
- Ascites, see *Ascites & Edema GEMS*
- Depression, see *Depression GEMS*
- Dyspnea, see *Dyspnea GEMS*
- Fatigue, see *Fatigue GEMS*
- Nausea, see *Nausea & Vomiting GEMS*
- Pain, see *Pain GEMS*
- Pruritus, see *Pruritus GEMS*

Table 1. West Haven Criteria for Grading Hepatic Encephalopathy[12]

Grade 1	Grade 3
• Trivial lack of awareness • Euphoria or anxiety • Shortened attention span • Impaired performance of addition	• Somnolence to semi-stupor, but responsive to verbal stimuli • Confusion • Gross disorientation
Grade 2	**Grade 4**
• Lethargy or apathy • Minimal disorientation for time or place • Subtle personality change • Inappropriate behavior • Impaired performance of subtraction	• Coma (unresponsive to verbal or noxious stimuli)

Clinical Pearls[2,4,9-12]

- The liver plays a key role in the metabolism of medications and low serum albumin related to cirrhosis reduces the amount of protein-drug binding thereby increasing drug exposure. Keep medication profiles as simple as possible. Patients with ESLD have a higher risk of adverse effects and toxicity related to medications.
- Patients with ESLD are at high risk of upper GI bleeding from esophageal varices and an overall increased risk of bleeding from failure of the liver to produce sufficient clotting factors. Always review the medication profile to remove medications associated with an increased risk of bleeding, GI ulceration, or with antiplatelet activity.
- Increased bowel movements necessary to reduce intestinal ammonia can be very burdensome on the patient and caregivers. Discuss caregiving needs and capabilities prior to initiating aggressive HE management plans.
- Systemic absorption of oral neomycin is about 3%, with doses above 15mg/kg/day (about 1000mg in a 70kg person) the risk of renal and oto-toxicity is increased.
- Additional medications: metronidazole (Flagyl®), vancomycin (Vancocin®), acarbose (Precose®), sodium benzoate-sodium phenylacetate (Ammonul®), sodium phenylbutyrate (Buphenyl®) and zinc have been used for HE but there is limited data regarding safety and effectiveness.

Table 2. Medications for Management of Hepatic Encephalopathy[13]

Medication (Brands)	Dosage Forms	Usual Dose Range
Non-absorbable disaccharides: alter intestinal pH to reduce ammonia, increase ammonia clearance via feces.		
Lactulose (Enulose®, Constulose®, Generlac®, Kristalose®)	Solution: 10 g/15mL Packets: 10g, 20g/pack	15-30mL (10-20g) BID-TID
Sorbitol	Solution: 70%	15-30mL BID-TID
• Adjust sorbitol or lactulose dose to maintain 1-3 BM/day. • Some patients may find sorbitol more palatable; patient preference may guide therapy.		
Antibiotics: decrease intestinal concentrations of ammoniagenic bacteria		
Neomycin	Tablet: 500mg	500-1000mg BID-TID
Rifaximin (Xifaxan®)	Tablet: 200mg, 550mg	400mg TID or 550mg BID
• Avoid neomycin in patients with renal failure. • Rifaximin 550mg tablets tend to be more cost effective dosing strategy.		

References

1. National Hospice & Palliative Care Organization (NHPCO). NHPCO's facts and figures: hospice care in America. 2014 edition. Alexandria, VA; NHPCO, October 2014. Available at http://www.nhpco.org/sites/default/files/public/Statistics_Research/2014_Facts_Figures.pdf
2. Roth K, Lynn J, Zhong Z, et al. Dying with end stage liver disease with cirrhosis: insights from SUPPORT. *J Am Geriatr Soc.* 2000;48(5Suppl):S122-S130.
3. Kamath PS, Kim WR. The model for end stage liver disease (MELD). *Hepatol.* 2007;45:797-805.
4. Thornton K. Evaluation and prognosis of patients with cirrhosis. In Module 2. Evaluation, staging, and monitoring of chronic hepatitis C. Hepatitis C Online; updated February 3, 2014. Available at http://www.hepatitisc.uw.edu/go/evaluation-staging-monitoring/evaluation-prognosis-cirrhosis/core-concept/all. Accessed December 18, 2014.
5. Pugh R, Murray-Lyon IM, Dawson JL, et al. Transection of the oesophagus for bleeding oesophageal varices. *Brit J Surg.* 1973;60(8):646-649.
6. Weisner R, Edwards E, Freeman R, et al. Model for end stage liver disease (MELD) and allocation of liver donors. *Gastroenterol.* 2003;124:91-6.
7. Centers for Medicare & Medicaid Services (CMS). Local coverage determination (LCD): hospice determining terminal status. Available at http://www.cms.gov/medicare-coverage- database/details/lcd-details.aspx. Accessed December 18, 2014.

8. Centers for Medicare & Medicaid Services (CMS). Medicare program; hospice care amendments. *Fed Register* 2005;70:FR70532-70548. Available at https://federalregister.gov/a/05-23078. Accessed December 18, 2014.

9. Poonja Z, Brisebois A, van Zanten SV, et al. Patients with cirrhosis and denied liver transplants rarely receive adequate palliative care or appropriate management. *Clin Gastroent Hepatol*. 2014;12:692-698.

10. Cox-North P, Doorenbos A, Shannon SE, et al. Transition to end-of-life care in end-stage liver disease. *J Hosp Palliat Nurs*. 2013;15(4):209-215.

11. Yates WR. Psychiatric disorders in liver disease. *J Pharm Pract*. 2007;20(5):373-376.

12. Blei AT, Cordoba J, Practice Parameters Committee of the American College of Gastroenterology. Hepatic encephalopathy. *Am J Gastroenterol*. 2001;96(7):1968-1976.

13. Lexi-Drugs Online. Hudson, OH; Lexi-Comp, Inc. Accessed December 18, 2014.

End Stage Renal Disease

Introduction

According to NHPCO statistics, patients with a terminal diagnosis of end stage renal disease (ESRD) make up about 3% of hospice admissions annually.[1] Patients may wish to continue to receive dialysis concurrently with hospice care. If the patient's terminal diagnosis is not related to ESRD, the patient may receive covered services under both the Medicare ESRD benefit and the Medicare hospice benefit.[2,3] Patients also have the right to refuse dialysis. The decision to continue, refuse, or to withdraw from, dialysis should be guided by the patient's goals of care. Considerations including comorbid diseases, severity of ESRD-related symptoms, residual renal function, and impact on quality of life, all contribute to a well informed and shared decision-making process.[4]

Prognosis after Dialysis Withdrawal vs Non-dialysis Management in ESRD

Patients withdrawing from dialysis tend to have a much shorter prognosis (average of 8-10 days) than those forgoing dialysis, 68% survival at one year after a stage 5 (GFR<15ml/min/1.73m^2) kidney disease diagnosis.[5-7]

A recent study of nearly 2,000 patients who had discontinued dialysis determined average survival times and independent predictors of survival.[6] Patients with higher PPS scores (i.e., PPS > 20%) at hospice admission tend to have longer length of stay. Predictors of shorter length of stay were: admission to hospice in hospital or inpatient unit, male patients, white patients, patients with peripheral edema, and patients on oxygen at hospice admission.[6]

A systematic review examined prognosis in stage 5 kidney disease with conservative management and no dialysis. [7] Patients with severe neurological impairment, another non-renal terminal disease, the very elderly, and patients with multiple comorbid diseases may refuse to initiate dialysis. Median survival with conservative management ranges from 6 to almost 24 months. [7] Patients with multiple comorbidities and poor performance status had the shortest survival time. [7] Prolonged survival was predicted by female patients, fewer comorbidities, higher serum albumin, an nephrologist referral prior to stage 5 diagnosis.[7]

Calculating Creatinine Clearance (CrCL) Estimation (Cockcroft-Gault)

Men:

$$CrCl = \frac{[140 - \text{age}(yrs)] \times [\text{weight}(kg)]}{72 \times \text{SCr}\,(mg/dL)}$$

Women:

$$CrCl = \frac{[140 - \text{age}(yrs)] \times [\text{weight}(kg)]}{72 \times \text{SCr}\,(mg/dL)} \times 0.85$$

Chronic Kidney Disease Staging[8]

Stage	Description	GFR (mL/min/1.73m^2)
1	Kidney damage with normal or increased GFR	>90
2	Kidney damage with mild decreased GFR	60-89
3	Moderate decreased GFR	30-59
4	Severe decreased GFR	15-29
5	Kidney failure	<15 (or dialysis)

GFR=glomerular filtration rate
Kidney damage=pathologic abnormalities or markers of damage

Guidance for Determination of Hospice Eligibility: Renal Failure[2]

A patient with acute or chronic renal failure has:

1. The patient is not seeking dialysis or renal transplant
2. Creatinine clearance is <10 mL/min (<15 mL/min for diabetics)
3. Serum creatinine > 8.0 mg/dL (>6.0 mg/dL for diabetics)

Supporting documentation for chronic renal failure includes:

o Gastrointestinal bleeding
o Uremia
o Oliguria (urine output is less than 400 mL in 24 hours)
o Intractable hyperkalemia (greater than 7.0 mEq/L) not responsive to treatment

- o Uremic pericarditis
- o Hepatorenal syndrome
- o Intractable fluid overload, not responsive to treatment

Supporting documentation for acute renal failure includes:
- o Mechanical ventilation
- o Malignancy (other organ system)
- o Chronic lung disease
- o Advanced cardiac disease
- o Advanced liver disease

In the absence of one or more of the above criteria, rapid decline or comorbidities may also support the physician's determination of a life expectancy of < 6 months and hospice eligibility. Certification or recertification is based upon a physician's clinical judgment. According to the Benefits Improvement and Protection Act of 2000 (BIPA), hospice certification of terminal illness "shall be based on the physician's or medical director's clinical judgment regarding the normal course of the individual's illness."[9]

Prevalent Symptoms[6,7,13-16]

All patients with ESRD report a high symptom burden. The median number of symptoms reported was similar between patients with ESRD and patients with a terminal cancer diagnosis. Most common symptoms reported were weakness, fatigue, poor appetite, pruritus, drowsiness, dyspnea, pain, edema, and insomnia. According to patient reports, lack of energy and pain are the most distressing symptoms with the most impact on quality of life. Many of these symptoms may be related to electrolyte disturbances or elevated levels of metabolic products from medications and muscle breakdown (e.g., creatinine). See chapters below for additional information on symptom management.

- Anorexia, see *Anorexia GEMS*
- Dyspnea, see *Dyspnea GEMS*
- Edema, see *Ascites & Edema GEMS*
- Fatigue, see *Fatigue GEMS*
- Insomnia, see *Insomnia GEMS*
- Pain, see *Pain GEMS*
- Pruritus, see *Pruritus GEMS*

Clinical Pearls[7,13-16]

- Consider patient comorbid conditions, in addition to ESRD, when assessing patient symptoms. For example, many patients with ESRD also have diabetes and may have diabetic peripheral neuropathy as a component of their pain.
- Oxycodone, methadone, and fentanyl tend to be safer pain medications to use in patients with ESRD because these opioids do not have problematic metabolites that may accumulate causing neurotoxicity.
- Patients with chronic kidney disease have a threefold higher rate of medication-related adverse reactions compared to patients with normal renal function. Absorption, distribution, metabolism, and excretion of medications are all altered in ESRD. Simplify medication profiles as much as possible to reduce medication-related risk.
- Avoid use of NSAIDs, meperidine, codeine in ESRD. Due to metabolite accumulation and opioid toxicity, use morphine, hydromorphone, and tramadol cautiously with lower starting doses, close monitoring.
- Gabapentin and pregabalin effectively treat neuropathy in ESRD; doses must be reduced and dosing intervals extended to ensure safe use and lower risk of adverse effects.
- When assessing the risk vs benefit of using erythropoietin-stimulating agents (ESA) to manage anemia in ESRD, consider the patient's current clinical status; perceived improvement in fatigue, dyspnea, or weakness; and tolerability of ESA side effects (hypertension, headache, pruritus, nausea, arthralgia). Additionally, patients continuing ESA therapy will require ongoing lab monitoring of hemoglobin and hematocrit as well as iron supplementation.
- Metoclopramide may be useful in treating nausea and gastroparesis in ESRD, but requires dose reduction. Initiate therapy at half of the usual dose.
- Information on renal dosing requirements and dialysis clearance of commonly used medications in included in the *Drug Monograph* section.

Table 1. Erythropoiesis-Stimulating Agents (ESA)[10]

ESA products stimulate the division and differentiation of erythroid precursor cells and induce the release of reticulocytes from the bone marrow into the bloodstream, where they mature to erythrocytes. An increase in reticulocyte counts is followed by a rise in hematocrit and hemoglobin (Hgb) levels.		
Generic	**Brand Example**	**Usual Dosing and Comments**
Epoetin alfa	Procrit®, Epogen®	50-100 units/kg given IV or SC three times/week with dialysis • For non-dialysis patients: use only if Hgb < 10 g/dL, patient is symptomatic with anemia, and to avoid blood transfusions. • Do not increase dose more than once every 4 weeks. • Adjust dose if Hgb does not increase by 1 g/dL • If inadequate response in 12 weeks, further increases are unlikely to provide benefit and will increase risks; discontinue ESA therapy.
Darbepoetin alfa	Aranesp®	0.45 mcg/kg given IV or SC once weekly or 0.75 mcg/kg every 2 weeks with dialysis. • For non-dialysis patients: use only if Hgb < 10 g/dL, patient is symptomatic with anemia, and to avoid blood transfusions. • Use 0.45 mcg/kg once every 4 weeks. • Adjust dose if Hgb does not increase by 1 g/dL • If inadequate response in 12 weeks, further increases are unlikely to provide benefit and will increase risks; discontinue ESA therapy.
Ongoing lab monitoring is required for safe use of ESA therapy. If the patient refuses lab work, or no longer desires blood draws, recommend discontinuing the ESA.		

Patient and Caregiver Talking Points about ESAs

- ESAs may be effective for improving symptoms of anemia related to ESRD including fatigue, weakness, and dyspnea when used with the goal of improving functional status and quality of life. However, as a patient declines, many factors contribute to a patient's fatigue, not just hemoglobin levels, therefore an ESA may not be able to alleviate patient's symptoms as well as before.
- The goal of ESA use is to target the treatment of patient's symptoms, not just a laboratory value. If the patient does not perceive a benefit, then multiple injections and blood draws may negatively affect quality of life.
- Use of an ESA will not prolong life. If an ESA is stopped and patient declines, the underlying disease state has progressed and would likely do so regardless of the ESA.
- Patients who are bedbound do not expend as much energy as a healthy, ambulatory person and can be comfortable despite lower hemoglobin levels.
- Medications are available to manage anemia-related symptoms that may be experienced during ESA use and after an ESA has been stopped.
- ESAs have common side-effects including fever, headache, itching, rash, nausea and vomiting, joint pain, and cough. ESAs increase patient risk for more thromboembolism leading to heart attack, stroke, and death.

Table 2. Renal Medication Management Considerations[10-12]

CALCIMIMETIC: Increases the sensitivity of the calcium-sensing receptor on the parathyroid gland, lowering parathyroid hormone (PTH), serum calcium, and serum phosphorus levels, preventing progressive bone disease associated with mineral metabolism disorders. Treatment of 2nd hyperparathyroidism in patients with CKD.

Generic	Brand Example	Usual Dosing
Cinacalcet	Sensipar	30mg PO Daily, titrate to maintain iPTH level 150-300 pg/mL

PHOSPHATE BINDERS: Reduce the fraction of dietary phosphate absorbed by patients with ESRD by binding to dietary phosphate to form insoluble complexes that are excreted. Reduces serum phosphorous concentrations to help prevent ectopic calcifications. Reduction or control of serum phosphorus in patients with CKD on dialysis; adjusted to maintain phosphorus levels in goal range of 3.5-5.5 mg/dL. *All phosphate binders must be administered with meals.*

Generic	Brand Example	Usual Dosing
Calcium acetate	PhosLo®	1334mg PO with each meal
	Phoslyra®	1334mg/10mL PO with each meal
Ferric citrate	Zerenex®	420mg PO BID with meals (also acts as iron supplement)
Lanthanum	Fosrenal®	500-1000mg PO TID with meals
Sevelamer HCl	Renagel®	800-1600mg PO TID with meals
Sevelamer carbonate	Renvela®	800-1600mg PO TID with meals
Sucroferric oxyhydroxide	Velphoro®	500mg PO TID with meals (also acts as iron supplement)

VITAMIN D ANALOGS: Metabolized to active forms of vitamin D or biologically active analogs (eg, calcitriol, paricalcitriol) which act directly on the parathyroid glands to suppress synthesis and secretion of parathyroid hormone. Treatment of hyperparathyroidism secondary to active vitamin D metabolite deficiency in CKD.

Generic	Brand Example	Usual Dosing
Calcitriol	Rocaltrol	0.25mg PO Daily
Doxecalciferol	Hectorol	1mcg PO Daily
Ergocalciferol	Calciferol	50,000 IU/week, then monthly based on 25(OH)-D levels
Paricalcitol	Zemplar	1mcg PO Daily

References

1. National Hospice & Palliative Care Organization (NHPCO). NHPCO's facts and figures: hospice care in America. 2014 edition. Alexandria, VA; NHPCO, October 2014. Available at http://www.nhpco.org/sites/default/files/public/Statistics_Research/2014_Facts_Figures.pdf

2. National Hospice & Palliative Care Organization (NHPCO). Determining hospice eligibility for chronic kidney disease – Medicare hospice benefit. NHPCO; 2009.

3. Centers for Medicare & Medicaid (CMS). Medicare Policy Benefit Manual. Chapter 11- End stage renal disease (ESRD). Rev.177, 12-13-13. CMS; December 13, 2013. Available at http://www.cms.gov/Regulations-and-Guidance/Guidance/Manuals/downloads/bp102c11.pdf

4. Tamura MK, Cohen LM. Should there be an expanded role for palliative care in end-stage renal disease? *Curr Opin Nephrol Hypertens.* 2010;19:556-560.

5. Murtagh FE, Higginson IJ. Death from renal failure 80 years on: how far have we come? *J Palliat Med* 2007;10(6):1236-1238.

6. O'Connor NR, Dougherty M, Harris PS, Casarett DJ. Survival after dialysis discontinuation and hospice enrollment for ESRD. *Clin J Am Soc Nephrol.* 2013; 8:2117-2122

7. O'Connor NR, Kumar P. Conservative management of end-stage renal disease without dialysis: a systematic review. *J Pain Symptom Manage.* 2012; 15(2):228-235.

8. National Kidney Foundation. KDOQI Clinical practice guidelines for chronic kidney disease: evaluation, classification, and stratification. *Am J Kidney Dis* 2002;39(suppl1):S1-S266. Available at http://www2.kidney.org/professionals/KDOQI/guidelines_ckd/toc.htm. Accessed November 14, 2014.

9. Centers for Medicare and Medicaid Services (CMS). Medicare program; hospice care amendments. *Fed Register* 2005;70:FR70532-70548. Available at https://federalregister.gov/a/05-23078. Accessed December 18, 2014.

10. Lexi-Drugs Online. Hudson, OH; Lexi-Comp, Inc. Accessed December 29, 2011.

11. Monthly Prescribing Reference. Haymarket Media, Inc. Available at http://www.empr.com Accessed December 29, 2011.

12. Uhlig K, Berns JS, Kestenbaum B, et al. KDOQI US commentary on the 2009 KDIGO clinical practice guideline for the diagnosis, evaluation, and treatment of CKD-mineral and bone disorder (CKD-BMD) *Am J Kidney Dis* 2010;55(5):773-799. Available at http://www.kidney.org/professionals/KDOQI/pdf/KDOQI-CKD-MBD-Commentary.pdf

13. Murtagh FE, Addington-Hall J, Edmonds P, et al. Symptoms in the month before death for stage 5 chronic kidney disease patients managed without dialysis. *J Pain Symptom Manage* 2010;40(3):342-352.

14. Kidney End of Life Coalition. Palliative care and hospice [Internet]. Available at http://www.kidneyeol.org/Palliative-Care---Hospice.aspx. Accessed November 14, 2014.

15. Murtagh FE, Addington-Hall J, Edmonds P, et al. Symptoms in advanced renal disease: a cross sectional survey of symptom prevalence in stage 5 chronic kidney disease managed without dialysis. *J Palliat Med* 2007;10(6): 1266-1276.

16. Moss AH. Improving end-of-life care for dialysis patients. *Am J Kidney Dis.* 2005;45(1):209-212.

End Stage Parkinson's Disease

Introduction[1-5]
Parkinson's disease (PD) is the most common cause of Parkinsonism, a syndrome manifested by resting tremor, rigidity, bradykinesia, and postural instability. Degeneration of dopaminergic neurons in the substantia nigra contributes to the motor dysfunction of patients with PD. Non-dopaminergic pathways may be responsible for common non-motor symptoms of sleep, sensory, and autonomic disturbances (e.g., orthostatic hypotension, constipation, anosmia, mood disorder, and cognitive impairment). The average age at onset of symptoms is 65 years. About 1% of annual hospice admissions are patients with a primary diagnosis of Parkinson's disease.

Prognosis[4-10]
PD is a chronic, progressive neurodegenerative disease with a life expectancy of 15 to 20 years from time of diagnosis. Severity of motor symptoms appears to be an independent predictor of mortality in patients with PD. According to a recent study by Goy et al in veterans with PD, body mass index (BMI) < 18.5 and changes to, or reduction of, dopaminergic medications may signal a prognosis of 6 to 12 months and hospice referral may be considered. Additionally, clinician led discussions with patient and family member about how to recognize changes in functional ability, cognition, or emotional well-being could be used along with traditional clinical signs of progression to help signal the need for hospice and palliative care. Pneumonia may be the cause of death in about 45% of patients with PD.

Guidance for Determination of Hospice Eligibility: Parkinson's Disease[9,10]
Critical nutritional impairment demonstrated by all of the following in the preceding 12 months:
- o   Oral intake of nutrients and fluids insufficient to sustain life
- o   Continuing weight loss
- o   Dehydration or hypovolemia
- o   Absence of artificial feeding methods

Rapid disease progression as evidenced by:
- o   Progression from independent ambulation to wheelchair or bed-bound status
- o   Progression from normal to barely intelligible or unintelligible speech
- o   Progression from normal to pureed diet
- o   Progression from independence in most or all Activities of Daily Living (ADLs) to needing major assistance by caretaker in all ADLs

Supporting evidence:
- o   Dyspnea at rest
- o   Patient requires supplemental oxygen at rest
- o   Patient declines artificial ventilation
- o   Recurrent aspiration pneumonia (with or without tube feedings)
- o   Upper urinary tract infection (e.g., pyelonephritis)
- o   Sepsis
- o   Recurrent fever after antibiotic therapy
- o   Stage 3 or Stage 4 pressure ulcer(s)

In the absence of one or more of the above criteria, rapid decline or comorbidities may also support the physician's determination of a life expectancy of < 6 months and hospice eligibility. Certification or recertification is based upon a physician's clinical judgment. According to the Benefits Improvement and Protection Act of 2000 (BIPA), hospice certification of terminal illness "shall be based on the physician's or medical director's clinical judgment regarding the normal course of the individual's illness."[10]

Prevalent Symptoms[3,5,6,11-19]
Patients with PD experience many of the common symptoms associated with end of life. Parkinson's specific motor symptoms include dyskinesia, motor fluctuations ("on" "off" periods), tremor, rigidity, and postural instability. Motor symptoms become increasingly difficult to manage as PD progresses. In patients with advanced PD, there is a higher risk of medication-related adverse effects when doses are increased as the motor symptoms become refractory (see Figure 1). Non-motor symptoms such as orthostatic hypotension, gastroparesis, cognitive impairment, and urinary disturbances can be very difficult to manage medically. The need to weigh the benefit of

therapy for non-motor symptoms against the increased risk of adverse effects in a frail patient is a challenge for hospice clinicians (Table 3).

- Agitation, see *Agitation & Delirium GEMS*
- Anxiety, see *Anxiety GEMS*
- Constipation, see *Constipation GEMS*
- Depression, see *Depression GEMS*
- Dysphagia, see *Dysphagia GEMS*
- Fatigue, see *Fatigue GEMS*
- Insomnia, see *Insomnia GEMS*
- Nausea, see *Nausea & Vomiting GEMS*
- Pain, see *Pain GEMS*
- Sialorrhea, see *Secretions GEMS*

Table 1. Parkinson's Disease Related Terms[3,5]

Term	Definition
"Off" period	Time period when patient's response to medication wears off and PD symptoms return (e.g. rigidity, freezing gait); "off" period increases as PD progresses; also known as "end-of-dose deterioration" or "wearing off" phenomenon; may be accompanied by painful dystonic muscle cramping.
"On" period	Time period when patient has a good response to the medication; "on" period of therapeutic response decreases as PD progresses.
Diphasic dyskinesia	Alternate pattern of dystonia/dyskinesia – improvement – dystonia/dyskinesia (D-I-D) associated with beginning and end of dose rather than peak of dose.
Dopamine dysregulation	Cause of impulsive and compulsive behaviors such as hypersexuality, binge eating, repetitive/purposeless behaviors (punding).
Dyskinesia	Involuntary, choreiform movements and dystonia frequently related to dopaminergic medication dosing peaks; risk of injury and social embarrassment.
Freezing	Transient, lasting several seconds, patient's feet have sensation of being "glued to the ground"; caused by inadequate dopamine levels in CNS.
Motor fluctuations	Alternations between "on" and "off" periods.

Figure 1. Motor Fluctuations, Dyskinesia, and Medications in Parkinson's Disease[3,6,19]

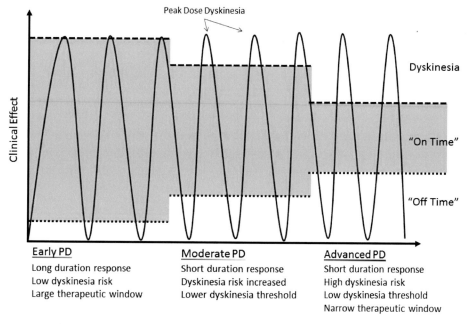

- - - - Dyskinesia threshold
· · · · · · · ·Therapeutic response threshold

Table 2. Medication Management in Parkinson's Disease[3,14]

Medication Class	Effectiveness	Indication	Adverse Effects
Levodopa-DI Levodopa-carbidopa (Sinemet) Levodopa-carbidopa-entacapone (Stalevo)	Most effective for motor symptoms, all stages of disease; therapeutic window narrows as disease progresses	All motor symptoms, mono or adjunct therapy	Nausea, orthostatic hypotension, dyskinesia, hallucinations
Dopamine Agonists Pramipexole (Mirapex) Ropinirole (Requip) Rotigotine (Neupro) Apomorphine (Apokyn)	Effective for motor symptoms for most stages of disease; therapeutic window narrows as disease progresses	All motor symptoms, mono or adjunct therapy	Nausea, orthostatic hypotension, hallucinations, edema, sleepiness, impulse control disorders
MAOB-I Selegiline (Eldepryl, Zelapar) Rasagiline (Azilect)	Effective for early or mild motor symptoms	Motor symptoms, motor fluctuations, mono or adjunct therapy	Dizziness, headache, confusion, arthralgia, exacerbation of levodopa adverse effects
COMT-I Entacapone (Comtan) Tolcapone (Tasmar)	Effective to control motor fluctuations, as adjunctive therapy with levodopa-DI	Motor fluctuations, adjunct therapy	Dark colored urine, exacerbation of levodopa adverse effects
Anticholinergic Trihexyphenidyl (Artane) Benztropine (Cogentin)	Possibly effective, conflicting data and higher risk of adverse effects	Tremor	Hallucinations, confusion, blurred vision, dry mouth, nausea, constipation
Other Amantadine	Possibly effective, conflicting data	Gait dysfunction and dyskinesia	Hallucinations, cognitive impairment, blurred vision, dry mouth, urinary retention, constipation

DI=decarboxylase inhibitor, MAOB-I = monoamine oxidase-B inhibitor, COMT-I catechol O-methyl transferase inhibitor

Clinical Pearls[14,17,18,20]

- Nausea is a common adverse effect of dopamine agonist medications; consider reducing the dose of dopamine agonists prior to determine if the nausea is relieved or improved prior to initiating an anti-emetic.
- Avoid dopamine antagonists such as haloperidol or metoclopramide for nausea especially if the patient is still ambulatory; consider use of low dose promethazine (e.g., 6.25mg) if an anti-emetic is needed.
- Trimethobenzamide (Tigan) has traditionally been used to manage nausea in patients with PD, however, the anticholinergic side effects (dry mouth, constipation, sedation, dizziness) can be difficult to tolerate. Trimethobenzamide also has a risk of orthostatic hypotension and extrapyramidal symptoms.
- Apomorphine (Apokyn) is a newer treatment to manage hypomobility episodes in patients with advanced PD. Apomorphine is given by subcutaneous injection and is only available through specialty pharmacies. Apomorphine can cause severe nausea and vomiting, however 5-HT3 antagonists (e.g. ondansetron) are contraindicated for concomitant use.
- Excess dopaminergic activity is associated with delirium, hallucinations, and impulse control disorders; consider reduction in dose of dopaminergic medications prior to initiating any antipsychotic medication to control behaviors.
- Always taper dopaminergic medications and levodopa; abrupt discontinuation can cause symptoms similar to neuroleptic malignant syndrome (e.g. hyperpyrexia, confusion, rigidity).

Table 3. Approach to Autonomic Disturbances in Parkinson's Disease[14-17]

Symptom	Medications that may improve symptoms[a]	Non-pharmacological options	Medications to avoid or use cautiously
Gastrointestinal Dysfunction[11]	*Constipation:* Senna (Senokot®) Bisacodyl (Dulcolax®) *Delayed gastric emptying:* Erythromycin (Ery-Tab®)	• Avoid high-fat foods and large portions. • Increase physical activity as tolerated. • Increase hydration.	*Dopamine antagonists:* metoclopramide (Reglan®)
	• Tolerance to effect of erythromycin for gastroparesis may develop after a few weeks of therapy. Give with food (non-dairy) to reduce nausea and GI upset. • If possible, discontinue or reduce dose of medications that cause constipation.		
Orthostatic hypotension[9]	Midodrine (ProAmatine®) Pyridostigmine (Mestinon®) Fludrocortisone (Florinef®)	• Increase fluid & salt intake. • Elevate head of the bed. • Wear compression stockings. • Reduce alcohol intake. • Slow postural changes.	Antihypertensives Diuretics
	• Discontinue use of any medication for OH when patient is no longer ambulatory. • Avoid use of midodrine within 4 hours of bedtime to reduce risk of supine hypertension. • Fludrocortisone must be combined with adequate salt and fluid intake for effectiveness. Discontinue if significant edema or weight gain. • Pyridostigmine may only be effective in mild OH. Discontinue if bothersome side effects develop nausea, diarrhea, urinary incontinence.		
Sialorrhea[10]	Hyoscyamine (Levsin®) Glycopyrrolate (Robinul®) Atropine (Isopto® Atropine) Scopolamine patch (Transderm-Scop®)	• Sugar-free candy or chewing gum can increase the swallowing reflex. • Chew food slowly and carefully. • Carry handkerchief or small towel to aid in removal of excess saliva.	*Systemic anticholinergics:* Trihexyphenidyl (Artane®) Benztropine (Cogentin®) Diphenhydramine (Benadryl®)
	• Use of anticholinergic agents may improve some symptoms (overactive bladder, sialorrhea) while worsening others (constipation, urinary retention). • Glycopyrrolate has lower risk of CNS effects (sedation, confusion) than other medications. • Avoid use of multiple anticholinergic medications.		
Urinary difficulties[10]	*Overactive bladder:* Oxybutynin (Oxytrol®) Tolterodine (Detrol®) *Urinary retention:* Bethanechol (Urecholine®)	*Overactive bladder:* • Schedule voiding. • Provide incontinence supplies. *Urinary retention:* • Evaluate use of urinary catheter.	*Systemic anticholinergics:* Trihexyphenidyl (Artane®) Benztropine (Cogentin®) Diphenhydramine (Benadryl®)
	• Use of anticholinergic agents may improve some symptoms (overactive bladder, sialorrhea) while worsening others (constipation, urinary retention). • Avoid use of competing medications (e.g., bethanechol and oxybutynin). • Patients using acetylcholinesterase inhibitors (donepezil, galantamine, rivastigmine, pyridostigmine) may be experiencing incontinence as a medication side effect. Discontinue prior to initiating medications for overactive bladder.		

References

1. National Hospice & Palliative Care Organization (NHPCO). NHPCO's facts and figures: hospice care in America. 2014 edition. Alexandria, VA; NHPCO, October 2014. Available at http://www.nhpco.org/sites/default/files/public/Statistics_Research/2014_Facts_Figures.pdf.
2. Caffrey C, Sengupta M, Moss A, et al. Home health care and discharged hospice care patients: United States, 2000 and 2007. National Health Statistics Reports; no.38. Hyattsville, MD:National Center for Health Statistics. 2011. Available at http://www.cdc.gov/nchs/data/nhsr/nhsr038.pdf.
3. Connolly BS, Lang AE. Pharmacological treatment of Parkinson disease: a review. *JAMA*. 2014;311(16):1670-1683.
4. Goy ER, Bohlig A, Carter J, Ganzini L. Identifying predictors of hospice eligibility in patients with Parkinson disease. *Am J Hosp Palliat Med*. 2015;32(1):29-33.
5. Olanow C, Schapira AV. Chapter 372. Parkinson's disease and other movement disorders. In: Longo DL, Fauci AS, Kasper DL, Hauser SL, Jameson J, Loscalzo J. eds. *Harrison's Principles of Internal Medicine, 18e*. New York, NY: McGraw-Hill; 2012.
6. Goudreau JL. Medical management of advanced Parkinson's disease. *Clin Geriatr Med*. 2006;22:753-772.
7. Hubbard G, McLachlan K, Forbat L, Munday D. Recognition by family members that relatives with neurodegenerative disease are likely to die within a year: a meta-ethnography. *Palliat Med*. 2012;26(2):108-122.
8. Pennington S, Snell K, Lee M, Walker R. The cause of death in idiopathic Parkinson's disease. *Parkinsonism Relat Disord*. 2010;16(7):434-437.
9. Centers for Medicare & Medicaid Services (CMS). Local coverage determination (LCD): hospice determining terminal status. Available at http://www.cms.gov/medicare-coverage- database/details/lcd-details.aspx. Accessed December 18, 2014.
10. Centers for Medicare & Medicaid Services (CMS). Medicare program; hospice care amendments. *Fed Register* 2005;70:FR70532-70548. Available at https://federalregister.gov/a/05-23078.
11. Stubendorff K, Aarsland D, Minthon L, Londos E. The impact of autonomic dysfunction on survival in patients with dementia with Lewy Bodies and Parkinson's disease with dementia. *PLoS ONE*. 2012;7(10):e45451. doi:10.1371/journal.pone.0045451.
12. Chou KL, Evatt M, Hinson V, Kompoliti K. Sialorrhea in Parkinson's disease: a review. *Mov Disord*. 2007;22(16):2306-2313.
13. Marjama-Lyons J, Koller W. Tremor-predominant Parkinson's disease: approaches to treatment. *Drugs Aging*. 2000;16(4):273-278.
14. Lexi-Comp Online. Lexi-Drugs Online. Hudson, Ohio: Lexi-Comp, Inc. June 20, 2014.
15. Sanchex-Ferro A, Benito-Leon J, Gomez-Esteban JC. The management of orthostatic hypotension in Parkinson's disease. *Front Neurol*. 2013;4(64):doi10.3389/fneur.2013.00064.
16. Pfeiffer R. Gastrointestinal and urinary dysfunction in PD. Parkinson's Disease Foundation Newsletter. 2007: [cited 20 June 2014]. Available from: http://www.pdf.org/en/spring07_gastrointestinal_and_urinary_dysfunction_in_pd
17. Woitalla D, Goetze O. Treatment approaches of gastrointestinal dysfunction in Parkinson's disease, therapeutical options and future perspectives. *J Neurol Sci*. 2011;310:152-158.
18. Riedel O, Klotsche J, SpottkeA, Deuschl G, Forstl H, Henn F, et al. Frequency of dementia, depression, and other neuropsychiatric symptoms in 1,449 outpatients with Parkinson's disease. *J Neurol*. 2010;257:1073-1082.
19. Fahn S. How do you treat motor complications in Parkinson's disease: medicine, surgery, or both? *Ann Neurol*. 2008;64(suppl):S56-S64.
20. Rayner AV, O'Brien JG, Schoenbachler B. Behavior disorders of dementia: recognition and treatment. *Am Fam Physician*. 2006;73(4):647-652.

Stroke

Introduction[1,2]

According to NHPCO statistics, patients with a terminal diagnosis of stroke or coma compose just over 5% of hospice admissions annually.[1] Approximately 50% of deaths from stroke occur in hospitals, 35% in nursing facilities, and about 15% in homes.[2] A recent statement from the American Heart Association/American Stroke Association recommends that all patients and families with stroke that affects daily functioning and reduces life expectancy or quality of life should have access to palliative care.[2]

Table 1. Common Types of Stroke[2-4]

Type	Characteristics
Ischemic stroke	About 84% of all strokes and highest percentage of deaths from stroke (73%); resulting from atherothrombotic/embolic, cardioembolic, or small blood vessel disease; caused by inadequate delivery of oxygen or glucose to the brain; degree and duration of reduced blood flow, hypoxia, or hypoglycemia determines if temporary dysfunction (transient ischemic attacks) or extensive damage (cerebral infarction and necrosis)
Intracerebral hemorrhage (ICH)	About 10% of all strokes and causes about 16% of death from strokes; primarily resulting from hypertensive disease and subsequent rupture of arteries within brain tissue; bleeding into the brain can cause damage to exposed brain tissue; accumulation of extravascular blood and resulting edema causes increased intracranial pressure (ICP)
Subarachnoid hemorrhage (SAH)	About 6% of all strokes and causes about 4% of death from strokes; usually resulting from aneurysm or arteriovenous malformation (AVM); vessel ruptures cause by bleeding near the surface of the brain into the subarachnoid space; hydrocephalus may occur from obstruction of cerebrospinal fluid (CSF) outflow

Prognosis[2,5]

Decisions to withdraw life-sustaining treatments in patients with severe ICH may bias prognostic models. Patient and family understanding of short-term mortality risk and longer-term cognitive and functional impacts do not always coincide with the clinician's definition of good outcomes. Discussions on prognosis should include aspects of recovery that are most important to the patient and family (e.g., ability to walk, communication, extent of paralysis, cognitive status). Stroke risk prognostic scores may improve clinician's ability to accurately predict clinical outcomes during acute hospitalization for stroke. No prognostic tools have been specifically developed or validated for determining end-of-life care with in the chronic stage of stroke.

Comparison of Prognostic Tools[5-9]

- iScore[6]
  - Predicts 30-day and 1-year mortality for patients with ischemic stroke
  - Components include age, gender, stroke severity and subtype, presence of underlying risk factors (atrial fibrillation, CHF, previous myocardial infarction, smoking status), comorbid conditions (cancer, renal disease), pre-stroke disability, blood glucose on hospital admission
  - Online calculator available at http://www.sorcan.ca/iscore/index.html

- Glasgow Coma Score (GCS)[7]
  - Describes level of impaired consciousness (mild, moderate, severe, coma)
  - Scoring system with 3 components
    - Best motor response (obeys command, localizing, flexing, extending, none)
    - Best verbal response (oriented, confused, inappropriate, incomprehensible, none)
    - Eye opening (spontaneous, to speech, to pain, none)
  - Online calculator available at http://www.sorcan.ca/iscore/gcs.html

- ICH Score[8]
  - Predicts 30-day mortality for patients with ICH
  - Components include GCS, ICH volume, presence of intraventricular hemorrhage (IVH), origin of ICH, age (≥ 80 year)
  - Online calculator available at http://www.mdcalc.com/intracerebral-hemorrhage-ich-score/

- Hunt and Hess Scale[9]
  - Clinical severity grading scale for patients with SAH to provide an impression on which to provide an early estimate of prognosis
  - Aneurysmal SAH grading 1 (minimal deficit) to 5 (deep coma, moribund)

Guidance for Determination of Hospice Eligibility: Stroke or Coma[10,11]
Stroke, chronic stage - prognosis less than 6 months demonstrated by:
- Palliative performance status of < 40%
- Inability to maintain sufficient fluid and calorie intake
  - 10% weight loss during the previous 6 months
  - Serum albumin < 2.5 g/dL
  - Pulmonary aspiration despite speech pathology intervention
  - Sequential calorie counts documenting inadequate intake
  - Dysphagia severe enough to prevent nutrition and fluid intake to sustain life in a patient that declines or does not receive artificial nutrition and hydration

Coma, Acute Stroke - prognosis less than 6 months demonstrated by presence of ≥ 3 of following criteria by day 3 of coma:
- Abnormal brain stem response
- Absent verbal response
- Absent withdrawal response to pain
- Serum creatinine > 1.5 mg/dL

In context of progressive clinical decline, at least 1 of following within the past 12 months:
- Aspiration pneumonia
- Pyelonephritis or other upper urinary tract infection
- Septicemia
- Pressure ulcers, multiple, stage 3-4
- Fever, recurrent after antibiotics

In the absence of one or more of the above criteria, rapid decline or comorbidities may also support the physician's determination of a life expectancy of < 6 months and hospice eligibility. Certification or recertification is based upon a physician's clinical judgment. According to the Benefits Improvement and Protection Act of 2000 (BIPA), hospice certification of terminal illness "shall be based on the physician's or medical director's clinical judgment regarding the normal course of the individual's illness."[11]

Prevalent Symptoms
- Anxiety, see *Anxiety GEMS*
- Delirium, see *Agitation & Delirium GEMS*
- Depression, see *Depression GEMS*
- Dysphagia, see *Dysphagia GEMS*
- Dyspnea, see *Dyspnea GEMS*
- Fatigue, see *Fatigue GEMS*
- Infection, see *Infection GEMS*
- Pain, see *Pain GEMS*
- Seizures, see *Seizures GEMS*

Clinical Pearls[2,12, 13, 14]

- Harris et al, found patients admitted to hospice with stroke and a PPS score of ≥ 40% were least likely to die when compared to other common hospice terminal diagnoses. Continued disease progression in stroke can be difficult to predict, even patients with a PPS of 40% and a primary diagnosis of stroke had an overall mortality rate of < 50%.
- About 30% of newly diagnosed seizures in the elderly appear to be stroke-related; there is no way to predict which patients will have recurrent seizures following stroke.
- Anti-epileptic drugs (AED) for primary prevention of post-stroke seizures are not recommended. AED use may be considered for patients having 2 or more post-stroke seizures. Most AEDs have a risk of drug interactions and adverse effects, select an AED based on comorbidities and concomitant medication use. Lamotrigine (Lamictal®), gabapentin (Neurontin®), or levetiracetam (Keppra®) are preferred.
- Family meetings are a critical intervention for palliative care and hospice teams for hospitalized patients, helping to explain prognosis, ensure treatment is consistent with the patient's goals of care, and bring all family members together in decision-making.
- Follow package instructions or request pharmacist assistance when converting patients from warfarin, heparin, or low molecular weight heparin to newer oral anticoagulants (apixaban, edoxaban, rivaroxaban, dabigatran).

Table 2. Comparison of Anticoagulant and Antiplatelet Medications for Stroke Prevention[14]

Medication (Brand)	Comment
Apixaban (Eliquis)	Inhibits factor Xa to inhibit platelet activation and fibrin clot formation; to reduce risk of stroke in patients with non-valvular atrial fibrillation (AF); reduce dose in renal failure or in patients > 80 years and weight < 60 kg; avoid in severe liver disease
Aspirin (Various OTC)	Inhibits platelet aggregation by decreasing formation of prostaglandin derivatives; prevention and treatment of ischemic stroke and risk reduction for stroke in patients with non-valvular AF; normal platelet function returns 7-10 days after discontinuing
Aspirin-dipyridamole (Aggrenox)	Inhibits platelet aggregation to reduce risk of stroke in patients who have had a stroke; avoid in severe renal or liver disease
Clopidogrel (Plavix)	Inhibits platelet aggregation by preventing activation of GPIIb/IIIa receptor complex; to reduce risk of stroke in patients who have had a stroke; normal platelet function returns 7-10 days after discontinuing; risk of prolonged bleeding in liver disease
Dabigatran (Pradaxa)	Direct thrombin inhibitor to thrombin-induced platelet aggregation and fibrin clot formation; to reduce risk of stroke in patients with non-valvular AF; avoid in renal failure (CrCL < 30 mL/min)
Edoxaban (Savaysa)	Selective factor Xa inhibitor, inhibits free factor Xa and prothrombinase activity and thrombin-induced platelet activation; to reduce risk of stroke in patients with non-valvular AF; avoid in severe renal disease (CrCl <15 mL/min) or moderate to severe liver disease
Rivaroxaban (Xarelto)	Inhibits factor Xa to inhibit platelet activation and fibrin clot formation; to reduce risk of stroke in patients with non-valvular AF; avoid in severe renal or liver disease
Ticlodipine (Ticlid)	Inhibits platelet aggregation to reduce risk of stroke in patients who have had a stroke; can cause life-threatening hematological reactions, reserve use for patients intolerant to other antiplatelet medications
Warfarin (Coumadin)	Vitamin K antagonist - depletes vitamin K reserves to reduce synthesis of active clotting factors; prevention and treatment of thromboembolic disorders; INR monitoring required; avoid use in severe liver disease

References

1. National Hospice & Palliative Care Organization (NHPCO). NHPCO's facts and figures: hospice care in America. 2014 edition. Alexandria, VA; NHPCO, October 2014. Available at http://www.nhpco.org/sites/default/files/public/Statistics_Research/2014_Facts_Figures.pdf.
2. Holloway RG, Arnold RM, Creutzfeldt CJ, Lewis EF, et al. Palliative and end-of-life care in stroke: a statement for healthcare professionals from the American Heart Association/American Stroke Association. *Stroke*. 2014;45:1887-1916. Available at http://stroke.ahajournals.org/content/45/6/1887.

3. National Institute of Neurological Disorders and Stroke (NINDS). Disorders A-Z. Bethesda, MD; National Institutes of Health. Available http://www.ninds.nih.gov/disorders/disorder_index.htm.

4. Zivin JA. Approach to cerebrovascular disease. In: Goldman L, Schafer AL, eds. *Goldman's Cecil Medicine*. 24th ed. Philadelphia, PA: Elsevier Saunders; 2012:2304-2310.

5. Saposnik G. The art of estimating outcomes and treating patients with stroke in the 21st century. *Stroke*. 2014;45:1603-1605.

6. Saposnik G, Kapral MK, Liu Y, Hall R, et al. iScore: a risk score to predict death early after hospitalization for an acute ischemic stroke. *Circulation*. 2011;123:739-749.

7. Teasdale G, Jennett B. Assessment of coma and impaired consciousness: a practical scale. *Lancet*. 1974;304(7872):81-84.

8. Hemphill JC, Bonovich DC, Besmertis L, Manley GT, Johnson SC. The ICH score: a simple reliable grading scale for intracerebral hemorrhage. *Stroke*. 2001;32:891-897.

9. Rosen DS, Macdonald RL. Subarachnoid hemorrhage grading scales: a systematic review. *Neurocrit Care*. 2005;2:110-118.

10. Centers for Medicare & Medicaid Services (CMS). Local coverage determination (LCD): hospice determining terminal status. Available at http://www.cms.gov/medicare-coverage- database/details/lcd-details.aspx. Accessed December 18, 2014.

11. Centers for Medicare & Medicaid Services (CMS). Medicare program; hospice care amendments. *Fed Register* 2005;70:FR70532-70548. Available at https://federalregister.gov/a/05-23078.

12. Harris PS, Stalam T, Ache KA, Harrold JE, et al. Can hospices predict which patients will die within six months? *J Palliat Med*. 2014;17(8):895-898.

13. Ryvlin P, Montavont A, Nighoghossian N. Optimizing therapy of seizures in stroke patients. *Neurology*. 2006;67(12, suppl.4):S3-S9.

14. Lexi-Drugs Online. Hudson, OH; Lexi-Comp, Inc. Accessed December 18, 2014.

15. Simmons BB, Parks SM. Intracerebral hemorrhage for the palliative care provider: what you need to know. *J Palliat Med*. 2008;11(10):1336-1339.

Section IV:

Appendices

- Benzodiazepine Equivalency Information
- Confused Drug Names (Look-alike and Sound-alike)
- Corticosteroid Equivalency Information
- Do Not Crush or Chew List
- Drugs That Prolong the QT Interval
- Extrapyramidal Symptoms (EPS) from Medications
- Insulin Comparison Table
- Medication Route Considerations
- Medications Associated with Anticholinergic Side Effects
- Palliative Performance Scale
- Subcutaneous Access Devices
- Withdrawal of Ventilator Life Support

Benzodiazepine Equivalency Information

Due to the distinct pharmacokinetic profile of each benzodiazepine, direct dosage conversions between agents are not available. The table below compares the commonly used benzodiazepines. Oral and parenteral dosing is equivalent for diazepam, lorazepam, and midazolam. For example, lorazepam 0.5 mg given orally is equivalent to lorazepam 0.5 mg given intravenously.

Benzodiazepine Pharmacokinetics and Approximate Equivalent Dosing

Medication	Dosage Forms	Onset of Action	Duration of Action	Active Metabolite?[a]	Approximate Equivalent Dose
alprazolam (Xanax)	Tablets Oral solution	30-60 min	5-6 hours	Yes[b]	0.5 mg
clonazepam (Klonopin)	Tablets Wafers	30-60 min	12 hours	No[b]	0.25 mg
diazepam (Valium, Diastat)	Tablets Oral solution Injectable Rectal gel	30-60 min (PO) 1-5 min (IV)	4-6 hours	Yes[b]	5 mg
lorazepam (Ativan)	Tablets Oral solution Injectable	30-60 min (PO) 5-20 min (IV)	6-8 hours	No	1mg
midazolam* (Versed)	Oral syrup Injectable	10-20 min (PO) 1-5 min (IV) 5-15 min (SQ)	2-3 hours	Yes[b]	1-2 mg*

Due to rapid onset of action and relatively short duration of action, midazolam equivalent dosing is not generally reported in the literature. The approximate equivalent dose provided here is based on clinical experience.

a: Presence of an active metabolite may extend the pharmacological activity of the drug past the desired clinical effect, increasing the likelihood of adverse effects of confusion, lethargy, ataxia, etc.

b: Undergoes oxidative metabolism. All benzodiazepines are metabolized in the liver and renally excreted. Avoid benzodiazepines that undergo oxidative metabolism in liver disease as this type of metabolism may be significantly impaired.

References
1. Lexi-Comp Online. Lexi-Drugs Online, Hudson, Ohio: Lexi-Comp, Inc, January 31, 2014
2. Benzodiazepine toolkit. *Pharmacist's Letter/Prescriber's Letter* 2011;27(4):270406
3. Olkkola K, Ahonen J. Midazolam and other benzodiazepines. *Handb Exp Pharmacol* 2008;182:335-360

Confused Drug Names

Unfortunately, many drug names can look or sounds like other drug names, which may lead to potentially harmful medication errors. The list below was adapted from the Institute for Safe Medication Practice's (ISMP) list of Confused Drug Names. Events involving these look-alike and sound-alike drug name pairs were reported to the ISMP National Medication Errors Reporting Program.[1]

Drug Name	Confused Drug Name	Drug Name	Confused Drug Name
Accupril	Aciphex	Flonase	Flovent
Aciphex	Aricept	FLUoxetine	PARoxetine
Actonel	Actos	FLUoxetine	Loxitane
Adacel (Tdap)	Daptacel (DTaP)	glipiZIDE	glyBURIDE
Adderall	Inderal	guaiFENesin	guanFACINE
Advair	Advicor	HumaLOG	HumuLIN
Allegra	Viagra	HumuLIN 70/30	HumaLOG 75/25
ALPRAZolam	LORazepam	hydrALAZINE	hydrOXYzine
amantadine	amiodarone	HYDROcodone	oxyCODONE
aMILoride	amLODIPine	HYDROmorphone	morphine
antacid	Atacand	Inspra	Spiriva
Anzemet	Avandamet	Keppra	Kaletra
ARIPiprazole	RABEprazole	ketorolac	Ketalar
Asacol	Os-Cal	ketorolac	methadone
Avandia	Coumadin	LaMICtal	LamISIL
Avinza	Evista	lamoTRIgine	lamiVUDine
B&O (belladonna & opium)	Beano	Lanoxin	levothyroxine
Benadryl	benazepril	Lanoxin	naloxone
buPROPion	busPIRone	Lasix	Luvox
captopril	carvedilol	Maxzide	Microzide
carBAMazepine	OXcarbazepine	Mephyton	methadone
ceFAZolin	cefTRIAXone	Metadate	methadone
CeleBREX	CeleXA	metFORMIN	metroNIDAZOLE
CeleBREX	Cerebyx	methadone	methylphenidate
CeleXA	ZyPREXA	metolazone	methimazole
cetirizine	sertraline	metoprolol succinate	metoprolol tartrate
chlordiazePOXIDE	chlorproMAZINE	Miralax	Mirapex
clonazePAM	cloNIDine	Motrin	Neurontin
clonazePAM	LORazepam	MS Contin	OxyCONTIN
cloNIDine	KlonoPIN	Mucinex	Mucomyst
Colace	Cozaar	niCARdipine	NIFEdipine
cycloSERINE	cycloSPORINE	NIFEdipine	niMODipine
Cymbalta	Symbyax	OLANZapine	QUEtiapine
Depakote	Depakote ER	opium tincture	paregoric
desipramine	disopyramide	oxyCODONE	OxyCONTIN
dexmethylphenidate	methadone	Pamelor	Tambocor
dimenhyDRINATE	diphenhydrAMINE	PARoxetine	piroxicam

Drug Name	Confused Drug Name	Drug Name	Confused Drug Name
Ditropan	Diprivan	Paxil	Plavix
DOBUTamine	DOPamine	PENTobarbital	PHENobarbital
DULoxetine	FLUoxetine	Prandin	Avandia
flavoxATE	fluvoxaMINE	prednisoLONE	predniSONE
PriLOSEC	PROzac	Toradol	Foradil
Protonix	protamine	traMADol	traZODone
quiNIDine	quiNINE	TRENtal	TEGretol
Restoril	RisperDAL	valACYclovir	valGANciclovir
risperiDONE	rOPINIRole	Valcyte	Valtrex
Roxanol	Roxicodone	Xanax	Zantac
Roxanol	Roxicet	Zegerid	Zestril
Rozerem	Razadyne	Zestril	Zetria
Salagen	selegiline	Zestril	ZyPREXA
sulfADIAZINE	sulfaSALAzine	Zocor	Cozaar
SUMAtriptan	ZOLMitriptan	Zocor	ZyrTEC
tiaGABine	tiZANidine	Zostrix	Zovirax
Tobradex	Tobrex	Zyban	Diovan
Topamax	Toprol-XL	Zyvox	Zovirax

- Table adapted and used with permission from the Institute for Safe Medication Practices ©2014
- Report medication errors or near misses to the ISMP Medication Errors Reporting Program (MERP) at 1-800-FAIL-SAF(E) or online at www.ismp.org

What prescribers can do:[2,3]

- Maintain awareness of look-alike and sound-alike drug names as published by various safety agencies.
- Clearly specify the dosage form, drug strength, and complete directions on prescriptions. These variables may help staff differentiate products.
- With name pairs known to be problematic, reduce the potential for confusion by writing prescriptions using both brand and generic name.
- Include the purpose of medication on prescriptions. In most cases drugs that sound or look similar are used for different purposes.
- Alert patients to the potential for mix-ups, especially with known problematic drug names. Advise ambulatory care patients to insist on pharmacy counseling when picking up prescriptions, and to verify that the medication and directions match what the prescriber has told them.
- Encourage inpatients to question nurses about medications that are unfamiliar or look or sound different than expected.
- Give verbal or telephone orders only when truly necessary, and never for chemotherapeutics. Include the drug's intended purpose to ensure clarity. Encourage staff to read back all order, spell the product name, and state its indication.

What organizations and practitioners can do:[2,3]

- Maintain awareness of look alike and sound-alike drug names as published by various safety agencies. Regularly provide information to professional staff.
- Whenever possible, determine the purpose of the medication before dispensing or drug administration. Most products with look or sound-alike names are used for different purposes.
- When possible, list brand and generic names on medication administration records and automated dispensing cabinet computer screens. Such redundancy could help someone identify an error.

- Encourage reporting of errors and potentially hazardous conditions with look and sound-alike product names and use the information to establish priorities for error reduction. Also maintain awareness of problematic product names and error prevention recommendations provided by ISMP (www.ismp.org), FDA (www.fda.gov), and USP (www.usp.org).

References

1. Institute for Safe Medication Practices (ISMP). ISMP's list of confused drug names (updated through April 2014). ISMP, 2014. Available at http://ismp.org/Tools/confuseddrugnames.pdf. Accessed February 18, 2015.
2. Institute for Safe Medication Practices (ISMP). What's in a name? Ways to prevent dispensing errors linked to name confusion. *ISMP Medication Safety Alert!* 2002;7:12. Available at http://www.ismp.org/Newsletters/acutecare/articles/20020612_2.asp. Accessed January 31, 2014
3. The Joint Commission (TJC). Look-alike, sound-alike drug names. Sentinel Event Alert 2001:19. Available at http://www.jointcommission.org/sentinel_event_alert_issue_19_look-alike_sound-alike_drug_names/ Accessed January 31, 2014
4. Santell JP, Cousins DD. Medication Errors Related to Product Names. *Joint. Commission J Qual Pt. Safety* 2005; 31:649-54.

Corticosteroid Equivalency Information

The following table compares systemic corticosteroids based upon two sets of data: equivalent dose and potency of mineralocorticoid and glucocorticoid activity. The equivalent dose information is used when switching from one steroid to another. The potency data is used to show the differences in activity of each corticosteroid, using cortisol as a standard (i.e. cortisol has a glucocorticoid activity of 1 and predniSONE has an activity of 4; this means prednisone has four times the activity of cortisol). The potency data should NOT be used to switch from one corticosteroid to another.

- *Mineralocorticoid Activity (MA):* Once the mineralocorticoid receptor is activated, the body will retain sodium and water. The higher the mineralocorticoid activity of a systemic steroid the more water and sodium the patient will retain. This could lead to an increase in edema, chest congestion, dyspnea, acute decompensated heart failure, and hypertension.[1,2]
- *Glucocorticoid Activity (GA):* Once the glucocorticoid receptor is activated, the inflammatory and immune responses decrease. The higher the glucocorticoid activity of a systemic steroid the more anti-inflammatory effects the drug will have. However, this could lead to hyperglycemia, mood changes, muscle weakness, slow wound healing, and increased risk of bruising.[3,4]

Table 1. Approximate Systemic Corticosteroid Equivalency[1,5-10]

Systemic Corticosteroid		Equivalent Dose (mg)	GA	MA	Duration of Action (h)	Peak Effect (h)
Generic	Brand					
Mineralocorticoid						
fludrocortisone	Florinef®	-	15	150	18-36	1.5
Short Acting						
cortisone	Cortone®	25	0.8	0.8	8-12	2
hydrocortisone	Cortef®	20	1	1	8-12	1
Intermediate Acting						
predniSONE	Deltasone®	5	4	0.8	12-36	2
prednisoLONE	Orapred®	5	4	0.8	12-36	1-2
triamcinolone	Kenalog®	4	5	0	12-36	1-2
methylPREDNISolone	Medrol®	4	5	0.5	12-36	1-2
Long Acting						
dexamethasone	Decadron®	0.75	30	0	36-54	1-2
betamethasone	Diprolene®	0.6	30	0	36-54	1-2
budesonide	Entocort® EC	1	N/A[†]	N/A[†]	Limited systemic absorption. Duration of action is unclear.	0.5-10
	Uceris®	1	N/A[†]	N/A[†]		7-19
Bodily Hormones						
cortisol*	-	-	1	1	-	-
aldosterone	-	-	0	400+	-	-

*A normal adult, not under stress, releases cortisol equivalent to 5 mg of predniSONE per day

†No specific activity data is available, however literature states high glucocorticoid activity and low mineralocorticoid activity

Inhaled to Systemic Corticosteroid Conversion[11]

No formal conversion from inhaled to systemic corticosteroids exists; however, studies suggest that a daily oral dose of prednisoLONE 7.5-10 mg appears to be equivalent to moderate to high doses of inhaled corticosteroids. Clinical presentation should be the basis of dose conversion. Different side effect profiles are present when switching from inhaled to systemic steroids. Common inhaled corticosteroid side effects include oral candidiasis and increased risk of respiratory infection, while common systemic side effects include GI upset, fluid retention, elevated blood glucose, and decreased wound healing.

Table 2. Approximate Inhaled Corticosteroid Equivalency (Age ≥ 12yrs)[8-10,12-14]

Inhaled Corticosteroid		High Daily Dose (mcg)	Moderate Daily Dose (mcg)	Low Daily Dose (mcg)
Generic	Brand			
Single Ingredient Products*				
ciclesonide	Alvesco®	>320	>160-320	80-160
mometasone	Asmanex®	>400	400	200
budesonide	Pulmicort® Flexhaler	>1,200	>600-1,200	180-600
fluticasone propionate	Flovent® Diskus	>500	>300-500	100-300
	Flovent® HFA	>440	>264-440	88-264
beclomethasone	QVAR®	>480	>240-480	80-240
flunisolide	Aerospan®	>640	>320-640	320
Combination Ingredient Products‡				
fluticasone propionate-salmeterol	Advair Diskus®	>500	>300-500	100-300
	Advair® HFA	>460	>270-460	90-270
mometasone-formoterol	Dulera®	>400	400	200
budesonide-formoterol	Symbicort®	>1,200	>600-1,200	180-600
fluticasone furoate-vilanterol	Breo Ellipta®	New to market; current potency data available. Currently only one formulation containing 100 mcg of fluticasone furoate (FF). FF 100 mcg once daily has similar efficacy to a moderate daily dose of fluticasone propionate/salmeterol (500mcg).		

*Some dosages outside of clinical practice; data from potency studies based upon a dose response curve indicate high, moderate, and low dosing for each specific drug.
‡Dose ranges based on the corticosteroid alone and the assumption that the patient is receiving the full dose of the inhaled corticosteroid. Take into account both ingredients and consider an appropriate substitution for the bronchodilator component when switching a patient to systemic steroids.

References

1. NADF: Tools for Life-Adrenal Hormone Replacements. Great Neck, NY: National Adrenal Disease Foundation. 1987-2007. Available at http://www.nadf.us/tools/adrenalhormone.htm
2. Gennaro AR, editor. Hormones and Hormone Antagonists. Chapter 77. In, *Remington: The Science and Practice of Pharmacy*. 20th ed. Baltimore: Lippincott Williams & Wilkins; 2000, p. 1358-94.
3. Duma D, Cidlowski J. Generating diversity in glucocorticoid receptor signaling: mechanisms, receptor isoforms, and post-translational modifications. *Horm Mol Biol Clin Invest* 2010;3(1):319-328.
4. Qi D, Rodrigues B. Glucocorticoids produce whole body insulin resistance with changes in cardiac metabolism. *Am J Physiol Endocrinol Metab* 2006;292:E 654-E667.
5. Entocort EC package insert. Wilmington, DE:AstraZeneca. Revised 2011.
6. ASCRS: Inflammatory Bowel Disease: Medical Management. Florida: American Society of Colon & Rectal Surgeons; 2013. Available at http://www.fascrs.org/physicians/education/core_subjects/2002/ifb_advances_medical_management/
7. Debono M, Ghobadi C, Rostami-Hodjegan A., et al. Modified-release hydrocortisone to provide circadian cortisol profiles. *J Clin Endocrinol Metab* 2009; 94(5):1548-1554.
8. LexiComp Online. Lexi-Drugs Online, Hudson, OH:Lexi-Drugs, Inc. October 14, 2013.
9. eAnswers. Facts & Comparisons Online, Indianapolis, IN: Wolter Kluwer Health. October 14, 2013.
10. Clinical Pharmacology Online, Tampa, Florida: Elsevier Gold Standard. October 14, 2013.
11. Mash BRJ, Bheekie A, Jones P. Inhaled versus oral steroids for adults with chronic asthma (Review). *Cochrane Collaboration*. 2009 (1):1-35.
12. Breo Ellipta medication guide. GlasxoSmithKline, 2013. Available at http://www.fda.gov/downloads/Drugs/DrugSafety/UCM352347.pdf
13. NHLBI: Guidelines for the Diagnosis and Management of Asthma. Bethesda, MD: National Heart, Lung, and Blood Institute. 2007. Managing Asthma Long term in youths ≥ 12yrs of age and adults. Available at http://www.nhlbi.nih.gov/guidelines/asthma/09_sec4_lt_12.pdf
14. Woodcock A, Bleecker E, Lotvall J, et al. Efficacy and safety of fluticasone furoate/vilanterol compared with fluticasone propionate/salmeterol combination in adult and adolescent patients with persistent asthma: a randomized trial. *Chest*. 2013;144 (4):1222-1229.

Do Not Crush or Chew List

All medications with formulations providing delayed-release, extended-release, or controlled-release properties must not be crushed. These dosage formulations frequently, but not always, include a suffix in the name (e.g., ER, DR, CR, LA, SR, XR, CC, CD, SA, or XL). Long-acting opioid medications are particularly dangerous when the dosage form is altered as tablet disruption can cause a potential fatal overdose of the drug (dose-dumping). Additionally, many long-acting opioid medications are prepared with abuse deterrent formulations (e.g., OxyCONTIN, Oxecta, Embeda, Zohydro, Hysingla) that will inactivate the opioid or render the tablet unusable if tampering or altering occurs.

Medications that are enteric-coated (EC) must not be crushed; however capsules containing enteric-coated microbeads may be sprinkled on soft food (e.g., applesauce or pudding) and swallowed without chewing or crushing the microbeads. The contents may be administered via enteral feeding tubes using sufficient water to flush and clear the tube. The list below provides guidance on medications that should not be crushed. Always consult a pharmacist for specific recommendations and additional information prior to altering any dosage form. This list was adapted and used with permission from the Institute for Safe Medication Practices (ISMP). Please refer to the ISMP website for the most current and complete list (www.ismp.org).

Do NOT Crush or Chew List

Brand	Generic	Dosage Form
AcipHex	RABEprazole	Tablet
Actiq	fentaNYL	Lozenge
Actonel	risedronate	Tablet
Afinitor	everolimus	Tablet
Aggrenox	aspirin + dipyridamole	Capsule
Allegra-D	fexofenadine+pseudoephedrine	Tablet
Altoprev	lovastatin	Tablet
Ampyra	dalfampridine	Tablet
Amrix	cyclobenzaprine	Capsule
Aplenzin	buPROPion	Tablet
Apriso	mesalamine	Capsule
Aptivus	tipranavir	Capsule
Aricept 23 mg	donepezil	Tablet
Arthrotec	diclofenac	Tablet
Asacol	mesalamine	Tablet
Atelvia	risedronate	Tablet
AVINza	morphine	Capsule
Avodart	dutasteride	Capsule
Azulfidine EN	sulfaSALAzine	Tablet
Bayer Regular	aspirin	Caplet
Bisa-Lax	combination	Tablet
Bisac-Evac	bisacodyl	Tablet
Boniva	ibandronate	Tablet
Carbatrol	carBAMazepine	Capsule
Cardizem	diltiazem	Tablet
Ceftin	cefuroxime	Tablet

Brand	Generic	Dosage Form
CellCept	mycophenolate	Capsule, Tablet
Charcoal Plus	charcoal, activated	Tablet
Chlor-Trimeton	chlorpheniramine	Tablet
Claritin-D	loratadine + pseudoephedrine	Tablet
Colace	docusate	Capsule
Colestid	colestipol	Tablet
Commit	nicotine	Lozenge
Concerta	methylphenidate	Tablet
Creon	pancrelipase	Capsule
Crixivan	indinavir	Capsule
Cymbalta	DULoxetine	Capsule
Cytovene	ganciclovir	Capsule
Cytoxan	cyclophosphamide	Tablet
Depakene	divalproex	Capsule
Depakote	divalproex	Tablet
Depakote Sprinkles	divalproex	Capsule
Dexilant	dexlansoprazole	Capsule
Diclegis	doxylamine + pyridoxine	Tablet
Doxidan	bisacodyl	Tablet
Drisdol	ergocalciferol	Capsule
Droxia	hydroxyurea	Capsule
Dulcolax	bisacodyl	Tablet; Capsule
E.E.S. 400	erythromycin	Tablet
E-Mycin	erythromycin	Tablet
Ecotrin (all)	aspirin	Tablet
Effer-K	potassium bicarbonate	Tablet
Effervescent Potassium	potassium	Tablet
Embeda	morphine sulfate	Capsule
Enablex	darifenacin	Tablet
Equetro	carBAMazepine	Capsule
Ergomar	ergotamine	Tablet
Erivedge	vismodegib	Capsule
Ery-Tab	erythromycin	Tablet
Erythromycin Base	erythromycin	Tablet
Erythromycin Stearate	erythromycin	Tablet
Evista	raloxifene	Tablet
Exalgo	HYDROmorphone	Tablet
Exjade	deferasirox	Tablet
Feen-a-mint	bisacodyl	Tablet
Feldene	piroxicam	Capsule
Fentora	fentaNYL	Tablet
Feosol	ferrous sulfate	Tablet

Brand	Generic	Dosage Form
Feratab	ferrous sulfate	Tablet
Fergon	ferrous gluconate	Tablet
Flomax	tamsulosin	Capsule
Fortamet	metFORMIN	Tablet
Fosamax	alendronate	Tablet
Gleevec	imatinib	Tablet
Glumetza	metFORMIN	Tablet
Gralise	gabapentin	Tablet
Horizant	gabapentin	Tablet
Hydrea	hydroxyurea	Capsule
Hysingla ER	Hydrocodone	Tablet
Imdur	isosorbide	Tablet
Intelence	etravirine	Tablet
Intuniv	guanFACINE	Tablet
Invega	paliperidone	Tablet
ISOtretinoin	ISOtretinoin	Capsule
Jakafi	ruxolitinib	Tablet
Jalyn	dutasteride + tamsulosin	Capsule
K-Dur	potassium	Tablet
K-Lyte	potassium	Tablet
K-Lyte CL	potassium	Tablet
K-Lyte DS	potassium	Tablet
K-Tab	potassium	Tablet
Kadian	morphine	Capsule
Kaletra	lopinavir + ritoavir	Tablet
Kapidex	dexlansoprazole	Capsule
Kapvay	cloNIDine	Tablet
Kazano	alogliptin + metFORMIN	Tablet
Ketek	telithromycin	Tablet
Klor-Con	potassium	Tablet
Letairis	ambrisentan	Tablet
Levbid	hyoscyamine	Tablet
Levsinex	hyoscyamine	Capsule
Lialda	mesalamine	Tablet
Lithobid	lithium	Tablet
Lovaza	omega-3 fatty acid esters	Capsule
Motrin	ibuprofen	Tablet
Moxatag	amoxicillin	Tablet
MS Contin	morphine	Tablet
Mucinex	guiaFENesin	Tablet
Mucinex D	guaiFENesin + pseudoephedrine	Tablet
Mucinex DM	guaiFENesin+dextromethorphan	Tablet

Brand	Generic	Dosage Form
Myfortic	mycophenolate	Tablet
Myrbetriq	mirabegron	Tablet
Naprelan	naproxen	Tablet
NexIUM	esomeprazole	Capsule
Niaspan	nicotinic acid	Tablet
Niaspan	niacin	Capsule; Tablet
Nitrostat	nitroglycerin	Tablet
Norvir	ritonavir	Tablet
Oleptro	traZODone	Tablet
Oracea	doxycycline	Capsule
Pancrelipase	pancrealipase	Capsule
Pentasa	mesalamine	Capsule
Plendil	felodipide	Tablet
Pradaxa	dabigatran	Capsule
Prevacid	lansoprazole	Capsule
Prevacid SoluTab	lansoprazole	Tablet
Prevacid Suspension	lansoprazole	Suspension
PriLOSEC	omeprazole	Capsule
PriLOSEC OTC	omeprazole	Tablet
Pristiq	desvenlafaxine	Tablet
Propecia	finasteride	Tablet
Proscar	finasteride	Tablet
Protonix	pantoprazole	Tablet
PROzac Weekly	FLUoxetine	Tablet
Ranexa	ranolazine	Tablet
Rapamune	sirolimus	Tablet
Rayos	predniSONE	Tablet
Renagel	sevelamer	Tablet
Renvela	sevelamer carbonate	Tablet
Revlimid	lenalidomide	Capsule
Ryzolt	traMADol	Tablet
Sensipar	cinacalcet	Tablet
Slo-Niacin	nicotinic acid	Tablet
Solodyn	minocycline	Tablet
Sprycel	dasatinib	Tablet
Strattera	atomoxetine	Capsule
Sular	nisoldipine	Tablet
Symax Duotab	hyoscyamine	Tablet
Tasigna	nilotinib	Capsule
Tecfidera	dimethyl fumarate	Capsule
Temodar	temozolomide	Capsule
Tessalon Perles	benzonatate	Capsule

Brand	Generic	Dosage Form
Theochron	theophylline	Tablet
Tiazac	diltiazem	Capsule
Topamax	topiramate	Tablet; Capsule
Toviaz	fesoterodine	Tablet
Tracleer	bosentan	Tablet
TRENtal	pentoxifylline	Tablet
Treximet	SUMAtriptan + naproxen	Tablet
Trilpix	fenofibric	Capsule
Tylenol Arthritis	acetaminophen	Tablet
Uceris	budesonide	Tablet
Ultrase	pancrealipase	Capsule
Uniphyl	theophylline	Tablet
Urocit-K	potassium citrate	Tablet
Uroxatral	alfuzosin	Tablet
Valcyte	valGANCiclovir	Tablet
Verelan	verapamil	Capsule
Verelan PM	verapamil	Capsule
Videx EC	didanosine	Capsule
Vimovo	naproxen + esomeprazole	Tablet`
Votrient	pazopanib	Tablet
Zegerid OTC	omeprazole + NaHCO3	Capsule
Zenpep	pancrealipase	Capsule
Zohydro ER	Hydrocodone ER	Capsule
Zolinza	vorinostat	Capsule
Zortress	everolimus	Tablet
Zyban	buPROPion	Tablet

Report medication errors or near misses to the ISMP Medication Errors Reporting Program (MERP) at 1-800-FAIL-SAF(E) or online at www.ismp.org.

References

1. Mitchell JF, Institute for Safe Medication Practices (ISMP). Oral dosage forms that should not be crushed, (updated through January 2014). ISMP 2014. Available at http://www.ismp.org/Tools/DoNotCrush.pdf. Accessed February 18, 2015.
2. Lexi-Comp Online. Lexi-Drugs Online, Hudon, Ohio: Lexi-Comp, Inc, January 31, 2015.

Drugs That Prolong the QT Interval

Each part of the cardiac electrical activity waveform is given an initial: P, Q, R, S, and T. When the QT interval is abnormal, the length of time between the Q and T of the waveform is prolonged, causing the heart to start a new contraction before recovering from the previous contraction. The measurement of the time between the Q and T parts of the waveform are reported as a corrected QT interval, or QTc. Normal QTc interval time is < 420 milliseconds (ms) for men and < 440 ms for females. Long QT syndrome can be inherited or acquired due to myocardial infarction, hypocalcemia, or medications. ***Please note, Table 1 is not intended to be comprehensive. Always review patient medication profiles with a pharmacist to confirm drug interaction risk and other medication safety considerations.***

Table 1. Drugs to Avoid in Congenital Long QT Syndrome (LQTS)

albuterol	alfluzosin	amantadine	amiodarone *
amitriptyline	amphetamine	arformoterol	atazanavir
atomoxetine	azithromycin *	chlorproMAZINE *	ciprofloxacin
citalopram *	clarithromycin *	clomiPRAMINE	cloZAPine
desipramine	dexmedetomidine	dexmethylphenidate	dextroamphetamine
diphenhydrAMINE	disopyramide *	DOBUTamine	dofetilide *
dolasetron	DOPamine	doxepin	ePHEDrine
EPINEPHrine	erythromycin *	escitalopram *	famotidine
felbamate	fingolimod	flecainide *	fluconazole
FLUoxetine	formoterol	foscarnet	fosphenytoin
furosemide	galantamine	gemifloxacin	granisetron
haloperidol *	hydrochlorothiazide	iloperidone	imipramine
indapamide	isoproterenol	isradipine	itraconazole
ketoconazole	levalbuterol	levofloxacin	lisdexamfetamine
lithium	metaproterenol	methadone *	methylphenidate
midodrine	mirabegron	mirtazapine	moexipril
moxifloxacin *	niCARdipine	norephinephrine	norfloxacin
nortriptyline	ofloxacin	OLANZapine	ondansetron *
paliperidone	PARoxetine	pasireotide	pentamidine *
phenylephrine	pimozide *	posaconazole	procainamide *
promethazine	pseudoephedrine	QUEtiapine	quiNIDine *
quiNINE	ranolazine	rilpivirine	risperiDONE
ritonavir	salmeterol	saquinavir	sertraline
sevoflurane *	solifenacin	sotalol *	tacrolimus
telaprevir	telavancin	telithromycin	terbutaline
tetrabenazine	thioridazine *	tiZANidine	tolterodine
traZODone	trimethoprim-sulfa	venlafaxine	voriconazole
ziprasidone			

Drugs with known risk of torsades de pointes.

References

1. Lexi-Comp Online. Lexi-Drugs Online. Hudson, Ohio: Lexi-Comp, Inc. January 31, 2015
2. CredibleMeds.org/AZCERT. Drugs to avoid for congenital long QT syndrome [Internet]. February 19, 2015. Available at http://crediblemeds.org/ Accessed February 20, 2015

Extrapyramidal Symptoms from Medications

Extrapyramidal symptoms (EPS) are a neurological side effect of antipsychotic medications. EPS can occur within the first few days or weeks of treatment, or it can appear after months and years of antipsychotic medication use. EPS are more common among patients taking conventional antipsychotic medications, compared to the newer atypical drugs. EPS can express as involuntary movements, tremors and rigidity, body restlessness, muscle contractions, and changes in breathing and heart rate. Symptoms include:

- Tardive dyskinesia: involuntary movements most often affecting the mouth, lips, and tongue (e.g. facial tics, rolling the tongue, licking the lips). The trunk or other parts of the body may also be affected. This side effect is usually managed or minimized by reducing the medication dosage or by changing type of medication. However, the symptoms may persist even when the medication is altered or discontinued.
- Tremors and rigidity (Parkinsonism): tremors, rigidity, temporary paralysis, and extreme slowness of movement, usually appearing in the first few days to weeks of medication use.
- Akathisia: characterized by an internal sense of motor restlessness often described as an inability to resist the urge to move. The most common form of akathisia involves pacing and an inability to sit still. This side effect is often very distressing to the patient and reduces the ability to perform everyday tasks.
- Acute dystonia: characterized by a spastic contraction of muscle groups, most often affecting the neck, eyes, and trunk. These involuntary muscle contractions can occur suddenly and are often very painful.
- Neuroleptic malignant syndrome (NMS): potentially fatal if not treated. NMS includes diffuse muscle rigidity, tremor, high fever, labile blood pressure, cognitive dysfunction, and autonomic disturbances. NMS onset can be sudden and often occurs within the first week of medication use. NMS can be effectively and rapidly treated with medication.

Table 1. Medications Associated with Extrapyramidal Effects[1-3]

Medication	Category
buPROPion (Wellbutrin)	Antidepressant, dopamine reuptake inhibitor
citalopram (Celexa)	Antidepressant, selective serotonin reuptake inhibitor
escitalopram (Lexapro)	Antidepressant, selective serotonin reuptake inhibitor
FLUvoxamine (Luvox)	Antidepressant, selective serotonin reuptake inhibitor
sertraline (Zoloft)	Antidepressant, selective serotonin reuptake inhibitor
DULoxetine (Cymbalta)	Antidepressant, serotonin norepinephrine reuptake inhibitor
amitriptyline (Elavil)	Antidepressant, tricyclic
ondansetron (Zofran)	Antiemetic, 5HT antagonist
prochloperazine (Compazine)	Antiemetic, phenothiazine
promethazine (Phenergan)	Antiemetic, phenothiazine
metoclopramide (Reglan)	Antiemetic, prokinetic
carBAMazepine (TEGretol)	Anti-epileptic
OLANZapine (ZyPREXA)	Antipsychotic, atypical
risperiDONE (RisperDAL)	Antipsychotic, atypical
ziprasidone (Geodon)	Antipsychotic, atypical
chlorproMAZINE (Thorazine)	Antipsychotic, conventional
haloperidol (Haldol)	Antipsychotic, conventional
diltiazem (Cardizem)	Calcium channel blocker
lithium (Lithobid)	Mood stabilizer

References

1. Madhusoodanan S, Alexeenko L, Sanders R, Brenner R. Extrapyramidal symptoms associated with antidepressants: a review of the literature and an analysis of spontaneous reports. *Ann Clin Psych* 2010;22(3):148-156.
2. Muench J, Hamer A. Adverse effects of antipsychotic medications. *Am Fam Phys* 2010;81(5):617-622.
3. Lexi-Comp Online. Lexi-Drugs Online. Hudson, Ohio: Lexi-Comp, Inc. January 31, 2015.

Insulin Products and Non-Insulin Injectables Comparison Table

Medications[1-3]	Onset (O)/Peak (P) of Action[C]	Duration of Action
Rapid Acting Insulin		
Afrezza (*inhaled* insulin) [Rx, A]	O: 50 min P: 15 min	2.5-3 hours
Apidra (insulin glulisine) [Rx, B]	O: 25 min P: 45 min	4-5.5 hours
HumaLOG (insulin lispro)[Rx, B]	O: 15-30 min P: 30 min-2.5 hours	3-6.5 hours
NovoLOG (insulin aspart) [Rx, B]	O: 10-20 min P: 40-50 min	3-5 hours
Short Acting (Regular) Insulin		
HumuLIN R	O: 30-60 min P: 1-5 hours	4-12 hours
NovoLIN R	O: 30 min P: 2.5-5 hours	8 hours
Intermediate Acting (NPH) Insulin		
HumuLIN N[A]	O: 1-2 hours P: 6-14 hours	Up to 24 hours
NovoLIN N	O: 90 min P: 4-12 hours	Up to 24 hours
Long Acting Insulin		
Lantus (insulin glargine) [Rx, B]	O: 1 hour P: none	11 to 24 hours
Levemir (insulin detemir) [Rx, B]	O: 1-2 hours P: none	6 to 24 hours
Insulin Mixtures		
NovoLOG Mix 70/30 [Rx, B]	O: 10-20 min P: 1-4 hours	Up to 24 hours
HumaLOG Mix 75/25 [Rx, B]	O: 15-30 min P: 1-6 hours	Up to 24 hours
HumaLOG Mix 50/50 [Rx, B]	O: 15-30 min P: 1-5 hours	Up to 24 hours
HumuLIN 70/30[B]	O: 30 min P: 2-16 hours	Up to 24 hours
NovoLIN 70/30	O: 30 min P: 2-12 hours	Up to 24 hours
Non-Insulin Injectable Agents	**Therapeutic Class**	**Meal Timing**
Byetta (exetanide) [Rx, B]	Incretin mimetic / GLP-1 agonist	60 min prior to meals BID
Symlin (pramlintide) [Rx, B]	Synthetic amylin analog	Immediately prior to meals
Tanzeum (abliglutide) [Rx, B]	Incretin mimetic / GLP-1 agonist	Once *weekly*, independent of meals
Trulicity (dulaglutide) [Rx, B]	Incretin mimetic / GLP-1 agonist	Once *weekly*, independent of meals
Victoza (liraglutide) [Rx, B]	Incretin mimetic / GLP-1 agonist	Once *daily*, independent of meals

Rx: Available by prescription only. Humulin R (500 units/mL presentation) is also prescription only.
A: Inhaled insulin (Technosphere insulin, TI); powder for inhalation with 4 and 8 unit dose cartridges.
B: Prefilled product dose administration device available (e.g. FlexPen, AutoPen, Opticlik, Pen-Injector)
C: Onset, peak, and duration of action based on subcutaneous administration

References
1. Lexi-Comp Online. Lexi-Drugs Online, Hudson, Ohio: Lexi-Comp; February 19, 2015.
2. Monthly Prescribing Reference. eMPR [Internet]. Haymarket Media. Available at http://www.empr.com Accessed July 29, 2014.
3. Comparison of insulins and injectable diabetes meds. Pharmacist's Letter/Prescriber's Letter 2010;26(3):260304.

Medication Route Considerations

Route	Considerations
Oral	• Painless. • Most convenient and safe route; most medications are available in oral dosage forms. • Consider taste, especially if crushing medications. • Easy to titrate. • Not recommended in patients with bowel obstruction. • Difficult to tolerate in patients with nausea or vomiting. • Lack of available liquid options may limit use in patients with dysphagia.
Feeding tube (PEG)	• Absorption of medications is influenced by the location of the distal end of the tube (stomach, duodenum, jejunum). • Feeding tubes may clog with frequent administration of crushed medications. • Many drug formulations cannot be crushed (extended release, enteric coated). • Routine flushing of tube before and after medication administration is required. • Medications with "empty stomach" administration instructions require holding of feedings for 1-2 hours before and after administrations. • Possibility of drug interactions with the enteral nutrition formula.
Inhalation	• Painless. • May require patient with adequate cognition and manual dexterity to time inhaler device actuation and controlled inspiration. • Nebulized medications are generally preferred over metered dose inhalers for inhalation therapy in hospice. • Local application of drug at the site of action (lungs).
Rectal	• Consider patient preference and privacy. • May be used for local (laxative) and systemic effect. • Medication absorption may have wide variability due to lipophilicity of drug, higher or lower placement in rectum, compounding base of suppositories. • Useful when unable to swallow or significant vomiting. • Use caution in neutropenic or thrombocytopenic patients. • Many medications have no literature to support rectal administration.
Sublingual	• Painless. • May need to add water or wet tablets if patient has dry mouth. • Consider volume of liquid, usually 1-2 mL can be held comfortably. • Not all medications are absorbed sublingually; dose may trickle back, swallowed with saliva. • Sublingual absorption of some medications may be enhanced if patient retains medication in sublingual space. • Surface area of sublingual space is small but lipophilic drugs can be absorbed rapidly (fentanyl, nitroglycerin).
Transdermal	• Painless. • Patient must be opioid tolerant; there are no short acting transdermal opioid preparations. • Difficult to titrate; due to long titration intervals (3-6 days per titration). • Most patches cannot be cut or folded. • May have increased absorption in febrile patients or young children. • Requires another route of administration for breakthrough pain dosing. • Approximately 8-12 hours for onset of analgesia (fentanyl). • Duration of action of patches varies considerably from 12 hours (lidocaine, nitroglycerin), 24 hours (rivastigmine), 72 hours (fentanyl, scopolamine), 3-4 days (oxybutynin), and up to 7 days (buprenorphine, clonidine). • Patients with multiple patches have a greatly increased risk of medication errors. • Not all drugs will penetrate intact skin; compounded topical preparations have no literature to support systemic absorption or effectiveness.

Medication Route Considerations - PARENTERAL

Route	Considerations
Intravenous	• Fastest and most reliable way of delivering a drug systemically. • Suitable for large volume infusions and mixtures of medications. • Rapid pain control for opioid administration. • Easy to titrate and adjust doses quickly. • Useful if severe vomiting, mucositis, bowel obstruction, or questionable GI absorption. • Consider using lidocaine gel or cream prior to inserting new IV line or accessing port. • Invasive; infusion pumps require equipment and electricity (if used in home, must consider alternative if loss of power). • Bolus dosing may have increased side effects (especially itching & vomiting), shortest duration, and shortest frequency.
Patient controlled analgesia (PCA)	• Can provide basal maintenance rate, as well as breakthrough doses. • Eliminates time between pain perception and relief. • Patient must understand the relationship between pushing the button and pain relief. • Caregivers must not administer doses by proxy (i.e., not to push button for the patient). • Maximum amounts can be set to minimize the risk of overdose or excessive use. • Monitor breakthrough doses received regularly; adjust maintenance dose as appropriate. • Invasive; requires equipment and electricity (if used in home, consider alternative if loss of power).
Intramuscular	• Painful. • Many drugs cannot be given IM because of pain, local tissue irritation, or erratic absorption; review suitability with a pharmacist. • Absorption altered in patients with decreased muscle mass. • Adequate blood flow to the injection site required to ensure absorption. • Minimize volume to minimize discomfort. • Volume of injection is limited by size of muscle mass available. Larger volume injections (>2mL) should be given into gluteal muscle.
Subcutaneous	• Small, portable pump available for continuous subcutaneous infusion (CSCI). • Bioavailability may be affected by body composition (fat, muscle) and hydration status. • Minimize volume to minimize discomfort (max volume: 2 mL). • Convenient and generally less painful than IM injection. • Not all injectable medications are safe for SC injection; see *Subcutaneous Access Devices* and review suitability with a pharmacist.
Epidural	• Short term use; may be tunneled subcutaneously. • Use only if consistent with patient and family goals. • Maximize use of less invasive route first. • May be beneficial for uncontrolled neuropathic pain, severe lower extremity pain, or if intolerable side effects from systemic analgesia.
Intrathecal	• Surgical procedure required for placement of implanted pump. • Longer term use; generally for chronic pain. • Implanted pumps must be refilled every 1-3 months. • Individualize dosing for oral opioids for breakthrough pain; start low and titrate as needed. • Create a plan for managing pump failure and acute pain crisis. • Contact patient's pain management clinic and/or manufacturer for information on specific device installed. • Must identify either pain management clinic or sterile compounding pharmacy to prepare medications for implanted pump refills.

References

1. Buxton IO, Benet LZ. Chapter 2. Pharmacokinetics: The Dynamics of Drug Absorption, Distribution, Metabolism, and Elimination. In: Brunton LL, Chabner BA, Knollmann BC. eds. *Goodman & Gilman's The Pharmacological Basis of Therapeutics, 12e.* New York, NY: McGraw-Hill; 2011. http://accesspharmacy.mhmedical.com. Accessed November 22, 2014.

2. Shargel L, Wu-Pong S, Yu AC. Chapter 20. Application of Pharmacokinetics to Clinical Situations. In: Shargel L, Wu-Pong S, Yu AC. eds. *Applied Biopharmaceutics & Pharmacokinetics, 6e.* New York, NY: McGraw-Hill; 2012.http://accesspharmacy.mhmedical.com. Accessed November 22, 2014.

3. Lee M, Phillips J. Transdermal patches: high risk for error? *Drug Topics.* 2002;Apr:54-55 Available at http://www.fda.gov/downloads/Drugs/DrugSafety/MedicationErrors/UCM080691.pdf Accessed November 14, 2014

4. Lovborg H, Holmlund M, Hagg S. Medication errors related to transdermal opioid patches: lessons from a regional incident reporting system. *BMC Pharmacol Toxicol.* 2014;15:31 Available at http://www.ncbi.nlm.nih.gov/pmc/articles/PMC4062292/ Accessed November 14, 2014

5. Kaestli LZ, Wasilewski-Rasca AF, Bonnabry P, Vogt-Ferrier N. Use of transdermal drug formulations in the elderly. *Drugs Aging.* 2008;25(4):269-280

6. Mathias NR, Hussain MA. Non-invasive systemic drug delivery: developability considerations for alternate routes of administration. *J Pharmaceut Sci.* 2010;99(1):1-20.

7. Kestenbaum MG, Vilches AO, Messersmith S, Connor SR, et al. Alternative routes to oral opioid administration in palliative care: a review and clinical summary. *Pain Med.* 2014;15(7):1129-1153

8. Ghafoor V, Epshteyn M, Carlson G, et al. Intrathecal drug therapy for long-term pain management. *Am J Health-Syst Pharm.* 2007;64:2447-61.

9. Hayes C, Jordan M, Hodson F, Ritchard L. Ceasing Intrathecal Therapy in Chronic Non-Cancer Pain: An Invitation to Shift from Biomedical Focus to Active Management. *PLoS One.* 2012;7(11):1-6.

Medications Associated with Anticholinergic Side Effects

The effects of anticholinergic medications are often considered when choosing medications for elderly patients. However, problematic anticholinergic side effects can occur in patients of any age. Common side effects of anticholinergic medications are dry mouth, constipation, and drowsiness. Symptoms of anticholinergic excess include restlessness, shaking, flushing, tachycardia, hallucinations, delirium, fever, dilated pupils, blurred vision, urinary retention, and difficulty speaking and swallowing. Monitor all patients for signs and symptoms when initiating or titrating medications with anticholinergic properties. Review medication profiles for total anticholinergic burden because the effect of these medications is cumulative and symptoms can worsen when multiple anticholinergic medications are used concurrently. A popular anticholinergic symptoms mnemonic is "blind as a bat, dry as a bone, red as a beet, mad as a hatter, and hot as a hare."

- blind as a bat: dilated pupils, blurred vision
- dry as a bone: dry mouth, dry eyes, decreased sweating
- red as a beet: flushed face
- mad as a hatter: delirium, confusion
- hot as a hare: increased body temperature

Table 1. Medications Associated with Anticholinergic Side Effects[1,2]

Category	Medications
Antiarrhythmics	disopyramide, procainamide, quiNIDine
Antidepressants	amitriptyline, doxepin, imipramine, nortriptyline, clomiPRAMINE, PARoxetine
Antidiarrheal	diphenoxylate-atropine
Antiemetics	promethazine, prochlorperazine, trimethobenzamide, meclizine
Antiepileptics	carBAMazepine, OXcarbazepine, valproic acid
Antihistamines	diphenhydrAMINE, chlorpheniramine, hydrOXYzine, cyproheptadine, dimenhyDRINATE
Antipsychotics	chlorproMAZINE, cloZAPine, fluPHENAzine, thiothixene
Muscle relaxants	metaxalone, cyclobenzaprine, orphenadrine, baclofen, carisoprodol, tiZANidine
Opioids	meperidine
Urinary, GI antispasmodics	oxybutynin, flavoxATE, dicyclomine, hyoscyamine, propantheline, darifenacin, fesoterodine, tolterodine, trospium, solifenacin

References

1. Lexi-Comp Online. Lexi-Drugs Online. Hudson, Ohio: Lexi-Comp, Inc. January 31, 2015.
2. Hester S. Drugs with anticholinergic activity. *Pharmacist's Letter/Prescriber's Letter* 2011;271206.

Palliative Performance Scale (PPSv2)

PPS Level	Ambulation	Activity & Evidence of Disease	Self-Care	Intake	Conscious Level
100%	Full	Normal activity & work; No evidence of disease	Full	Normal	Full
90%	Full	Normal activity & work; Some evidence of disease	Full	Normal	Full
80%	Full	Normal activity with effort; Some evidence of disease	Full	Normal or reduced	Full
70%	Reduced	Unable normal work/job Significant disease	Full	Normal or reduced	Full
60%	Reduced	Unable hobby/house work Significant disease	Occasional assistance necessary	Normal or reduced	Full or confusion
50%	Mainly Sit or Lie	Unable to do any work Extensive disease	Considerable assistance required	Normal or reduced	Full or confusion
40%	Mainly in Bed	Unable to do any activity Extensive disease	Mainly assistance	Normal or reduced	Full or drowsy, ± confusion
30%	Totally Bed Bound	Unable to do any activity Extensive disease	Total care	Normal or reduced	Full or drowsy, ± confusion
20%	Totally Bed Bound	Unable to do any activity Extensive disease	Total care	Minimal to sips	Full or drowsy, ± confusion
10%	Totally Bed Bound	Unable to do any activity Extensive disease	Total care	Mouth care only	Drowsy or coma, ± confusion
0	Death	-	-	-	-

©2001, Victory Hospice Society, BC, Canada www.victoriahospice.org

Instructions for Use of PPS (see also definition of terms)

1. PPS scores are determined by reading horizontally at each level to find a 'best fit' for the patient who is then assigned as the PPS% score.

2. Begin at the left column and read downwards until the appropriate ambulation level is reached, then read across to the next column and downwards again until the activity/evidence of disease is located. These steps are repeated until all five columns are covered before assigning the actual PPS for that patient. In this way, 'leftward' columns (columns to the left of any specific column) are 'stronger' determinants and generally take precedence over others.

Example 1: A patient who spends the majority of the day sitting or lying down due to fatigue from advanced disease and requires considerable assistance to walk even for short distances but who is otherwise fully conscious level with good intake would be scored at PPS 50%.

Example 2: A patient who has become paralyzed and quadriplegic requiring total care would be PPS 30%. Although this patient may be placed in a wheelchair (and perhaps seem initially to be at 50%), the score is 30% because he or she would be otherwise totally bed bound due to the disease or complication if it were not for caregivers providing total care including lift/transfer. The patient may have normal intake and full conscious level. Example 3: However, if the patient in example 2 was paraplegic and bed bound but still able to do some self-care such as feed themselves, then the PPS would be higher at 40 or 50% since he or she is not 'total care.'

3. PPS scores are in 10% increments only. Sometimes, there are several co? decision. Choosing a 'half-fit' value of PPS 45%, for example, is not correct. The combination of clinical judgment and 'leftward precedence' is used to determine whether 40% or 50% is the more accurate score for that patient.

4. PPS may be used for several purposes. First, it is an excellent communication tool for quickly describing a patient's current functional level. Second, it may have value in criteria for workload assessment or other measurements and comparisons. Finally, it appears to have prognostic value.

Definition of Terms for PPS

As noted below, some of the terms have similar meanings with the differences being more readily apparent as one reads horizontally across each row to find an overall 'best fit' using all five columns.

1. Ambulation: The items **'mainly sit/lie,'** **'mainly in bed,'** and **'totally bed bound'** are clearly similar. The subtle differences are related to items in the self-care column. For example, 'totally bed 'bound' at PPS 30% is due to either profound weakness or paralysis such that the patient not only can't get out of bed but is also unable to do any self-care. The difference between 'sit/lie' and 'bed' is proportionate to the amount of time the patient is able to sit up vs need to lie down. **'Reduced ambulation'** is located at the PPS 70% and PPS 60% level. By using the adjacent column, the reduction of ambulation is tied to inability to carry out their normal job, work occupation or some hobbies or housework activities. The person is still able to walk and transfer on their own but at PPS 60% needs occasional assistance.

2. Activity & Extent of disease: **'Some,'** **'significant,'** and **'extensive'** disease refer to physical and investigative evidence which shows degrees of progression. For example in breast cancer, a local recurrence would imply 'some' disease, one or two metastases in the lung or bone would imply 'significant' disease, whereas multiple metastases in lung, bone, liver, brain, hypercalcemia or other major complications would be 'extensive' disease. The extent may also refer to progression of disease despite active treatments. Using PPS in AIDS, 'some' may mean the shift from HIV to AIDS, 'significant' implies progression in physical decline, new or difficult symptoms and laboratory findings with low counts. 'Extensive' refers to one or more serious complications with or without continuation of active antiretrovirals, antibiotics, etc. The above extent of disease is also judged in context with the ability to maintain one's work and hobbies or activities. Decline in activity may mean the person still plays golf but reduces from playing 18 holes to 9 holes, or just a par 3, or to backyard putting. People who enjoy walking will gradually reduce the distance covered, although they may continue trying, sometimes even close to death (eg. trying to walk the halls).

3. Self-Care: **'Occasional assistance'** means that most of the time patients are able to transfer out of bed, walk, wash, toilet and eat by their own means, but that on occasion (perhaps once daily or a few times weekly) they require minor assistance. **'Considerable assistance'** means that regularly every day the patient needs help, usually by one person, to do some of the activities noted above. For example, the person needs help to get to the bathroom but is then able to brush his or her teeth or wash at least hands and face. Food will often need to be cut into edible sizes but the patient is then able to eat of his or her own accord.
'Mainly assistance' is a further extension of 'considerable.' usually eat with minimal or no help. This may fluctuate according to fatigue during the day. **'Total care'** means that the patient is completely unable to eat without help, toilet or do any self-care. Depending on the clinical situation, the patient may or may not be able to chew and swallow food once prepared and fed to him or her.

4. Intake: Changes in intake are quite obvious with **'normal intake'** referring to the person's usual eating habits while healthy. **'Reduced'** means any reduction from that and is highly variable according to the unique individual circumstances. **'Minimal'** refers to very small amounts, usually pureed or liquid, which are well below nutritional sustenance.

5. Conscious Level: **'Full consciousness'** implies full alertness and orientation with good cognitive abilities in various domains of thinking, memory, etc. **'Confusion'** is used to denote presence of either delirium or dementia and is a reduced level of consciousness. It may be mild, moderate or severe with multiple possible etiologies. **'Drowsiness'** implies fatigue, drug side effects, delirium or closeness to death and is sometimes included in the term stupor. **'Coma'** in this context is the absence of response to verbal or physical stimuli; some reflexes may or may not remain. The depth of coma may fluctuate throughout a 24 hour period.

Content used with permission from Victory Hospice Society, BC, Canada www.victoriahospice.org

Subcutaneous Access Devices

The subcutaneous (SQ) route of medication administration provides appropriate management of symptoms for patients who are unable to take medications through other routes of administration. The over-the needle catheter (e.g., BD Saf-T-Intima® or Smith's Jelco®) or the winged steel needle (e.g. Terumo Surflo® Winged Infusion Set or BD Safety Lok®) are commonly used to administer medications via the SQ route. Alternately, a button or patch type SQ infusion set may also be available (e.g., Neria® or Thalaset®). Always follow infusion set specific instructions for insertion and maintenance of the SQ site. Basic sample instructions for subcutaneous access device (SAD) procedures are below.

Indications

1. Circumstances that preclude or compromise oral administration:
   a. Dysphagia – due to neuromuscular weakness or mechanical obstruction
   b. Decreased level of consciousness
   c. Intestinal obstruction
   d. Nausea and vomiting
   e. Medication is not available in an oral form
2. Symptom control crisis requiring rapid and reliable medication administration and absorption.
3. Poor or variable compliance:
   a. Dementia
   b. Agitated delirium, with paranoia and non-compliance
   c. Personality issues

Inserting a subcutaneous access device (SAD)

Equipment needed:

- Alcohol swabs
- Antimicrobial solution (e.g. chlorhexidine, povidone-iodine, isopropyl alcohol)
- Skin barrier film (e.g. Skin Prep Protective Barrier Wipe), 25 gauge or 27 gauge SAD
  o Separate SAD for each medication to be injected/infused
- Transparent semipermeable membrane (TSM) dressing
- Needleless connector (also known as end cap, injection cap, or injection port)
- Catheter stabilization device or Tape
- Non-sterile gloves
- Sharps container

Procedures:

1. Wash hands, put on gloves.
2. Explain the procedure to the patient and caregiver.
3. Assemble the equipment at a convenient work area.
4. Assist the patient to a comfortable position.
5. Attach needleless connector (NC) to end of SAD.
6. Draw up approximately 0.25 mL of prescribed medication with syringe.
7. Inject medication into end NC until NC and SAD are filled.
8. Cleanse the selected site with antimicrobial solution. Allow to air dry. If povidone-iodine is used it must remain on skin at least 2 minutes.
9. Apply skin barrier film around area surrounding anticipated insertion site.
10. Insert SAD into subcutaneous space, with the bevel up, using a 45 degree angle.
11. Secure SAD with a catheter stabilizing device. Cover site, with TSM dressing, so that the skin over the needle is visible and the NC is accessible for injections.
12. At the site, write the time, date of insertion, medication and concentration, and your initials.
13. Discard disposable items in a plastic trash bag. Place the used needles and syringes in a sharps container.
14. Document procedure and patient's tolerance of procedure.
15. Before each medication injection, inspect the needle site for redness, or dislodgement of the needle.
16. If needle site is reddened, needle dislodged, or medication leaks from around needle, insert new SAD at a different body site.
17. Change SAD site based on clinical indication.

Signs of Infection, Cannula Misplacement, or Overuse of Site

Leaking, redness, exudate, localized heat, localized inflammation, pain, tenderness, hardness, burning, swelling, scarring, itching, bruising, unresolved blanching, or necrosis.

If Administering More than One Medication

Establish an additional SQ site for each new medication or if there is a change in the concentration of the current medication. Label and color code each site as to which medication is to be administered in that site.

Amount of Medication to Be Administered in a Single Injection

The maximum amount of medication to be administered at one time is 3-5 mL. This will allow for optimal absorption and comfort for the patient. *Do not flush the SAD.*

Instilling Medications through SAD (Intermittent Push)

Equipment needed:
- 3 mL syringes
- Alcohol swabs
- Medication
- Non-sterile gloves

Procedures:
1. Wash hands, put on gloves.
2. Explain procedure to patient and family
3. Cleanse injection cap that is attached to SAD tubing, with alcohol swabs.
4. Insert the syringe needle containing medication into the NC. Gently draw back on the plunger. If blood appears in the tubing, remove the syringe, discard medication, and remove the SAD. Restart the SAD in a different site in order to administer the medication.
5. If no blood appears in the SAD line, instill the medication into the SQ site. Discard used equipment.
6. Document medication given, any adverse effects or difficulties encountered, and patient tolerance of the procedure.

Initiating a Continuous SQ Infusion

Equipment needed:
- Alcohol swabs
- Medication in appropriate cassette/IV bag
- Continuous infusion pump
- 3 mL syringe with 1 mL normal saline

Procedures:
1. Wash hands, put on gloves.
2. Explain procedure to patient and family
3. Prime the tubing and set the program as ordered by the physician. Insert SQ catheter or use existing site.
4. Cleanse NC with alcohol swabs
5. Insert the syringe containing normal saline (0.5 mL) into the injection cap. Gently draw back on the plunger. If blood appears in the tubing, remove the SAD and discard. Restart the SAD in a different site.
6. If no blood appears in the SQ site extension tubing, attach the primed tubing and start the infusion.
7. Discard the syringe in the appropriate container and discard the other supplies used.
8. Ensure the "SQ Line" identification sticker is located by the SQ site.
9. Document the procedure, medication that is being administered, time of initiation of infusion, rate of infusion, bolus dose information (if included in the physician's order), and patient tolerance to the procedure.

Medications Acceptable for SQ Administration

0.9% or 0.45% Saline solution (NS or ½NS)	Glycopyrrolate	Methadone±
2.5% or 5% Dextrose solution (D5W)	Haloperidol	Midazolam*
Lactated Ringer's solution*	Heparin	Morphine
Dexamethasone	Hydromorphone	Naloxone
Dexmedetomidine*	Ketamine±	Octreotide*±
Diphenhydramine	Lidocaine*	Phenobarbital±
Fentanyl*	Lorazepam	Ranitidine
Furosemide	Metoclopramide	Scopolamine

studied for use in pediatrics; ±possible irritant use cautiously in pediatric patients

Medications *Not Recommended* for SQ Administration*

Chlorpromazine	Hypertonic solutions
Diazepam	Prochlorperazine
Hydroxyzine	Promethazine

irritating to SQ tissue, high risk of pain, injection site reaction, and/or tissue damage

Possible SQ Insertion Sites (Shaded areas below)

- Outer arm (do not use for hypodermoclysis)
- Abdomen (avoid in presence of tense abdominal distention such as ascites)
- Anterior thigh
- Sub-clavicular area (avoid when patient has lung disease or risk of pneumothorax)
- Upper back (use when other sites are unsuitable or when patient is confused)

Areas to AVOID for SQ Insertion

- Areas with lymphedema, edema, or decreased sensation (e.g. CVA)
- Areas with minimal SQ tissue
- Areas with broken skin
- Skin sites that have recently been irradiated
- Sites with infection or inflammation present
- Area with bony prominences
- Tumor sites
- Skin folds

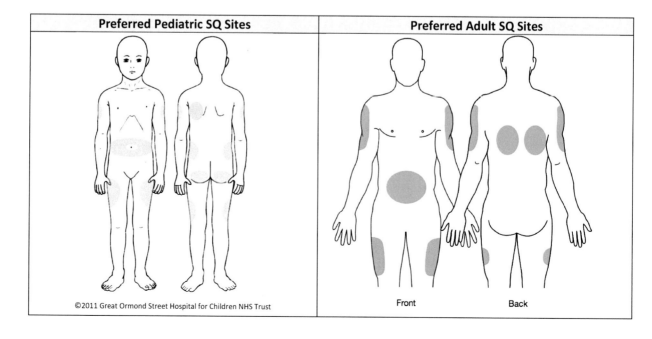

Preferred Pediatric SQ Sites	Preferred Adult SQ Sites

©2011 Great Ormond Street Hospital for Children NHS Trust

Front   Back

Subcutaneous Rehydration Therapy (SCRT, Hypodermoclysis)

Volume of subcutaneous fluid administered is dependent on age, weight, clinical condition of the patient. Maximum daily volume recommended for pediatrics is 25mL/kg/day, not to exceed a flow rate of 2mL/min

Pediatric SCRT Parameters

- Maximum recommended infusion rate: 2 mL/min
- Infants & children < 3 years: maximum 200 mL per infusion
- Children ≥ 3 years & adolescents: rate and volume should not exceed those of IV infusions
- Infusion of more than 3L in 24 hours not recommended in children or adults

If using gravity: Allow flow to freely adjust to gravity and rate of tissue absorption, approximately 1mL/min

Hyaluronidase: recombinant human hyaluronidase (Hylenex®, Vitrase®). If using, 15 units added to each 100mL of replacement fluids, *or* 150 units SQ bolus prior to initiation of SCRT isotonic fluids infusion of 1000 mL

Equipment needed:

- Alcohol swabs
- Medication in appropriate cassette/IV bag
- Continuous infusion pump, or gravity assist
- 3 mL syringe with 1 mL normal saline

Procedures:

1. Wash hands, put on gloves.
2. Explain procedure to patient and family.
3. Prime the tubing and set the program as ordered by the physician. Insert SQ catheter or use existing site.
4. Cleanse injection site cap with alcohol swabs
5. Insert the syringe containing normal saline (0.5 mL) into the injection cap. Gently draw back on the plunger. If blood appears in the tubing, remove the SAD and discard. Restart the SAD in a different site.
6. If no blood appears in the SQ site extension tubing, attach the primed tubing and start the infusion.
7. Discard the syringe in sharps container and discard the other supplies used.
8. Ensure the "SQ Line" identification sticker is located by the SQ site.
9. Gentle massage can be used to enhance absorption of fluid pocketing.
10. Document the procedure, medication that is being administered, time of initiation of infusion, rate of infusion, and patient tolerance to the procedure.

Hypodermoclysis Considerations

Advantages	Disadvantages
• Can prevent hospitalization of patients with dehydration • Procedure is safe, simple, and less expensive than intravenous (IV) hydration • May be performed in patients with collapsed, fragile, or thrombosed veins • Low risk of fluid overload • Patients experience a low incidence of pain or discomfort during administration • Low risk of infection or thrombophlebitis	• Limitation of solutions used (see chart on previous page) • Not recommended for patients with coagulopathies • Will not correct severe electrolyte abnormalities • Amount of fluid to be infused in 24 hours is limited (3L max recommended for adults) • Slight risk of pain and infection at infusion site • Fluid collection at injection site (resolve with gentle massage)

References

1. Fonzo-Christe C, Vukasovic C, Wasilewski-Rasca A, Bonnabry P. Subcutaneous administration of drugs in the elderly: survey of practice and systematic literature review. *Palliat Med* 2005;19(3):208-219.
2. Frisoli A, de Paula A, Feldman D, Nasri F. Subcutaneous hydration by hypodermoclysis: a practical and low cost treatment for elderly patients. *Drugs Aging* 2000;16(4):313-319.
3. Letizia M, Shenk M, Jones D. Intermittent subcutaneous injections for symptom control in hospice care: a retrospective investigation. *Hospice J* 2000;15(2):1-11.

4. Sasson M, Shvartzman P. Hypodermoclysis: an alternate infusion technique. *Am Fam Phys* 2001;64(9):1575-1578.
5. Remington R, Hultman T. Hypodermoclysis to treat dehydration: a review of the evidence. *J Am Geriatr Soc* 2007;55:2051-2055.
6. Pope B. How to administer subcutaneous and intramuscular injections. *Nursing* 2002;32(1):50-51.
7. Justad M. Continuous subcutaneous infusion: an efficacious, cost-effective analgesia alternative at the end of life. *Home Healthcare Nurse* 2009;27(3):140-147
8. Tobias J. Subcutaneous dexmedetomidine infusions to treat or prevent drug withdrawal in infants and childred. *J Opioid Manage* 2008;4(4):187-191
9. Breen M. Evaluation of two subcutaneous infusion devices in children receiving palliative care. *Paediatr Nurs* 2006;18(4):38-40
10. Tobias J. Subcutaneous administration of fentanyl and midazolam to prevent withdrawal after prolonged sedation in children *Crit Care Med* 1999;27(10):2262-2265
11. Nanto-Salonen K, Koskinen P, Sonninen P, Toppari J. Suppression of GH secretion in pituitary gigantism by continuous subcutaneous octreotide infusion in a pubertal boy. *Acta Paediatr* 1999;88(1):29-33.
12. Hosgood JR, Kimbrel JM, Protus BM, Grauer PA. Evaluation of subcutaneous phenobarbital administration in hospice patients. *Am J Hosp Palliat Med.* 2014;epub ahead of print DOI: 10.1177/1049909114555157.

Guidance for Withdrawal of Ventilator Life Support

General Principles for Withdrawing Life Sustaining Treatments[1-4]
- Death occurs as a complication of the underlying disease. The goal of comfort care is to relieve suffering in a dying patient, not to hasten death.
- Withdrawal of a life sustaining treatment is a medical procedure that requires the same degree of physician participation and quality as other procedures.
- Actions solely intended to hasten death (e.g., high doses of potassium or paralytic drugs) are morally unacceptable. However, pain and symptom relieving medication can be used when the doses required are intended to provide comfort even if those doses may hasten death.
- Withholding and withdrawing unnatural life sustaining treatments (e.g., ventilator) is morally and legally appropriate if the treatment is not benefiting the patient's quality of life.
- Discontinuation of all life prolonging treatments [e.g., nutrition, fluids, internal cardiac defibrillator (ICD), antibiotics, continuous venous to venous hemodialysis (CVVHD), and blood products] is recommended prior to ventilator withdrawal unless the family is not in agreement (see *Family Considerations*, next section).
- Assessing pain and discomfort in critically ill and intubated patients can be difficult. Monitor and document clinical findings and signs of discomfort in the medical record when initiating and titrating sedating medications to treat these symptoms: tachypnea, tachycardia, diaphoresis, grimacing, accessory muscle use, nasal flaring, and restlessness.
- Concerns about hastening death by over-sedating patients are understandable. Many patients develop tolerance to sedative medications. Clinicians should be wary of under-treating discomfort during the ventilator withdrawal.
- Patients who are "brain dead" do not need sedation during the ventilator withdrawal. When applicable, follow organ donation protocols.
- Paralytic drugs mask signs of discomfort. Discontinue all paralytic drugs and allow time for the patient to have sufficient motor activity to be able demonstrate signs of discomfort prior to ventilator withdrawal. Medications for sedation and analgesia should be readily available and may be needed to prevent undue anxiety, discomfort and pain.

Family Considerations
- Address any family concerns and perceptions about the process immediately.
- Counsel families on potential outcomes following withdrawal including use of pain and anxiety medications for comfort.
- Reassure the family that the patient's comfort is of primary concern.
- Explain that labored breathing and signs of breathlessness may occur, but that they can be managed.
- Confirm that you will have medication available to manage any discomfort.
- Ensure that the family knows that the patient will likely need to be kept asleep to control their symptoms.
- Explain that involuntary movements, noisy or irregular breathing, or gasping do not necessarily reflect suffering if the patient is sedated or in a coma.
- Document discussion with families and/or surrogates along with goals of care.
- Invite family into the room. Provide adequate room for the family to access the bedside.
- Encourage the family to make arrangements for special music or rituals or support during and following the procedure.
- Encourage the family to hold the patient's hand, hug the patient, and say "Goodbye."
- Have tissues, moist cloth, and lip balm available.

Prior to Ventilator Withdrawal

- Turn off all monitors and alarms.
- Assign respiratory therapy or nursing staff to override alarms which cannot be disabled.
- Discontinue all previous orders including routine vital signs, medication administration, enteral feeding, radiographs, and laboratory tests.
- Remove devices not necessary for comfort from the room, if possible (e.g., blood pressure cuffs, intermittent compression devices, cardiac monitoring devices, transfusers, and restraints).
- Have suction available, if the family is in agreement.
- Maintain intravenous access for administration of comfort medications, if possible.
- Have 4 to 5 pre-drawn doses of medications for sedation and pain at the bedside.

After Ventilator Withdrawal and Death Occurs

- Be prepared to spend additional time with the family discussing questions and concerns.
- Encourage the family to spend as much time at the bedside as they require.
- Provide acute grief support and follow-up bereavement support.
- Validate that it is completely acceptable for physicians and staff to share in the emotions of the family.
- Debrief the entire patient care team afterwards.

Additional Resources

- Weissman DE, von Gunten CF. Ventilator withdrawal protocol. Fast Fact 33. March 2009. Available at https://www.capc.org/fast-facts/33-ventilator-withdrawal-protocol/
- Weissman DE, von Gunten CF. Symptom control for ventilator withdrawal in the dying patient. Fast Fact 34. March 2009. Available at https://www.capc.org/fast-facts/34-symptom-control-ventilator-withdrawal-dying-patient/
- Weissman DE, von Gunten CF. Information for patients and families about ventilator withdrawal. Fast Fact 35. March 2009. Available at https://www.capc.org/fast-facts/35-information-patients-and-families-about-ventilator-withdrawal/

References

1. Szalados JE. Discontinuation of mechanical ventilation at end of life: the ethical and legal boundaries of physician conduct in termination of life support. *Crit Care Clinics* 2007;23(2):317-337.
2. Marr L, Weissman DE. Withdrawal of ventilatory support from the dying adult patient. *J Supp Onc.* 2004; 2:283-288Clinch A, Le B. Withdrawal of mechanical ventilation in the home: a case report and review of the literature. *Palliat Med* 2011;25(4):378-381.
3. Billings JA. Terminal extubation of the alert patient. *J Palliat Med* 2011; 14(7):800-801.
4. Lexi-Comp Online. Lexi-Drugs Online, Hudson, OH: Lexi-Comp, Inc; Accessed December 28, 2014.

Suggested Orders for Ventilator Withdrawal

Terminal Extubation Checklist
- ☐ Do Not Resuscitate-Comfort Care (DNRCC) order written and advanced directives are attached to patient chart.
- ☐ Rationale for comfort care, discussions with the attending physician, all pertinent services, consultants, and/or ethics committee as appropriate are documented in patient chart.
- ☐ Discussions with family (or attempts to contact family) and/or Durable Power of Attorney are documented in patient chart.
- ☐ Review entire protocol document with patient's care team prior to initiating withdrawal of ventilator life support

Symptom Control Medication Orders for Ventilator Withdrawal**

For pain or dyspnea for OPIOID NAÏVE patients (select one):

- ☐ Morphine:_____ (Dose, Route, Frequency)
  - ▪ Titration:_____
  - o Usual range
    - ▪ SL: 5-20 mg every 4 hours; patients with prior opioid exposure may require higher initial doses. Repeated doses (up to every 30 to 60 minutes needed) in small increments (e.g., 2.5-10 mg) may be preferred to larger and less frequent doses; dose should be adjusted based on patient response.
    - ▪ IV/SC: 2.5-5 mg every 3-4 hours; patients with prior opioid exposure may require higher initial doses. Repeated doses (up to every 5 minutes if needed) in small increments (e.g., 1-4 mg) may be preferred to larger and less frequent doses); dose should be adjusted based on patient response.
- ☐ Hydromorphone:_____(Dose, Route, Frequency)
  - ▪ Titration:_____
  - o Usual range:
    - ▪ IV/SC: 0.5-4 mg (based on 70 kg patient) every 4 hours as needed. More frequent dosing may be needed (e.g., every 1-2 hours); dose should be adjusted based on patient response.
- ☐ Fentanyl:_____ (Dose, Route, Frequency)
  - ▪ Titration:_____
  - o Usual range:
    - ▪ IV/SC: 25-100 mcg (based on 70 kg patient) **or** 0.35-1.5 mcg/kg every 30-60 minutes as needed. More frequent dosing may be needed (e.g., every 5-10 minutes); dose should be adjusted based on patient response.
- ☐ Other:_____ (Dose, Route, Frequency)
  - ▪ Titration:_____

*** Usual ranges are provided for general guidance only. Always assess individual patient-specific needs for symptom control medication selection and dosing.*

For anxiety, conscious sedation or other distressing symptoms (select one):

☐ Lorazepam:_____ (Dose, Route, Frequency)
- ▪ Titration:_____
  - o Usual range:
    - ▪ SL: 0.05 mg/kg; range: 0.02-0.09 mg/kg (Start with 1-2 mg/dose)
    - ▪ IV/SC: May use smaller doses (e.g., 0.01-0.03 mg/kg) and repeat every 20 minutes, as needed to titrate to effect

☐ Midazolam:_____ (Dose, Route, Frequency)
- ▪ Titration:_____
  - o Usual range:
    - ▪ Initial: IV/SC 0.5-2 mg or slow IV over at least 2 minutes; slowly titrate to effect by repeating doses every 2-3 minutes if needed; usual total dose: 2.5-5 mg; use decreased doses in elderly.
    - ▪ Some patients respond to doses as low as 1 mg; no more than 2.5 mg should be administered over a period of 2 minutes.
    - ▪ Additional doses of midazolam may be administered after a 2-minute waiting period and evaluation of sedation after each dose increment. A total dose >5 mg is generally not needed.

☐ Phenobarbital:_____ (Dose, Route, Frequency)
- ▪ Titration:_____
  - o Usual range:
    - ▪ Initial: IV/SC 100-300 mg may repeat in 20 minutes, as needed to titrate to effect. Maximum of 30 mg/kg

☐ Propofol:_____ (Dose, Route, Frequency)
- ▪ Titration:_____
  - o Usual range:
    - ▪ Initial: IV 5 mcg/kg/minute; increase by 5-10 mcg/kg/minute every 5-10 minutes until desired sedation level is achieved; usual maintenance 5-80 mcg/kg/minute

For terminal respiratory secretions, if treating (select one):

☐ Glycopyrrolate: _____ (Dose, Route, Frequency)
  - o Usual range:
    - ▪ SC/IV: 0.2 mg q4-6h prn; 4-10 mcg/kg/dose every 3-4 hours; maximum: 0.2 mg/dose or 0.8 mg/24 hours

☐ Atropine:_____ (Dose, Route, Frequency)
  - o Usual range:
    - ▪ SL : atropine 1% ophth soln: 2-4 drops q2-4h prn
    - ▪ SC/IV: 0.4 mg q2-4h prn: 0.4-0.6 mg; may repeat in 4 hours if necessary; 0.4 mg initial dose may be exceeded in certain cases and may repeat in 4 hours if necessary

☐ Other:_____ (Dose, Route, Frequency)

*** Usual ranges are provided for general guidance only. Always assess individual patient-specific needs for symptom control medication selection and dosing.*

Drug Dosing For Liver and Renal Disease

Acetaminophen (Tylenol)
Drug Class & Common Uses: Analgesic (Non-Opioid) - Nociceptive Pain, Fever
Hepatic Impairment: Administer with caution
Renal Impairment: For CrCl 10-50mL/min: administer every 6 hours; CrCl <10mL/min: administer every 8 hours
Dialyzable: No adjustment necessary

Acetazolamide (Diamox)
Drug Class & Common Uses: Carbonic Anhydrase Inhibitor - Diuretic, Increased ICP
Hepatic Impairment: Avoid use in liver disease
Renal Impairment: For CrCl 10-50mL/min: administer every 12 hours; CrCl < 10mL/min: avoid use
Dialyzable: Moderately dialyzable (25-50%)

Acetylcysteine (Acetadote)
Drug Class & Common Uses: Mucolytic - Expectorant
Hepatic Impairment: No Data
Renal Impairment: Dose as in normal renal function
Dialyzable: Dialyzed. Dose as in normal renal function

Aclidinium (Tudorza Pressair)
Drug Class & Common Uses: Anticholinergic - Long-Acting Bronchodilator
Hepatic Impairment: No dosage adjustment provided, not studied
Renal Impairment: No adjustment necessary
Dialyzable: No Data

Acyclovir (Zovirax)
Drug Class & Common Uses: Antiviral - Herpes Zoster, Herpes Labialis
Hepatic Impairment: No Data
Renal Impairment: For CrCl 10-25mL/min: administer every 8 hours; CrCl <10mL/min administer every 12 hours
Dialyzable: Dialyzed. Dose as in CrCl<10mL/min. Give dose after dialysis

Albuterol (Proventil, Ventolin, ProAir)
Drug Class & Common Uses: Short Acting Beta Agonist (SABA) - Bronchodilator, Asthma, COPD
Hepatic Impairment: No Data
Renal Impairment: Administer with caution
Dialyzable: No Data

Albuterol and Ipratropium (Combivent, DuoNeb)
Drug Class & Common Uses: Short Acting Beta Agonist (SABA) and Anticholinergic - Bronchodilator, COPD
Hepatic Impairment: No Data
Renal Impairment: No Data
Dialyzable: No Data

Alendronate (Fosamax)
Drug Class & Common Uses: Bisphosphonate - Osteoporosis, Bone Metastases
Hepatic Impairment: No dose adjustment required
Renal Impairment: Do not use if CrCl <35mL/min
Dialyzable: Not Dialyzed; Dose as in CrCl<35mL/min

Aliskiren (Tekturna)
Drug Class & Common Uses: Renin Inhibitor - Hypertension
Hepatic Impairment: No dosage adjustment necessary
Renal Impairment: Dose as in normal renal function.
Dialyzable: Unlikely to be dialyzed. Dose as in normal renal function.

Allopurinol (Aloprim, Zyloprim)
Drug Class & Common Uses: Antigout Agent (Uricosuric) - Gout, Hyperuricemia
Hepatic Impairment: Use with caution in patients with hepatic impairment
Renal Impairment: For CrCl 20-50mL/min: administer 200-300mg daily. CrCl 10-20mL/min: administer 100-200mg daily. CrCl <10mL/min: administer 100mg dailly or 100mg on alternating days.
Dialyzable: Dialyzed. Dose as in CrCl<10mL/min.

Alprazolam (Xanax)
Drug Class & Common Uses: Benzodiazepine - Anxiety, Nausea & Vomiting (Anticipatory), Dyspnea, Insomnia
Hepatic Impairment: 0.25mg 2-3 times daily; titrate gradually if needed and tolerated.
Renal Impairment: No Dosage adjustment
Dialyzable: No Data

Aluminum Hydroxide (ALternaGel)
Drug Class & Common Uses: Antacid - Dyspepsia, Phosphate Binder
Hepatic Impairment: No Data
Renal Impairment: Dose as in normal renal function
Dialyzable: Unknown dialyzability. Dose as in normal renal function.

Aluminum Hydroxide, Magnesium Hydroxide and Simethicone (Maalox, Maalox Plus)
Drug Class & Common Uses: Antacid - Dyspepsia, Antiflatulent
Hepatic Impairment: No Data
Renal Impairment: Dose as in normal renal function
Dialyzable: Unknown dialyzability. Dose as in normal renal function.

Amantadine (Symmetrel)
Drug Class & Common Uses: Antiviral - Parkinson's, Extrapyramidal Symptoms (EPS)
Hepatic Impairment: Administer with caution
Renal Impairment: For CrCl 35-50mL/min: administer 100mg every 24 hours. CrCl 15-35mL/min: administer 100mg every 48-72 hours. CrCl<15mL/min: administer 100mg every 7 days.
Dialyzable: Not dialyzed. Dose as in CrCl <10mL/min

Amiloride (Midamor)
Drug Class & Common Uses: Potassium-Sparing Diuretic - Fluid Retention
Hepatic Impairment: No Data
Renal Impairment: For CrCl 10-50mL/min: administer 50% of dose. CrCl <10mL/min: avoid use.
Dialyzable: Not applicable. Avoid.

Amiodarone (Cordarone)
Drug Class & Common Uses: Antiarrhythmic - Cardiovascular
Hepatic Impairment: If hepatic enzymes exceed 3 times normal or double in a patient with an elevated baseline, consider decreasing the dose or discontinuing amiodarone.
Renal Impairment: Dose as in normal renal function
Dialyzable: Not dialyzed. Dose as in normal renal function.

Amitriptyline (Elavil)
Drug Class & Common Uses: Antidepressant (Tricyclic) - Neuropathic Pain, Depression, Sialorrhea
Hepatic Impairment: Use with caution
Renal Impairment: Dose as in normal renal function
Dialyzable: Not dialyzed. Dose as in normal renal function.

Amlodipine (Norvasc)
Drug Class & Common Uses: Calcium Channel Blocker - Hypertension, Angina
Hepatic Impairment: For angina: 5mg daily; For hypertension: 2.5mg daily
Renal Impairment: Dose as in normal renal function
Dialyzable: Not dialyzed. Dose as in normal renal function.

Amlodipine and Olmesartan (Azor)
Drug Class & Common Uses: Calcium Channel Blocker and Angiotensin II Receptor Blocker - Hypertension
Hepatic Impairment: Initial therapy is not recommended
Renal Impairment: No guidelines for dosage adjustment
Dialyzable: No Data

Amoxicillin (Amoxil)
Drug Class & Common Uses: Antibiotic (Penicillin) - Respiratory Infection, Skin Infection, Urinary Tract Infection
Hepatic Impairment: No data
Renal Impairment: Dose as in normal renal function unless CrCl <10mL/min: administer 250mg-1g every 8 hours
Dialyzable: Dialyzed. Dose as in CrCl < 10mL/min

Amoxicillin and Clavulanate (Augmentin)
Drug Class & Common Uses: Antibiotic (Penicillin) - Respiratory Infection, Skin Infection, Urinary Tract Infection
Hepatic Impairment: No Data
Renal Impairment: For CrCl < 30mL/min: do not use 875mg tablets; CrCl 10-30mL/min: 250mg-500mg every 12 hours; CrCl < 10mL/min: 250mg-500mg every 24 hours
Dialyzable: Dialyzable (20% to 50%)

Apomorphine (Apokyn)
Drug Class & Common Uses: Dopamine Agonist - Parkinson's
Hepatic Impairment: Use caution
Renal Impairment: Dose as in normal renal function; start with 1mg.
Dialyzable: Unlikely to be dialyzed. Dose as in normal renal function; start with 1mg

Arformoterol (Brovana)
Drug Class & Common Uses: Long Acting Beta2 Agonist (LABA) - Asthma, COPD
Hepatic Impairment: No dosage adjustment required; monitor
Renal Impairment: No adjustment required
Dialyzable: No Data

Aripiprazole (Abilify)
Drug Class & Common Uses: Antipsychotic (Atypical) - Delirium, Agitation, Schizophrenia, Bipolar Disorder
Hepatic Impairment: No dosage adjustment required
Renal Impairment: Dose as in normal renal function
Dialyzable: Not dialyzed. Dose as in normal renal function.

Armodafinil (Nuvigil)
Drug Class & Common Uses: CNS Stimulant - Excessive Sedation
Hepatic Impairment: Severe hepatic impairment: reduce dose in half
Renal Impairment: Safety not established in severe renal impairment.
Dialyzable: No Data

Artificial Saliva (Biotene, Oasis)
Drug Class & Common Uses: Lubricant - Xerostomia
Hepatic Impairment: Not applicable
Renal Impairment: Not applicable
Dialyzable: Not applicable

Artificial Tears (Refresh, Lacri-Lube)
Drug Class & Common Uses: Lubricant - Dry Eyes
Hepatic Impairment: Not applicable
Renal Impairment: Not applicable
Dialyzable: Not applicable

Aspirin (Aspirin, Ecotrin)
Drug Class & Common Uses: Salicylate - Antiplatelet, Nociceptive Pain, Fever
Hepatic Impairment: Avoid use in severe liver disease
Renal Impairment: Dose as in normal renal function
Dialyzable: Dialyzed. Dose as in normal renal function

Atenolol (Tenormin)
Drug Class & Common Uses: Beta Blocker - Hypertension, Tachycardia
Hepatic Impairment: No Data
Renal Impairment: Dose as in normal renal function
Dialyzable: Dialyzed. Dose as in normal renal function

Atropine (Isopto Atropine)
Drug Class & Common Uses: Anticholinergic - Terminal Secretions, Sialorrhea
Hepatic Impairment: No Data
Renal Impairment: No Data
Dialyzable: No Data

Azilsartan and Chlorthalidone (Edarbyclor)
Drug Class & Common Uses: Angiotensin II Receptor Blocker and Diuretic - Cardiovascular
Hepatic Impairment: Severe impairment: use caution
Renal Impairment: Severe renal impairment (CrCl <30 mL): Safety and effectiveness not established.
Dialyzable: No Data

Azithromycin (Zithromax)
Drug Class & Common Uses: Antibiotic (Macrolide) - Respiratory Infection
Hepatic Impairment: Use with caution
Renal Impairment: Dose as in normal renal function
Dialyzable: Unknown dialyzability. Dose as in normal renal function.

Baclofen (Lioresal)
Drug Class & Common Uses: Muscle Relaxant - Hiccups, Muscle Spasm
Hepatic Impairment: No Data
Renal Impairment: For CrCl 20-50mL/min: administer 5mg three times daily and titrate according to response. CrCl 10-20mL/min: 5mg twice daily. CrCl <10mL/min: 5mg once daily
Dialyzable: Dialyzed. Dose as in CrCl < 10mL/min

Beclomethasone (Qvar)
Drug Class & Common Uses: Inhaled Corticosteroid - Asthma
Hepatic Impairment: No Data
Renal Impairment: No Data
Dialyzable: No Data

Belladonna and Opium (B & O Suppositories)
Drug Class & Common Uses: Anticholinergic and Opioid - Urinary Antispasmodic
Hepatic Impairment: No Data
Renal Impairment: No Data
Dialyzable: No Data

Benzonatate (Tessalon Perles)
Drug Class & Common Uses: Antitussive - Cough Suppressant
Hepatic Impairment: No Data
Renal Impairment: No Data
Dialyzable: No Data

Benztropine (Cogentin)
Drug Class & Common Uses: Anticholinergic - Anti-Parkinson's, Extrapyramidal Symptoms (EPS)
Hepatic Impairment: No Data
Renal Impairment: Start with low doses and adjust according to response
Dialyzable: Unknown dialyzability. Start with low doses and adjust according to response

Betamethasone (Diprolene)
Drug Class & Common Uses: Topical Corticosteroid - Pruritus, Rash
Hepatic Impairment: Extensive hepatic metabolism-may require adjustment
Renal Impairment: Dose as in normal renal function
Dialyzable: Unknown dialyzability. Dose as in normal renal function.

Bethanechol (Urecholine)
Drug Class & Common Uses: Cholinergic Agonist - Urinary Retention, Neurogenic Bladder
Hepatic Impairment: No Data
Renal Impairment: No Data
Dialyzable: No Data

Bisacodyl (Dulcolax)
Drug Class & Common Uses: Laxative (Stimulant) - Constipation
Hepatic Impairment: No Data
Renal Impairment: Dose as in normal renal function
Dialyzable: Unknown dialyzability. Dose as in normal renal function.

Bismuth Subsalicylate (Kaopectate)
Drug Class & Common Uses: Antidiarrheal - Mild Diarrhea, Dyspepsia
Hepatic Impairment: No Data
Renal Impairment: Administer with caution
Dialyzable: No Data

Bromocriptine (Parlodel)
Drug Class & Common Uses: Dopamine Agonist - Parkinson's
Hepatic Impairment: May be necessary, but no guidelines
Renal Impairment: Dose as in normal renal function
Dialyzable: Not dialyzed. Dose as in normal renal function.

Budesonide (Pulmicort)
Drug Class & Common Uses: Inhaled Corticosteroid - Asthma
Hepatic Impairment: Dosage reduction may be required; watch for hypercorticism
Renal Impairment: Dose as in normal renal function
Dialyzable: Unlikely to be dialyzed. Dose as in normal renal function.

Bumetanide (Bumex)
Drug Class & Common Uses: Loop Diuretic - Fluid Retention
Hepatic Impairment: No Data
Renal Impairment: Dose as in normal renal function
Dialyzable: Not dialyzed. Dose as in normal renal function.

Buprenorphine (Butrans)
Drug Class & Common Uses: Opioid (Mixed) - Nociceptive Pain
Hepatic Impairment: Injection, Sublingual: use caution, dosage adjustment recommended; Patch: mild-to-moderate impairment: no dosage adjustment; severe impairment: not studied, consider alternative therapy
Renal Impairment: For CrCl 10-20mL/min: dose as in normal renal function, but avoid very large doses. CrCl <10mL/min: Reduce dose by 25-50% initially and increase as tolerated; avoid very large single doses; Transdermal: Dose as in normal renal function.
Dialyzable: Dialyzed. Dose as in CrCl < 10mL/min

Calcitonin (Miacalcin, Fortical)
Drug Class & Common Uses: Hormone - Osteoporosis, Hypercalcemia of Malignancy, Bone Pain
Hepatic Impairment: No dosage adjustment
Renal Impairment: Dose as in normal renal function
Dialyzable: Unlikely to be dialyzed. Dose as in normal renal function.

Calcium Carbonate (Tums)
Drug Class & Common Uses: Antacid - Dyspepsia, Dietary Supplement
Hepatic Impairment: No Data
Renal Impairment: Dose as in normal renal function; titrate to response.
Dialyzable: Unknown dialyzability. Dose as in normal renal function.

Camphor and Menthol (Sarna)
Drug Class & Common Uses: Topical Emollient - Pruritus
Hepatic Impairment: No Data
Renal Impairment: No Data
Dialyzable: No Data

Capsaicin (Zostrix)
Drug Class & Common Uses: Topical Analgesic - Neuropathic pain
Hepatic Impairment: No Data
Renal Impairment: No Data
Dialyzable: No Data

Captopril (Capoten)
Drug Class & Common Uses: ACE Inhibitor - Cardiovascular
Hepatic Impairment: No Data
Renal Impairment: Start low - adjust according to response
Dialyzable: Dialyzed. Start low - adjust according to response

Carbamazepine (Tegretol)
Drug Class & Common Uses: Anticonvulsant - Neuropathic Pain, Hiccups, Seizures
Hepatic Impairment: Use with caution, metabolized primarily in the liver
Renal Impairment: Dose as in normal renal function
Dialyzable: Not dialyzed. Dose as in normal renal function.

Carisoprodol (Soma)
Drug Class & Common Uses: Muscle Relaxant - Muscle Spasm
Hepatic Impairment: Use with caution
Renal Impairment: Use with caution.
Dialyzable: Dialyzable

Carvedilol (Coreg, Coreg CR)
Drug Class & Common Uses: Beta Blocker - Hypertension, Heart Failure
Hepatic Impairment: Use contraindicated in severe dysfunction
Renal Impairment: Dose as in normal renal function
Dialyzable: Not dialyzed. Dose as in normal renal function. Start with low doses; titrate according to response.

Cefaclor (Ceclor)
Drug Class & Common Uses: Antibiotic (Cephalosporin) - Respiratory Infection
Hepatic Impairment: No Data
Renal Impairment: Dose as in normal renal function unless CrCl <10mL/min: Dose 250mg every 8 hours
Dialyzable: Dialyzed. Dose at 250mg-500mg every 8 hours

Cefpodoxime (Vantin)
Drug Class & Common Uses: Antibiotic (Cephalosporin) - Respiratory Infection
Hepatic Impairment: No dosage adjustment necessary
Renal Impairment: Dose as in normal renal function unless CrCl <10mL/min: administer 1g every 8-12 hours
Dialyzable: Dialyzed. Dose as in CrCl < 10mL/min

Cefuroxime Axetil (Ceftin)
Drug Class & Common Uses: Antibiotic (Cephalosporin) - Respiratory Infection
Hepatic Impairment: No Data
Renal Impairment: Dose as in normal renal function
Dialyzable: Dialyzed. Dose as in normal renal function

Celecoxib (Celebrex)
Drug Class & Common Uses: NSAID (Cox II Selective) - Nociceptive Pain, Bone Pain
Hepatic Impairment: Moderate impairment: reduce dose by 50%; Severe impairment: Use is not recommended
Renal Impairment: CrCl 30-50mL/min: Use with caution. CrCl 10-30mL/min: avoid use if possible. CrCl <10mL/min: only use if on dialysis
Dialyzable: Unlikely to be dialyzed. Dose as in normal renal function.

Cephalexin (Keflex)
Drug Class & Common Uses: Antibiotic (Cephalosporin) - Urinary Tract, Skin Infections
Hepatic Impairment: No Data
Renal Impairment: CrCl 10-50mL/min: administer 500mg every 8-12 hours; CrCl < 10mL/min: administer every 12-24 hours
Dialyzable: Dialyzable (20-50%)

Cetirizine (Zyrtec)
Drug Class & Common Uses: Antihistamine - Seasonal Allergies, Pruritus
Hepatic Impairment: Administer 5mg once daily
Renal Impairment: CrCl 10-50mL/min: dose as in normal renal function. CrCl <10mL/min: reduce to 5-10mg daily
Dialyzable: Not dialyzed. Dose as in CrCl <10mL/min

Cevimeline (Evoxac)
Drug Class & Common Uses: Cholinergic Agonist - Xerostomia
Hepatic Impairment: No Data
Renal Impairment: No Data
Dialyzable: No Data

Chlorpromazine (Thorazine)
Drug Class & Common Uses: Antipsychotic (Conventional) - Nausea & Vomiting (Chemoreceptor Trigger Zone), Delirium, Agitation, Anxiety, Hiccups
Hepatic Impairment: Avoid in severe dysfunction
Renal Impairment: Usual dosing unless CrCl <10mL/min: start with low dose; titrate to response
Dialyzable: Not dialyzed. Dose as in CrCl <10mL/min

Chlorzoxazone (Parafon Forte)
Drug Class & Common Uses: Muscle Relaxant - Muscle Spasm
Hepatic Impairment: No Data
Renal Impairment: No Data
Dialyzable: No Data

Cholestyramine (Questran, Prevalite)
Drug Class & Common Uses: Antilipemic Agent - Bile Acid Sequestrant, Hypercholesterolemia, Diarrhea, Pruritus
Hepatic Impairment: No adjustment necessary
Renal Impairment: Dose as in normal renal function
Dialyzable: Not dialyzed. Dose as in normal renal function.

Choline Magnesium Trisalicylate (Trilisate)
Drug Class & Common Uses: Salicylate - Nociceptive Pain, Bone Pain
Hepatic Impairment: No Data
Renal Impairment: Avoid use in severe renal impairment
Dialyzable: No Data

Ciclesonide (Alvesco)
Drug Class & Common Uses: Inhaled Corticosteroid - Asthma
Hepatic Impairment: No dosage adjustments necessary
Renal Impairment: No Data
Dialyzable: No Data

Cimetidine (Tagamet)
Drug Class & Common Uses: H2 Antagonist (H2RA) - Gastritis, Dyspepsia, GERD, Sexual Aggression
Hepatic Impairment: Reduce dose in severe impairment
Renal Impairment: Dose as in normal renal function unless CrCl <20mL/min: administer 50% of normal dose
Dialyzable: Dialyzed. Dose as in CrCl < 20mL/min

Cinacalcet (Sensipar)
Drug Class & Common Uses: Calcimimetic - Hyperparathyroid, Hypercalcemia
Hepatic Impairment: Dose adjustment based on serum calcium, phosphorus, or iPTH levels
Renal Impairment: Dose as in normal renal function
Dialyzable: Not dialyzed. Dose as in normal renal function

Ciprofloxacin (Cipro)
Drug Class & Common Uses: Antibiotic (Quinolone) - Urinary Tract Infection, Skin Infection, Respiratory Infection
Hepatic Impairment: No Data
Renal Impairment: Dose as in normal renal function unless CrCl 10-20mL/min: administer 50-100% of normal dose or CrCl <10mL/min: administer 50% of normal dose
Dialyzable: Not dialyzed. Oral dosing: 250mg-500mg every 12 hours. IV dosing: 200mg every 12 hours

Citalopram (Celexa)
Drug Class & Common Uses: Antidepressant (SSRI) - Depression, Anxiety
Hepatic Impairment: Reduce dose; 20mg maximum daily dose
Renal Impairment: Dose as in normal renal function unless CrCl <10mL/min: Use with caution
Dialyzable: Not dialyzed. Dose as in CrCl <10mL/min

Clarithromycin (Biaxin)
Drug Class & Common Uses: Antibiotic (Macrolide) - Respiratory Infection
Hepatic Impairment: No adjustment needed if renal function is normal
Renal Impairment: Usual dosing unless CrCl <30mL/min: administer 250-500mg every 12 hours
Dialyzable: Dialyzed. Dose as in CrCl < 10mL/min

Clobazam (Onfi)
Drug Class & Common Uses: Benzodiazepine - Epilepsy (Lennox-Gastaut)
Hepatic Impairment: Mild-to-moderate impairment: < 30kg: 5mg once daily for > 2 weeks, then 5mg twice daily for > 1 week, then 10mg twice daily; > 30kg: 5mg once daily for > 1 week, then 5mg twice daily for > 1 week, then 10mg twice daily for > 1 week, then 20mg twice daily
Renal Impairment: Dose as in normal renal function unless CrCl <10mL/min then start with low doses
Dialyzable: Not dialyzed. Dose as in CrCl <10mL/min

Clonazepam (Klonopin)
Drug Class & Common Uses: Benzodiazepine - Anxiety, Seizures
Hepatic Impairment: No Data
Renal Impairment: Start at low doses and increase according to response
Dialyzable: Not dialyzed. Start at low doses and increase according to response

Clonidine (Catapres)
Drug Class & Common Uses: Alpha2 Adrenergic Agonist - Hypertension
Hepatic Impairment: No Data
Renal Impairment: Dose as in normal renal response
Dialyzable: Not dialyzed. Dose as in normal renal function.

Clopidogrel (Plavix)
Drug Class & Common Uses: Antiplatelet (Thienopyridine) - Cardiovascular, Stroke, Thromboembolism
Hepatic Impairment: Use with caution; experience is limited
Renal Impairment: Dose as in normal renal function
Dialyzable: Unlikely to be dialyzed. Dose as in normal renal function.

Clotrimazole (Mycelex, Lotrimin)
Drug Class & Common Uses: Antifungal - Fungal Infection, Thrush
Hepatic Impairment: No Data
Renal Impairment: No Data
Dialyzable: No Data

Codeine
Drug Class & Common Uses: Opioid - Diarrhea, Cough, Nociceptive Pain
Hepatic Impairment: Use with caution; careful titration recommended
Renal Impairment: Dose as in normal renal function unless CrCl 10-20mL/min: administer 30mg up to every 4 hours and increase if tolerated. CrCl <10mL/min: administer 30mg up to eery 6 hours and increse if tolerated
Dialyzable: Not dialyzed. Dose as in CrCl <10mL/min

Codeine and Acetaminophen (Tylenol #3, #4)
Drug Class & Common Uses: Analgesic Combination (Opioid) - Nociceptive Pain, Cough, Diarrhea
Hepatic Impairment: Avoid chronic use in impairment
Renal Impairment: For CrCl 10-50mL/min: administer every 6 hours and reduce dosage by 25%, and CrCl <10mL/min: administer every 8 hours and reduce dosage by 50%
Dialyzable: No dosage adjustment necessary

Colchicine (Colcrys)
Drug Class & Common Uses: Antigout Agent - Gout
Hepatic Impairment: Use is contraindicated (fatal toxicity has been reported)
Renal Impairment: Usual dosing unless CrCl <10mL/min: 500mcg 3-4 times daily (maximum dose of 3mg)
Dialyzable: Not dialyzed. Dose as in CrCl <10mL/min

Colesevelam (Welchol)
Drug Class & Common Uses: Antilipemic Agent - Bile Acid Sequestrant, Hypercholesterolemia
Hepatic Impairment: No dosage adjustment necessary
Renal Impairment: No dosage adjustment necessary
Dialyzable: No Data

Cyclobenzaprine (Flexeril)
Drug Class & Common Uses: Muscle Relaxant - Muscle Spasm
Hepatic Impairment: IR: Mild impairment: initiate with 5mg; use with caution, titrate slowly and consider less frequency dosing; Moderate-to-severe: use not recommended; ER: Mild-to-severe: use not recommended
Renal Impairment: No Data
Dialyzable: No Data

Cyproheptadine (Periactin)
Drug Class & Common Uses: Antihistamine - Anorexia, Pruritus
Hepatic Impairment: No Data
Renal Impairment: No Data
Dialyzable: No Data

Dabigatran (Pradaxa)
Drug Class & Common Uses: Anticoagulant (Thrombin Inhibitor) - Stroke, Thromboembolism
Hepatic Impairment: No dosage adjustment required
Renal Impairment: CrCl > 30mL/min: use with caution, increased risk of bleeding especially in elderly patients. American College of Chest Physicians consider CrCl < 30mL/min a contraindication to dabigatran use.
Dialyzable: Not recommended

Dalfampridine (Ampyra)
Drug Class & Common Uses: Potassium Channel Blocker - Multiple Sclerosis
Hepatic Impairment: No dosage adjustment required
Renal Impairment: CrCl 51-80mL/min: use with caution - risk of seizure increases secondary to reduced clearance; CrCl < 50mL/min: contraindicated
Dialyzable: No Data

Dantrolene (Dantrium)
Drug Class & Common Uses: Muscle Relaxant - Malignant Hyperthermia, Spasticity
Hepatic Impairment: Contraindicated in patients with active liver disease
Renal Impairment: No Data
Dialyzable: No Data

Darbepoetin Alfa (Aranesp)
Drug Class & Common Uses: Erythropoiesis Stimulating Agent (ESA) - Anemia
Hepatic Impairment: No Data
Renal Impairment: Dose as in normal renal function
Dialyzable: Not dialyzed. Dose as in normal renal function.

Darifenacin (Enablex)
Drug Class & Common Uses: Anticholinergic - Overactive Bladder, Urinary Spasms
Hepatic Impairment: Moderate impairment do not exceed 7.5mg/day
Renal Impairment: Dose as in normal renal function
Dialyzable: Unlikely to be dialyzed. Dose as in normal renal function.

Denosumab (Xgeva, Prolia)
Drug Class & Common Uses: Bone Modifying Monoclonal Antibody - Osteoporosis, Bone Metastases
Hepatic Impairment: No dosage adjustment provided, not studied
Renal Impairment: CrCl < 30mL/min: monitor due to increased risk of hypocalcemia
Dialyzable: No Data

Desipramine (Norpramin)
Drug Class & Common Uses: Antidepressant (Tricyclic) - Neuropathic Pain, Depression
Hepatic Impairment: Administer with caution
Renal Impairment: Administer with caution
Dialyzable: Supplemental dose is not necessary

Dexamethasone (Decadron)
Drug Class & Common Uses: Corticosteroid - Appetite, Bone Pain, Visceral Pain, Nerve Compression Pain, Pruritus, Seizures, Respiratory Inflammation, Increased Intracranial Pressure, Bowel Obstruction, Excessive Sedation
Hepatic Impairment: Administer with caution
Renal Impairment: Dose as in normal renal function
Dialyzable: Not dialyzed. Dose as in normal renal function

Dextroamphetamine (Dexedrine)
Drug Class & Common Uses: CNS Stimulant - Depression, Excessive Sedation
Hepatic Impairment: No Data
Renal Impairment: No Data
Dialyzable: No Data

Dextromethorphan (Delsym, Robafen)
Drug Class & Common Uses: Antitussive - Cough Suppressant
Hepatic Impairment: Not Data
Renal Impairment: No Data
Dialyzable: No Data

Dextromethorphan and Quinidine (Nuedexta)
Drug Class & Common Uses: NMDA Antagonist - Pseudobulbar Affect (PBA)
Hepatic Impairment: No dosage adjustment required; increase in adverse reactions observed with moderate impairment
Renal Impairment: No dosage adjustment required for mild-to-moderate impairment; not studied with severe impairment
Dialyzable: No Data

Diazepam (Valium, Diastat)
Drug Class & Common Uses: Benzodiazepine - Seizures, Anxiety, Muscle spasms, Dyspnea
Hepatic Impairment: Decrease maintenance dose by 50%
Renal Impairment: Dose as in normal renal function unless CrCl <20mL/min: use small doses and titrate to response
Dialyzable: Not dialyzed. Dose as in CrCl <20mL/min

Diclofenac (Voltaren, Flector, Pennsaid)
Drug Class & Common Uses: NSAID (Mixed COX) - Nociceptive Pain, Bone Pain
Hepatic Impairment: Use with caution
Renal Impairment: Dose as in normal renal function unless CrCl 10-20mL/min: avoid use if possible, and avoid use if CrCl <10mL/min
Dialyzable: Not dialyzed. Dose as in normal renal function.

Dicloxacillin (Dynapen)
Drug Class & Common Uses: Antibiotic (Penicillin) - Respiratory Infection, Skin Infection
Hepatic Impairment: No Data
Renal Impairment: Dosage adjustment not necessary
Dialyzable: Not dialyzable (0-5%); supplemental dose is not necessary

Dicyclomine (Bentyl)
Drug Class & Common Uses: Anticholinergic - Nausea & Vomiting, Abdominal Spasm, Cramping, Visceral Pain
Hepatic Impairment: Administer with caution
Renal Impairment: Administer with caution
Dialyzable: No Data

Digoxin (Lanoxin)
Drug Class & Common Uses: Cardiac Glycosides - Heart Failure, Atrial Fibrillation
Hepatic Impairment: No Data
Renal Impairment: For CrCl 10-50mL/min: administer 125-250mcg per day; monitor levels. For CrCl <10mL/min: dose commonly 62.5mcg daily or on alternating days; monitor levels
Dialyzable: Not dialyzed. Dose as in CrCl <10mL/min

Diltiazem (Cardizem, Tiazac)
Drug Class & Common Uses: Calcium Channel Blocker - Hypertension, Angina, Atrial Fibrillation
Hepatic Impairment: Administer with caution
Renal Impairment: Dose as in normal renal function
Dialyzable: Not dialyzed. Dose as in normal renal function

Diphenhydramine (Benadryl)
Drug Class & Common Uses: Antihistamine - Allergies, Extrapyramidal Symptoms (EPS), Pruritus, Insomnia, Anxiety
Hepatic Impairment: No Data
Renal Impairment: No Data
Dialyzable: No Data

Diphenoxylate and Atropine (Lomotil)
Drug Class & Common Uses: Antidiarrheal - Diarrhea
Hepatic Impairment: Administer with caution
Renal Impairment: Administer with caution
Dialyzable: No Data

Dipyridamole (Persantine)
Drug Class & Common Uses: Antiplatelet - Cardiovascular
Hepatic Impairment: Administer with caution
Renal Impairment: Dose as in normal renal function
Dialyzable: Not dialyzed. Dose as in normal renal function.

Docusate (Colace)
Drug Class & Common Uses: Laxative (Stool Softener) - Constipation
Hepatic Impairment: No Data
Renal Impairment: No Data
Dialyzable: No Data

Docusate and Senna (Senokot-S, Senna S)
Drug Class & Common Uses: Laxative (Stool Softener and Stimulant) - Constipation
Hepatic Impairment: No Data
Renal Impairment: No Data
Dialyzable: No Data

Dolasetron (Anzemet)
Drug Class & Common Uses: 5HT3 Receptor Antagonist - Nausea & Vomiting
Hepatic Impairment: No dosage adjustment required
Renal Impairment: Dose as in normal renal function
Dialyzable: Unknown dialyzability. Dose as in normal renal function.

Donepezil (Aricept)
Drug Class & Common Uses: Acetylcholinesterase Inhibitor - Dementia
Hepatic Impairment: No Data
Renal Impairment: Dose as in normal renal function
Dialyzable: Unlikely to be dialyzed. Dose as in normal renal function.

Doxazosin (Cardura)
Drug Class & Common Uses: Alpha1 Blocker - Hypertension, Urinary hesitancy, BPH
Hepatic Impairment: Use with caution in mild-mod; do not use in severe
Renal Impairment: Dise as in normal renal function
Dialyzable: Not dialyzed. Dose as in normal renal function.

Doxepin (Silenor)
Drug Class & Common Uses: Antidepressant (Tricyclic) - Neuropathic Pain, Pruritus, Depression
Hepatic Impairment: Use a lower dose and adjust gradually
Renal Impairment: C
Dialyzable: No Data

Doxycycline (Vibramycin, Doryx)
Drug Class & Common Uses: Antibiotic (Tetracycline) - Respiratory Infection, Skin Infection
Hepatic Impairment: No Data
Renal Impairment: Dose as in normal renal function
Dialyzable: Poorly dialyzed; no supplemental dose or dosage adjustment necessary

Dronabinol (Marinol)
Drug Class & Common Uses: Cannabinoid - Anorexia, Nausea & Vomiting
Hepatic Impairment: Caution; usual dose should be reduced in patients with severe liver failure
Renal Impairment: No dosage adjustment required
Dialyzable: No Data

Dronedarone (Multaq)
Drug Class & Common Uses: Antiarrhythmic - Cardiovascular
Hepatic Impairment: Mild-to-moderate: no dosage adjustment necessary; severe: contraindicated
Renal Impairment: No dosage adjustment necessary
Dialyzable: No Data

Duloxetine (Cymbalta)
Drug Class & Common Uses: Antidepressant (SNRI) - Neuropathic Pain, Depression, Anxiety, Fibromyalgia
Hepatic Impairment: Not recommended for use in liver disease.
Renal Impairment: For CrCl 30-50mL/min: Dose as in normal renal function; start with a low dose. CrCl 10-30mL/min: start at low dose and increase according to response. CrCl <10mL/min: start at very low dose and increase according to response
Dialyzable: Not dialyzed. Dose as in CrCl <10mL/min

Enalapril (Vasotec)
Drug Class & Common Uses: ACE Inhibitor - Cardiovascular
Hepatic Impairment: No dosage adjustment necessary
Renal Impairment: Dose as in normal renal function unless CrCl <20mL/min: start with 2.5mg per day and increase according to response
Dialyzable: Dialyzed. Dose as in CrCl < 20mL/min

Eplerenone (Inspra)
Drug Class & Common Uses: Potassium Sparing Diuretic - Fluid Retention
Hepatic Impairment: Contraindicated in severe liver disease
Renal Impairment: Contraindicated in moderate to severe renal impairment, CrCl<50mL/min
Dialyzable: Avoid use in ESRD and hemodialysis

Epoetin Alfa (Procrit, Epogen)
Drug Class & Common Uses: Erythropoiesis Stimulating Agent (ESA) - Anemia
Hepatic Impairment: No Data
Renal Impairment: Dose as in normal renal function
Dialyzable: Not dialyzed. Dose as in normal renal function.

Erythromycin (E-Mycin, Erytab)
Drug Class & Common Uses: Antibiotic (Macrolide) - Respiratory Infection, Skin Infection, Gastric Stasis
Hepatic Impairment: Administer with caution
Renal Impairment: Dose as in normal renal function unless CrCl <10mL/min: use 50% to 75% of normal dose; maximum of 2g daily
Dialyzable: Not dialyzed. Dose as in CrCl<10mL/min

Escitalopram (Lexapro)
Drug Class & Common Uses: Antidepressant (SSRI) - Depression, Anxiety
Hepatic Impairment: 10mg once daily
Renal Impairment: Dose as in normal renal function unless CrCl <30mL/min: start with a low dose and titrate slowly
Dialyzable: Not dialyzed. Dose as in CrCl <10mL/min

Esomeprazole (Nexium)
Drug Class & Common Uses: Proton Pump Inhibitor (PPI) - Dyspepsia, GERD, GI Ulcers
Hepatic Impairment: Severe impairment: dose should not exceed 20mg/day
Renal Impairment: Dose as in normal renal function
Dialyzable: Not dialyzed. Dose as in normal renal function

Estazolam (Prosom)
Drug Class & Common Uses: Benzodiazepine - Insomnia
Hepatic Impairment: Adjustment may be necessary
Renal Impairment: Administer with caution
Dialyzable: No Data

Eszopiclone (Lunesta)
Drug Class & Common Uses: Non-Benzodiazepine Hypnotic - Insomnia
Hepatic Impairment: Use caution. Reduce to maximum 1mg in severe impairment.
Renal Impairment: No dosage adustment required.
Dialyzable: No Data

Exetanide (Byetta)
Drug Class & Common Uses: Antidiabetic Agent (GLP-1)
Hepatic Impairment: No dose adjustment required
Renal Impairment: Not recommended if CrCl <30mL/min
Dialyzable: No Data

Famotidine (Pepcid)
Drug Class & Common Uses: H2 Antagonist (H2RA) - Gastritis, Dyspepsia, GERD
Hepatic Impairment: No Data
Renal Impairment: Dose as in normal renal function unless CrCl 10-20mL/min: administer 50% of normal dose. CrCl <10mL/min: administer 20mg at night (maximum)
Dialyzable: Not dialyzed. Dose as in CrCl <10mL/min

Febuxostat (Uloric)
Drug Class & Common Uses: Antigout Agent (Xanthine Oxidase Inhibitor) - Gout, Hyperuricemia
Hepatic Impairment: Mild-to-moderate impairment: no adjustment needed; Severe: not studied, use caution
Renal Impairment: CrCl 30-89mL/min: no adjustment needed; CrCl < 30mL/min: insufficient data, use caution
Dialyzable: Not Studied

Fenofibrate, Fenofibric Acid (TriCor, Trilipix)
Drug Class & Common Uses: Antilipemic Agent (Fibric Acid) - Hypercholesterolemia, Hyperuricemia
Hepatic Impairment: Use is contraindicated
Renal Impairment: For CrCl 20-60mL/min: administer 134mg daily. CrCl 10-20mL/min: administer 67mg daily. CrCl <10mL/min: avoid use
Dialyzable: Not dialyzed. Avoid.

Fentanyl Transdermal (Duragesic)
Drug Class & Common Uses: Opioid - Nociceptive Pain
Hepatic Impairment: Kinetics may be altered in hepatic disease
Renal Impairment: For CrCl 20-50mL/min: dose as in normal renal function; titrate according to response. CrCl 10-20mL/min: administer 75% of normal dose; titrate according to response. CrCl <10mL/min: administer 50% of normal dose; titrate according to response
Dialyzable: Not dialyzed. Dose as in CrCl <10mL/min

Fentanyl Transmucosal (Actiq, Fentora, Lazanda)
Drug Class & Common Uses: Opioid - Nociceptive Pain
Hepatic Impairment: Kinetics may be altered in hepatic disease
Renal Impairment: C
Dialyzable: No Data

Filgrastim (Neupogen)
Drug Class & Common Uses: Colony Stimulating Factor - Neutropenia
Hepatic Impairment: No Data
Renal Impairment: Dose as in normal renal response and titrate to dose response
Dialyzable: Not dialyzed. Dose as in CrCl <10mL/min

Fluconazole (Diflucan)
Drug Class & Common Uses: Antifungal - Infection (Systemic Fungal)
Hepatic Impairment: Use with caution in patients with pre-existing hepatic impairment
Renal Impairment: Dose as in normal renal function unless CrCl <10mL/min: administer 50% of normal dose
Dialyzable: Dialyzed. Administer 50% of normal dose daily, or 100% of normal dose 3 times a week after dialysis.

Flunisolide (Aerospan, Nasalide)
Drug Class & Common Uses: Inhaled Corticosteroid - Asthma, Allergic Rhinitis
Hepatic Impairment: No Data
Renal Impairment: No Data
Dialyzable: No Data

Fluocinonide (Lidex)
Drug Class & Common Uses: Topical Corticosteroid - Pruritus, Rash
Hepatic Impairment: No Data
Renal Impairment: No Data
Dialyzable: No Data

Fluoxetine (Prozac)
Drug Class & Common Uses: Antidepressant (SSRI) - Depression, Anxiety
Hepatic Impairment: Lower dose or less frequent dosing should be used in hepatic impairment; Cirrhosis: lower dose or less frequent dosing; Cirrhosis without ascites: 50% of dose
Renal Impairment: Dose as in normal renal function unless CrCl <10mL/min: use low dose or on alternate days and increase according to response
Dialyzable: Not dialyzed. Dose as in CrCl <10mL/min

Flurazepam (Dalmane)
Drug Class & Common Uses: Benzodiazepine - Insomnia
Hepatic Impairment: Administer with caution
Renal Impairment: Administer with caution
Dialyzable: No Data

Fluticasone (Flovent)
Drug Class & Common Uses: Inhaled Corticosteroid - Asthma
Hepatic Impairment: Administer with caution
Renal Impairment: No Data
Dialyzable: No Data

Fluticasone and Salmeterol (Advair)
Drug Class & Common Uses: Long Acting Beta2 Agonist (LABA) and Corticosteroid - Asthma, COPD
Hepatic Impairment: No dosage adjustment required; monitor
Renal Impairment: No Data
Dialyzable: No Data

Fosinopril (Monopril)
Drug Class & Common Uses: ACE Inhibitor - Cardiovascular
Hepatic Impairment: Decrease dose and monitor effects
Renal Impairment: For CrCl 20-50mL/min: administer 28mg/kg every 8 hours. CrCl 10-20mL/min: administer 15mg/kg every 8 hours. CrCl <10mL/min: administer 6mg/kg every 8 hours
Dialyzable: Dialyzed. Dose as in CrCl <10mL/min

Furosemide (Lasix)
Drug Class & Common Uses: Loop Diuretic - Fluid Retention, Refractory Dyspnea
Hepatic Impairment: Monitor potassium and fluid levels in cirrhosis, particularly with high doses.
Renal Impairment: Dose as in normal renal function. Additional doses may be required for CrCl <20mL/min
Dialyzable: Not dialyzed. Dose as in CrCl <10mL/min

Gabapentin (Neurontin, Gralise)
Drug Class & Common Uses: Anticonvulsant - Neuropathic Pain, Hiccups, Agitation
Hepatic Impairment: No dosage adjustment required; not hepatically metabolized
Renal Impairment: Start at low dose and increase according to response. For CrCl <15mL/min: administer 300mg on alternate days or 100mg at night initially, increase according to tolerability.
Dialyzable: Dialyzed. Maintenance dose of 100-300mg after each session and increase according to tolerability

Galantamine (Razadyne)
Drug Class & Common Uses: Acetylcholinesterase Inhibitor - Dementia
Hepatic Impairment: Moderate: 16mg/day; Severe: not recommended
Renal Impairment: Dose as in normal renal function but for CrCl <10mL/min start with lower doses
Dialyzable: Dialyzed. Dose as in CrCl <10mL/min

Glipizide (Glucotrol)
Drug Class & Common Uses: Oral Hypoglycemic - Hyperglycemia
Hepatic Impairment: IR: 2.5mg/day; ER: use of lower initial and maintenance dose should be considered
Renal Impairment: For CrCl <50mL/min administer 2.5mg initially then titrate according to response
Dialyzable: Unlikely to be dialyzed. Dose as in CrCl <10mL/min

Glyburide (Diabeta)
Drug Class & Common Uses: Oral Hypoglycemic - Hyperglycemia
Hepatic Impairment: Use caution and avoid in severe disease
Renal Impairment: CrCl < 50mL/min: not recommended
Dialyzable: No Data

Glycerin (Pedia-Lax, Sani-Supp)
Drug Class & Common Uses: Laxative (Osmotic) - Constipation
Hepatic Impairment: No Data
Renal Impairment: No Data
Dialyzable: No Data

Glycopyrrolate (Robinul, Cuvposa)
Drug Class & Common Uses: Anticholinergic - Nausea & Vomiting, Abdominal Spasm, Cramping, Bowel Obstruction, Terminal Secretions, Visceral Pain
Hepatic Impairment: No Data
Renal Impairment: Elimination impaired in renal failure; dosage adjustment recommended
Dialyzable: No Data

Granisetron (Kytril, Sancuso)
Drug Class & Common Uses: 5HT3 Receptor Antagonist - Nausea & Vomiting
Hepatic Impairment: No dosage adjustment necessary
Renal Impairment: Dose as in normal renal function
Dialyzable: Unknown dialyzability. Dose as in normal renal function.

Guaifenesin (Robitussin, Mucinex)
Drug Class & Common Uses: Expectorant - Cough, Thick Secretions
Hepatic Impairment: No Data
Renal Impairment: No Data
Dialyzable: No Data

Guaifenesin and Codeine (Robitussin AC)
Drug Class & Common Uses: Expectorant and Suppressant - Cough
Hepatic Impairment: Administer with caution
Renal Impairment: Administer with caution
Dialyzable: No Data

Guaifenesin and Dextromethorphan (Robitussin DM)
Drug Class & Common Uses: Expectorant and Suppressant - Cough
Hepatic Impairment: No Data
Renal Impairment: No Data
Dialyzable: No Data

Haloperidol (Haldol)
Drug Class & Common Uses: Antipsychotic (Conventional) - Nausea & Vomiting (Chemoreceptor Trigger Zone), Delirium, Agitation, Anxiety, Bowel Obstruction, Hiccups
Hepatic Impairment: No Data
Renal Impairment: Dose as in normal renal function unless CrCl <10mL/min then start with lower doses; accumulation with repeated dosage
Dialyzable: Not dialyzed. Dose as in CrCl <10mL/min

Heparin (Heparin)
Drug Class & Common Uses: Anticoagulant - Thromboembolism, IV Patency
Hepatic Impairment: No dosage adjustment required; adjust therapeutic heparin according to aPTT or anti-Xa activity
Renal Impairment: Dose as in normal renal function
Dialyzable: Not Dialyzed. Dose as in normal renal function

Hydralazine (Apresoline)
Drug Class & Common Uses: Vasodilator - Hypertension, Heart Failure
Hepatic Impairment: No Data
Renal Impairment: For CrCl <50mL/min start at low dose and adjust in accordance with response
Dialyzable: Note dialyzed. Dose as in CrCl <10mL/min

Hydrochlorothiazide (Microzide)
Drug Class & Common Uses: Thiazide Diuretic - Fluid Retention
Hepatic Impairment: Administer with caution in patients with severe hepatic dysfunction; in cirrhosis, avoid electrolyte and acid/base imbalances
Renal Impairment: For CrCl < 10mL/min: avoid use
Dialyzable: No Data

Hydrocodone and Acetaminophen (Lortab, Vicodin, Norco)
Drug Class & Common Uses: Analgesic Combination (Opioid) - Nociceptive Pain
Hepatic Impairment: Administer with caution; avoid chronic use in hepatic impairment
Renal Impairment: Administer with caution in patients with renal impairment
Dialyzable: No Data

Hydrocodone and Chlorpheniramine (Tussionex Pennkinetic ER)
Drug Class & Common Uses: Antitussive - Cough Suppressant
Hepatic Impairment: Administer with caution in patients with severe hepatic impairment
Renal Impairment: Administer with caution in patients with severe renal impairment
Dialyzable: No Data

Hydrocodone and Homatropine (Hydromet, Tussigon)
Drug Class & Common Uses: Antitussive - Cough Suppressant
Hepatic Impairment: Administer with caution in patients with severe hepatic impairment
Renal Impairment: Administer with caution in patients with severe renal impairment
Dialyzable: No Data

Hydrocodone and Ibuprofen (Vicoprofen)
Drug Class & Common Uses: Analgesic Combination (Opioid) - Nociceptive Pain
Hepatic Impairment: Administer with caution in patients with severe hepatic impairment
Renal Impairment: Administer with caution and monitor renal function closely
Dialyzable: No Data

Hydrocortisone (Cortaid)
Drug Class & Common Uses: Topical Corticosteroid - Pruritus, Rash
Hepatic Impairment: Administer with caution in patients with hepatic impairment, including cirrhosis
Renal Impairment: Dose as in normal renal function
Dialyzable: Unlikely to be dialyzed. Dose as in normal renal function

Hydrocortisone (Cortef)
Drug Class & Common Uses: Corticosteroid - Bone Pain, Nerve Compression Pain, Respiratory Inflammation, Visceral Pain
Hepatic Impairment: No adjustment required
Renal Impairment: Dose as in normal renal function
Dialyzable: Unlikely to be dialyzed. Dose as in normal renal function

Hydromorphone (Dilaudid, Exalgo)
Drug Class & Common Uses: Opioid - Dyspnea, Nociceptive Pain
Hepatic Impairment: Dose adjustment should be considered; Exalgo: in patients with moderate to severe hepatic impairment, start with reduced dose and monitor closely, consider alternative analgesic
Renal Impairment: For CrCl <20mL/min reduce dose - start with lowest dose and titrate according to response
Dialyzable: Unknown dialyzability. Dose as in CrCl <10mL/min

Hydroxyzine (Atarax, Vistaril)
Drug Class & Common Uses: Antihistamine - Pruritus, Anxiety, Nausea & Vomiting (Vestibular)
Hepatic Impairment: Decrease interval to every 24 hours in patients with primary biliary cirrhosis
Renal Impairment: Dose as in normal renal function unless CrCl < 20mL/min then start with small dose at night and increase to 2-3 times a day if necessary
Dialyzable: Not dialyzed. Dose as in CrCl <10mL/min

Hyoscyamine (Levsin)
Drug Class & Common Uses: Anticholinergic - Nausea & Vomiting, Abdominal Spasm, Cramping, Bowel Obstruction, Terminal Secretions, Visceral Pain
Hepatic Impairment: No Data
Renal Impairment: Administer with caution in patients with renal impairment
Dialyzable: No Data

Ibuprofen (Motrin)
Drug Class & Common Uses: NSAID (Mixed COX) - Fever, Nociceptive Pain, Bone Pain
Hepatic Impairment: Avoid in severe impairment
Renal Impairment: Dose as in normal renal function but avoid if possible if CrCl 20-50mL/min. For CrCl <10mL/min dose as in normal renal function but only if on dialysis
Dialyzable: Not dialyzed. Dose as in normal renal function.

Imipramine (Tofranil)
Drug Class & Common Uses: Antidepressant (Tricyclic) - Neuropathic Pain, Depression
Hepatic Impairment: Administer with caution
Renal Impairment: Dose as in normal renal function
Dialyzable: Not dialyzed. Dose as in normal renal function.

Indacaterol (Arcapta)
Drug Class & Common Uses: Long Acting Beta2 Agonist (LABA) - Asthma, COPD
Hepatic Impairment: No dosage adjustment required; monitor
Renal Impairment: No adjustment required
Dialyzable: No Data

Indomethacin (Indocin)
Drug Class & Common Uses: NSAID (Mixed COX) - Fever, Nociceptive Pain, Bone Pain
Hepatic Impairment: Use with caution
Renal Impairment: Dose as in normal renal function, but avoid use if possible if CrCl 20-50mL/min. If CrCl <10mL/min dose as in normal renal function but only use if CKD 5 and on dialysis
Dialyzable: Not dialyzed. Dose as in normal renal function

Insulin, Intermediate-Acting, [Regular or NPH (Humulin R or N, Novolin R or N)]
Drug Class & Common Uses: Insulin - Hyperglycemia
Hepatic Impairment: Close monitoring and adjustment of therapy is required
Renal Impairment: CrCl 10-50mL/min: administer 75% of dose; CrCl < 10mL/min: administer 25-50% of dose; monitor blood glucose closely
Dialyzable: Not significantly removed by dialysis. Supplemental dose is not necessary.

Insulin, Long Acting [Levemir (detemir), Lantus (glargine)]
Drug Class & Common Uses: Insulin - Hyperglycemia
Hepatic Impairment: Close monitoring and adjustment of therapy is required
Renal Impairment: CrCl 10-50mL/min: administer 75% of dose; CrCl < 10mL/min: administer 25-50% of dose; monitor blood glucose closely
Dialyzable: Not significantly removed by dialysis. Supplemental dose is not necessary.

Insulin, Rapid-Acting [Apidra (glulisine), Novolog (aspart), Humalog (lispro)]
Drug Class & Common Uses: Insulin - Hyperglycemia
Hepatic Impairment: Close monitoring and adjustment of therapy is required
Renal Impairment: CrCl 10-50mL/min: administer 75% of dose; CrCl < 10mL/min: administer 25-50% of dose; monitor blood glucose closely
Dialyzable: Not significantly removed by dialysis. Supplemental dose is not necessary.

Ipratropium (Atrovent)
Drug Class & Common Uses: Anticholinergic - Short-Acting Bronchodilator
Hepatic Impairment: No Data
Renal Impairment: Dose as in normal renal function
Dialyzable: Not dialyzed. Dose as in normal renal function

Irbesartan (Avapro)
Drug Class & Common Uses: Angiotensin II Receptor Blocker - Cardiovascular
Hepatic Impairment: No Data
Renal Impairment: Dose as in normal renal function
Dialyzable: Not dialyzed. Initial dose 75mg daily and gradually increase

Isosorbide Dinitrate (Isordil)
Drug Class & Common Uses: Antianginal (Nitrate) - Cardiovascular
Hepatic Impairment: No Data
Renal Impairment: Dose as in normal renal function
Dialyzable: Not dialyzed. Dose as in normal renal function

Isosorbide Mononitrate (Imdur)
Drug Class & Common Uses: Antianginal (Nitrate) - Cardiovascular
Hepatic Impairment: No dosage adjustment necessary
Renal Impairment: Dose as in normal renal function
Dialyzable: Dialyzed. Dose as in normal renal function

Itraconazole (Sporonox)
Drug Class & Common Uses: Antifungal - Infection (Systemic Fungal)
Hepatic Impairment: Administer with caution
Renal Impairment: Dose as in normal renal function
Dialyzable: Not dialyzed. Dose as in normal renal function

Ketamine (Ketolar)
Drug Class & Common Uses: NMDA Antagonist - Neuropathic Pain, Refractory Pain, Depression
Hepatic Impairment: No Data
Renal Impairment: Dose as in normal renal function
Dialyzable: Not dialyzed. Dose as in normal renal function

Ketoconazole
Drug Class & Common Uses: Antifungal - Infection (Systemic Fungal)
Hepatic Impairment: Dose reductions should be considered in severe liver disease
Renal Impairment: Dose as in normal renal function
Dialyzable: Not dialyzed. Dose as in normal renal function

Ketorolac (Toradol)
Drug Class & Common Uses: NSAID (Mixed COX) - Nociceptive Pain, Bone Pain
Hepatic Impairment: Administer with caution
Renal Impairment: For CrCl 20-50mL/min: Maximum 60mg daily. For CrCl <20mL/min: Avoid
Dialyzable: Unlikely to be dialyzed. Dose as in CrCl <10mL/min

Lacosamide (Vimpat)
Drug Class & Common Uses: Anticonvulsant - Partial-onset Seizures
Hepatic Impairment: Use caution when titrating dose; Mild-to-moderate: max 300mg/day; Severe: Avoid
Renal Impairment: Use caution when titrating dose; Mild-to-moderate: no dose adjustment necessary; Severe (CrCl < 30mL/min): max dose 300mg/day
Dialyzable: removed by hemodialysis; after 4-hour HD treatment, a supplemental dose of up to 50%

Lactobacillus spp (Bacid, Culturelle, Lactinex)
Drug Class & Common Uses: Probiotics
Hepatic Impairment: No dosage adjustment necessary
Renal Impairment: Dose as in normal renal function
Dialyzable: Not dialyzed, no oral absorption

Lactulose (Enulose, Kristalose)
Drug Class & Common Uses: Laxative (Osmotic) - Constipation, Hepatic Encephalopathy
Hepatic Impairment: No Data
Renal Impairment: Dose as in normal renal function
Dialyzable: Not dialyzed. Dose as in normal renal function

Lansoprazole (Prevacid)
Drug Class & Common Uses: Proton Pump Inhibitor (PPI) - Dyspepsia, GERD, GI Ulcers
Hepatic Impairment: Consider dose reduction in severe hepatic impairment
Renal Impairment: Dose as in normal renal function
Dialyzable: Not dialyzed. Dose as in normal renal function

Lanthanum (Fosrenol)
Drug Class & Common Uses: Phosphate Binder
Hepatic Impairment: No dosage adjustment necessary
Renal Impairment: Dose as in normal renal function
Dialyzable: Not dialyzed. Dose as in normal renal function

Levalbuterol (Xopenex)
Drug Class & Common Uses: Short Acting Beta Agonist (SABA) - Bronchodilator, Asthma, COPD
Hepatic Impairment: No Data
Renal Impairment: No Data
Dialyzable: No Data

Levocetirizine (Xyzal)
Drug Class & Common Uses: Antihistamine - Rhinitis, Urticaria, Seasonal Allergies
Hepatic Impairment: No dosage adjustment required
Renal Impairment: For CrCl 30-50mL/min: 5mg every 48 hours. For CrCl <30mL/min: 5mg every 72 hours
Dialyzable: Not dialyzed. Dose as in CrCl <10mL/min

Levodopa and Carbidopa (Sinemet)
Drug Class & Common Uses: Dopamine Precursor - Parkinson's
Hepatic Impairment: Administer with caution
Renal Impairment: Administer with caution
Dialyzable: No Data

Levofloxacin (Levaquin)
Drug Class & Common Uses: Antibiotic (Quinolone) - Respiratory Infection
Hepatic Impairment: No Data
Renal Impairment: Initial dose 250-500mg then if CrCl 20-50mL/min reduce dose by 50%. If CrCl 10-20mL/min after initial dose: 125mg every 12-24 hours. If CrCl <10mL/min after initial dose: 125mg every 24-48 hours
Dialyzable: Not dialyzed. Dose as in CrCl <10mL/min

Levothyroxine (Synthroid)
Drug Class & Common Uses: Thyroid Replacement - Hypothyroidism
Hepatic Impairment: No Data
Renal Impairment: Dose as in normal renal function
Dialyzable: Not dialyzed. Dose as in normal renal function

Lidocaine (Lidoderm, Xylocaine)
Drug Class & Common Uses: Local Anesthetic - Topical Pain, Neuropathic Pain, Pruritus, Mucositis
Hepatic Impairment: Administer with caution
Renal Impairment: Dose as in normal renal function
Dialyzable: Not dialyzed. Dose as in normal renal function

Lidocaine (Xylocaine)
Drug Class & Common Uses: Local Anesthetic - Refractory Cough, Mucositis
Hepatic Impairment: No Data
Renal Impairment: Dose as in normal renal function
Dialyzable: Not dialyzed. Dose as in normal renal function

Lidocaine and Prilocaine (EMLA)
Drug Class & Common Uses: Local Anesthetic - Topical Pain
Hepatic Impairment: Smaller areas of treatment are recommended in patients with hepatic dysfunction
Renal Impairment: Smaller areas of treatment are recommended in patients with renal dysfunction
Dialyzable: No Data

Linaclotide (Linzess)
Drug Class & Common Uses: GI Miscellaneous - Constipation
Hepatic Impairment: No dosage adjustment required
Renal Impairment: No dosage adjustment required
Dialyzable: Not dialyzed. Dose as in normal renal function

Liraglutide (Victoza)
Drug Class & Common Uses: Antidiabetic Agent (GLP-1)
Hepatic Impairment: Mild to severe impairment: Use caution
Renal Impairment: Mild to severe impairment: use caution
Dialyzable: No Data

Lisinopril (Prinivil, Zestril)
Drug Class & Common Uses: ACE Inhibitor - Cardiovascular
Hepatic Impairment: No Data
Renal Impairment: Administer initial dose at 2.5mg daily and titrate according to response
Dialyzable: Administer initial dose at 2.5mg daily and titrate according to response

Loperamide (Imodium AD)
Drug Class & Common Uses: Antidiarrheal - Diarrhea
Hepatic Impairment: Administer with caution
Renal Impairment: Dose as in normal renal function unless CrCl <10mL/min then maximum dose usuall 12mg daily depending on tollerability
Dialyzable: Unlikely to be dialyzed. Dose as in CrCl <10mL/min

Loratadine (Claritin)
Drug Class & Common Uses: Antihistamine - Seasonal Allergies, Pruritus
Hepatic Impairment: 5-10mg every other day
Renal Impairment: Dose as in normal renal function
Dialyzable: Not dialyzed. Dose as in normal renal function

Lorazepam (Ativan)
Drug Class & Common Uses: Benzodiazepine - Anxiety, Agitation, Insomnia, Nausea & Vomiting (Anticipatory), Dyspnea, Seizures, Sedation
Hepatic Impairment: No dosage adjustment required
Renal Impairment: Dose as in normal renal function
Dialyzable: Not dialyzed. Dose as in normal renal function

Losartan (Cozaar)
Drug Class & Common Uses: Angiotensin II Receptor Blocker - Cardiovascular
Hepatic Impairment: Reduce initial dose to 25mg/day
Renal Impairment: Dose as in normal renal function unless CrCl <20mL/min then administer initial dose at 25mg and titrate according to response
Dialyzable: Not dialyzed. Dose as in CrCl <20mL/min

Low Molecular Weight Heparin (Lovenox, Fragmin)
Drug Class & Common Uses: Anticoagulant (Factor Xa Inhibitor) - Thromboembolism
Hepatic Impairment: No Data
Renal Impairment: CrCl > 30mL/min: no specific adjustment, monitor closely for bleeding; CrCl < 30mL/min: DVT prophylaxis - 30mg SC once daily, DVT treatment - 1mg/kg SC once daily, STEMI - 1mg/kg SC once daily
Dialyzable: Dialysis: Not FDA approved, serious bleeding complications have been reported, if used, monitor frequently; Hemodialysis: supplemental dose is not necessary

Lubiprostone (Amitiza)
Drug Class & Common Uses: Chloride Channel Activator - Constipation
Hepatic Impairment: Mild-Mod: 16mcg/dose; Severe: 8mcg/dose
Renal Impairment: No dosage adjustment necessary
Dialyzable: No Data

Magnesium Hydroxide (Milk of Magnesia)
Drug Class & Common Uses: Laxative (Osmotic) - Constipation
Hepatic Impairment: No Data
Renal Impairment: CrCl < 30ml/min: monitor serum magnesium levels; Patients in severe renal failure should not receive magnesium due to toxicity from accumulation
Dialyzable: No Data

Meclizine (Antivert)
Drug Class & Common Uses: Antihistamine - Nausea & Vomiting (Vestibular)
Hepatic Impairment: No Data
Renal Impairment: No Data
Dialyzable: No Data

Megestrol (Megace)
Drug Class & Common Uses: Progestin - Appetite Stimulant, Cachexia
Hepatic Impairment: No Data
Renal Impairment: No data available; Urinary excretion of megestrol acetate administered in doses of 4-90mg ranged from 57% to 78% within 10 days
Dialyzable: No Data

Meloxicam (Mobic)
Drug Class & Common Uses: NSAID (Mixed COX) - Nociceptive Pain, Bone Pain
Hepatic Impairment: Use with caution
Renal Impairment: Dose as in normal renal function unless CrCl < 20mL/min then avoid if possible. If CrCl <10mL/min, only use if on dialysis
Dialyzable: Not dialyzed. Dose as in normal renal function

Memantine (Namenda)
Drug Class & Common Uses: NMDA Antagonist - Dementia
Hepatic Impairment: Mild to moderate: no dosage adjustment required. Severe: Use with caution
Renal Impairment: Mild-moderate impairment: No adjustment; Severe: 5-29 mL/min: Initial: 5mg once daily; after at least 1 week of therapy and if tolerated, may titrate up to a target dose of 5mg twice daily
Dialyzable: No Data

Meperidine (Demerol)
Drug Class & Common Uses: Opioid - Nociceptive Pain, Rigors
Hepatic Impairment: Severe impairment: Use with caution, consider lower initial dose; dose reduction more important for oral than IV route
Renal Impairment: Avoid use in renal impairment
Dialyzable: No Data

Metaxalone (Skelaxin)
Drug Class & Common Uses: Muscle Relaxant - Muscle Spasm
Hepatic Impairment: Mild to moderate: use with caution; Severe: contraindicated
Renal Impairment: Mild to moderate: use with caution; Severe: contraindicated
Dialyzable: No Data

Metformin (Glucophage)
Drug Class & Common Uses: Oral Hypoglycemic - Hyperglycemia
Hepatic Impairment: Avoid use
Renal Impairment: If CrCl 40-50mL/min: 25-50% of dose. If 10-40mL/min: 25% of dose. If CrCl <10mL/min: Avoid
Dialyzable: Dialyzed. Avoid.

Methadone (Methadose)
Drug Class & Common Uses: Opioid (NMDA Antagonist) - Nociceptive Pain, Neuropathic Pain
Hepatic Impairment: Avoid in severe disease
Renal Impairment: Usual dosing unless CrCl <10mL/min then administer 50% of dose, titrate to response
Dialyzable: Not dialyzed. Dose as in CrCl <10mL/min

Methylcellulose (Citrucel)
Drug Class & Common Uses: Laxative (Bulk Producing) - Constipation, Diarrhea
Hepatic Impairment: No Data
Renal Impairment: No Data
Dialyzable: No Data

Methylnaltrexone (Relistor)
Drug Class & Common Uses: Opioid Antagonist - Opioid-Induced Constipation
Hepatic Impairment: Use in severe impairment has not been studied.
Renal Impairment: CrCl < 30mL/min: Administer 50% of normal dose
Dialyzable: No Data

Methylphenidate (Ritalin)
Drug Class & Common Uses: CNS Stimulant - Depression, Excessive Sedation
Hepatic Impairment: No Data
Renal Impairment: No Data
Dialyzable: No Data

Metoclopramide (Reglan, Metozolv)
Drug Class & Common Uses: Antiemetic - Nausea & Vomiting (Gastric Stasis) Hiccups, Partial Bowel Obstruction
Hepatic Impairment: No Data
Renal Impairment: Dose as in normal renal function
Dialyzable: Dialyzed. Dose as in normal renal function

Metolazone (Zaroxolyn)
Drug Class & Common Uses: Thiazide Diuretic - Fluid Retention
Hepatic Impairment: No Data
Renal Impairment: Dose as in normal renal function
Dialyzable: Dialyzed. Dose as in normal renal function

Metoprolol (Lopressor, Toprol XL)
Drug Class & Common Uses: Beta Blocker - Hypertension, Heart Failure
Hepatic Impairment: Reduced dose may be necessary
Renal Impairment: Usual dosing unless CrCl <20mL/min then start with low dose, titrate to response
Dialyzable: Not dialyzed. Dose as in CrCl <20mL/min

Metronidazole (Flagyl)
Drug Class & Common Uses: Antibiotic - C. difficile Associated Diarrhea, Wound Odor, Vaginosis
Hepatic Impairment: Severe liver disease: reduce dose
Renal Impairment: Dose as in normal renal function
Dialyzable: Dialyzed. Dose as in normal renal function

Mexiletine (Mexitil)
Drug Class & Common Uses: Antiarrhythmic - Cardiovascular
Hepatic Impairment: Reduce dose to 25-30% of usual dose
Renal Impairment: Usual dosing unless CrCl <10mL/min then use 50-75% of normal dose, titrate to response
Dialyzable: Not dialyzed. Dose as in CrCl <10mL/min

Miconazole (Aloe Vesta, Baza AF, Lotrimin AF, Monistat)
Drug Class & Common Uses: Topical Antifungal - Rash, Fungal Infection
Hepatic Impairment: No Data
Renal Impairment: Dose as in normal renal function
Dialyzable: Not dialyzed. Dose as in normal renal function

Midazolam (Versed)
Drug Class & Common Uses: Benzodiazepine - Delirium, Agitation, Hiccups, Sedation
Hepatic Impairment: Use caution with hepatic impairment.
Renal Impairment: Dose as in normal renal function unless CrCl <10mL/min then use sparingly and titrate according to response. Only bolus doses, not continuous infusion
Dialyzable: Not dialyzed. Dose as in CrCl <10mL/min

Milnacipran (Savella)
Drug Class & Common Uses: Antidepressant (SNRI) - Fibromyalgia
Hepatic Impairment: Severe impairment: Use with caution
Renal Impairment: CrCl ≤ 29mL/min: reduce maintenance dose to 25mg twice daily; dose may be increased to 50mg based on tolerance. ESRD: use not recommended
Dialyzable: No Data

Mineral Oil (Fleet Mineral Oil Enema)
Drug Class & Common Uses: Laxative (Lubricant) - Constipation
Hepatic Impairment: No Data
Renal Impairment: No Data
Dialyzable: No Data

Mirtazapine (Remeron)
Drug Class & Common Uses: Antidepressant (Misc) - Anorexia, Insomnia, Depression
Hepatic Impairment: Use with caution; no dosage adjustment reported; decrease in clearance by 30% is observed in hepatic impairment
Renal Impairment: Usual dosing unless CrCl <10mL/min then start at low dose and monitor closely
Dialyzable: Unlikely to be dialyzed. Dose as in CrCl <10mL/min

Modafinil (Provigil)
Drug Class & Common Uses: CNS Stimulant - Excessive Sedation
Hepatic Impairment: Severe hepatic impairment: reduce dose in half
Renal Impairment: Usual dosing unless CrCl <10mL/min then start at 50% normal dose, titrate to response
Dialyzable: Unknown dialyzability. Dose as in CrCl <10mL/min

Mometasone and Formoterol (Dulera)
Drug Class & Common Uses: Long Acting Beta2 Agonist (LABA) and Corticosteroid - Asthma
Hepatic Impairment: No dosage adjustment recommended; systemic exposure appears to increase with increasing impairment
Renal Impairment: No Data
Dialyzable: No Data

Montelukast (Singulair)
Drug Class & Common Uses: Leukotriene Receptor Antagonist - Asthma, Rhinitis
Hepatic Impairment: Mild-to-moderate impairment: no adjustment necessary; Severe: not studied
Renal Impairment: Dose as in normal renal function
Dialyzable: Not dialyzed. Dose as in normal renal function

Morphine ER (Avinza, Kadian, MS Contin)
Drug Class & Common Uses: Opioid - Nociceptive Pain
Hepatic Impairment: Unchanged in mild liver disease; excessive sedation may occur in cirrhosis
Renal Impairment: If CrCl 20-50mL/min administer 75% of dose. If CrCl <20mL/min use small doses and extend dosing intervals. Titrate according to response
Dialyzable: Dialyzed - active metabolite removed significantly. Dose as in CrCl <20mL/min

Morphine IR (Roxanol, Duramorph)
Drug Class & Common Uses: Opioid - Nociceptive Pain, Dyspnea, Angina
Hepatic Impairment: Unchanged in mild liver disease; excessive sedation may occur in cirrhosis
Renal Impairment: If CrCl 20-50mL/min administer 75% of dose. If CrCl <20mL/min use small doses and extend dosing intervals. Titrate according to response
Dialyzable: Dialyzed - active metabolite removed significantly. Dose as in CrCl <20mL/min

Moxifloxacin (Avelox)
Drug Class & Common Uses: Antibiotic (Quinolone) - Respiratory Infection
Hepatic Impairment: No dosage adjustment required in mild, moderate, or severe insufficiency. Use with caution in patients with secondary risk of QT prolongation.
Renal Impairment: Dose as in normal renal function
Dialyzable: Unknown dialyzability. Dose as in normal renal function.

Mupirocin (Bactroban)
Drug Class & Common Uses: Topical Antibiotic - Skin Infection
Hepatic Impairment: No Data
Renal Impairment: No Data
Dialyzable: No Data

Nabumetone (Relafen)
Drug Class & Common Uses: NSAID (Mixed COX) - Nociceptive Pain, Bone Pain
Hepatic Impairment: Administer with caution, closely monitor patients with any abnormal LFT
Renal Impairment: Dose as in normal renal function but avoid if possible. For CrCl <20mL/min dose at 0.5-1 gram daily. Only use if on dialysis if CrCl <10mL/min
Dialyzable: Not dialyzed. Dose as in CrCl <10mL/min

Nadolol (Corgard)
Drug Class & Common Uses: Beta Blocker - Hypertension, Migraine, Esophageal Varices
Hepatic Impairment: No dosage adjustment necessary
Renal Impairment: Start with low doses and adjust according to response
Dialyzable: Dialyzed. Start low - adjust according to response

Naproxen (Naprosyn)
Drug Class & Common Uses: NSAID (Mixed COX) - Fever, Nociceptive Pain, Bone Pain
Hepatic Impairment: Administer with caution in patients with decreased hepatic function
Renal Impairment: Avoid if possible. If CrCl <10mL/min only use if on dialysis
Dialyzable: Not dialyzed. Dose as in CrCl <10mL/min

Naproxen and Esomeprazole (Vimovo)
Drug Class & Common Uses: NSAID (Mixed COX) and Proton Pump Inhibitor (PPI) - Nociceptive Pain
Hepatic Impairment: Severe liver disease: Use not recommended
Renal Impairment: No Data
Dialyzable: No Data

Neomycin
Drug Class & Common Uses: Antibiotic (Aminoglycoside) - Hepatic Encephalopathy, *C. difficile* associated Diarrhea
Hepatic Impairment: No adjustment needed
Renal Impairment: Dose as in normal renal function. Use with caution, and monitor closely
Dialyzable: Dialyzed. Dose as in normal renal function

Neomycin, Polymyxin and Bacitracin (Neosporin)
Drug Class & Common Uses: Topical Antibiotic - Skin Infection
Hepatic Impairment: No Data
Renal Impairment: No Data
Dialyzable: No Data

Nitrofurantion (Macrodantin)
Drug Class & Common Uses: Antibiotic - Urinary Tract Infection
Hepatic Impairment: No Data
Renal Impairment: Dose as in normal renal function. Use with caution. Use is contraindicated if CrCl <50mL/min
Dialyzable: Dialyzed. Avoid use - contraindicated

Nitroglycerin (Nitrostat)
Drug Class & Common Uses: Antianginal (Nitrate) - Cardiovascular
Hepatic Impairment: No Data
Renal Impairment: No Data
Dialyzable: No Data

Nizatidine (Axid)
Drug Class & Common Uses: H2 Antagonist (H2RA) - Gastritis, Dyspepsia, GERD
Hepatic Impairment: Administer with caution, dosage adjustment recommended
Renal Impairment: If CrCl 20-50mL/min administer 150-300mg daily. If CrCl <20mL/min administer 150mg daily
Dialyzable: Not dialyzed. Dose as in CrCl <20mL/min

Normal Saline (0.9%, 3%, 7%)
Drug Class & Common Uses: Normal Saline - Dyspnea, Thick Secretions, Irrigation Solution, Mucosal Moisturizer
Hepatic Impairment: No Data
Renal Impairment: Administer with caution
Dialyzable: No Data

Nortriptyline (Pamelor)
Drug Class & Common Uses: Antidepressant (Tricyclic) - Neuropathic Pain, Depression
Hepatic Impairment: Lower doses and slower titration are recommended
Renal Impairment: Dose as in normal renal function. If CrCl <10mL/min start with small dose.
Dialyzable: Not dialyzed. Dose as in CrCl <10mL/min

Nystatin (Mycostatin)
Drug Class & Common Uses: Antifungal - Fungal Infection, Thrush
Hepatic Impairment: No Data
Renal Impairment: Dose as in normal renal function
Dialyzable: Not dialyzed. Dose as in normal renal function

Nystatin and Triamcinolone (Mycolog)
Drug Class & Common Uses: Topical Antifungal and Corticosteroid - Rash, Fungal infection
Hepatic Impairment: No Data
Renal Impairment: No Data
Dialyzable: No Data

Octreotide (Sandostatin)
Drug Class & Common Uses: Somatostatin Analog - GI Hypersecretion, Bowel Obstruction, Diarrhea, Visceral Pain
Hepatic Impairment: Administer with caution; dosage adjustment required in patients with established cirrhosis
Renal Impairment: Dose as in normal renal function
Dialyzable: Dialyzed. Dose as in normal renal function

Olanzapine (Zyprexa)
Drug Class & Common Uses: Antipsychotic (Atypical) - Delirium, Agitation, Schizophrenia, Bipolar Disorder
Hepatic Impairment: Dosage adjustment may be necessary; monitor
Renal Impairment: Initial dose 5mg daily and titrate as necessary
Dialyzable: Not dialyzed. Dose initially at 5mg per day and titrate as necessary

---

Olmesartan (Benicar)
Drug Class & Common Uses: Angiotensin II Receptor Blocker - Cardiovascular
Hepatic Impairment: No initial dosage adjustment necessary
Renal Impairment: Dose as in normal renal function. If CrCl 10-20mL/min start with low doses. If CrCl <10mL/min then administer initial dose at 10mg daily and gradually increase
Dialyzable: Not dialyzed. Dose as in CrCl <10mL/min

Olmesartan and Hydrochlorothiazide (Benicar HCT)
Drug Class & Common Uses: Angiotensin II Receptor Blocker and Diuretic - Cardiovascular
Hepatic Impairment: No dosage adjustment required
Renal Impairment: CrCl < 30mL/min: use not recommended
Dialyzable: No Data

Olmesartan, Amlodipine and Hydrochlorothiazide (Tribenzor)
Drug Class & Common Uses: Angiotensin II Receptor Blocker and Calcium Channel Blocker and Diuretic - Hypertension
Hepatic Impairment: Mild to moderate impairment: Use with caution; Severe impairment: start amlodipine at 2.5mg (half tablet)
Renal Impairment: CrCl ≤ 30mL/min: Use of combination not recommended; contraindicated in anuria
Dialyzable: No Data

Omeprazole (Prilosec OTC, Prilosec)
Drug Class & Common Uses: Proton Pump Inhibitor (PPI) - Dyspepsia, GERD, GI Ulcers
Hepatic Impairment: Consider dosage adjustment
Renal Impairment: Dose as in normal renal function
Dialyzable: Not dialyzed. Dose as in normal renal function

Omeprazole and Sodium Bicarbonate (Zegerid)
Drug Class & Common Uses: Proton Pump Inhibitor (PPI) - Dyspepsia, GERD, GI Ulcers
Hepatic Impairment: Consider dosage reduction if chronic use anticipated
Renal Impairment: Dose as in normal renal function
Dialyzable: No Data

Ondansetron (Zofran)
Drug Class & Common Uses: 5HT3 Receptor Antagonist - Nausea & Vomiting
Hepatic Impairment: Severe impairment: 8mg max
Renal Impairment: Dose as in normal renal function
Dialyzable: Not dialyzed. Dose as in normal renal function

Oxandrolone (Oxandrin)
Drug Class & Common Uses: Androgen - Appetite Stimulant, Cachexia
Hepatic Impairment: Administer with caution
Renal Impairment: Administer with caution
Dialyzable: No Data

Oxybutynin (Ditropan, Oxytrol, Gelnique)
Drug Class & Common Uses: Anticholinergic - Overactive Bladder, Urinary Spasms
Hepatic Impairment: Administer with caution
Renal Impairment: Dose as in normal renal function
Dialyzable: Dialyzed. Dose as in normal renal function

Oxycodone SR (OxyContin)
Drug Class & Common Uses: Opioid - Nociceptive Pain
Hepatic Impairment: Severe impairment: Decrease dose to 1/3-1/2 usual starting dose
Renal Impairment: Dose as in normal renal function unless CrCl <10mL/min then start with small doses.
Dialyzable: Unknown dialyzability. Dose at CrCl <10mL/min

Oxycodone (Roxicodone)
Drug Class & Common Uses: Opioid - Nociceptive Pain, Dyspnea
Hepatic Impairment: Reduce dosage in patients with liver dysfunction; titrate carefully
Renal Impairment: Dose as in normal renal function unless CrCl <10mL/min then start with small doses.
Dialyzable: Unknown dialyzability. Dose at CrCl <10mL/min

Oxycodone and Acetaminophen (Percocet, Endocet)
Drug Class & Common Uses: Analgesic Combination (Opioid) - Nociceptive Pain
Hepatic Impairment: Severe liver disease: reduce dose
Renal Impairment: No Data
Dialyzable: No Data

Oxymetazoline (Afrin)
Drug Class & Common Uses: Decongestant - Respiratory, Bleeding
Hepatic Impairment: No Data
Renal Impairment: No Data
Dialyzable: No Data

Pamidronate (Aredia)
Drug Class & Common Uses: Bisphosphonate - Osteoporosis, Bone Metastases
Hepatic Impairment: No dose adjustment required. Use in severe impairment has not been studied.
Renal Impairment: Do not use if CrCl <30mL/min. Use clinical judgement to determine if clinical benefit will outweigh risks for patients with renal insufficiency.
Dialyzable: No Data

Pancrelipase (Viokace, Zenpep, Creon, Ultresa)
Drug Class & Common Uses: Pancreatic Enzyme - GI Malabsorption, Visceral Pain
Hepatic Impairment: No Data
Renal Impairment: Dose as in normal renal function
Dialyzable: Unlikely to be dialyzed. Dose as in normal renal function

Pantoprazole (Protonix)
Drug Class & Common Uses: Proton Pump Inhibitor (PPI) - Dyspepsia, GERD, GI Ulcers
Hepatic Impairment: No dosage adjustment necessary
Renal Impairment: Dose as in normal renal function
Dialyzable: Not dialyzed. Dose as in normal renal function

Paregoric (Camphorated Opium)
Drug Class & Common Uses: Opioid - Diarrhea
Hepatic Impairment: No Data
Renal Impairment: No Data
Dialyzable: No Data

Paroxetine (Paxil, Pexeva, Brisdelle)
Drug Class & Common Uses: Antidepressant (SSRI) - Depression, Anxiety
Hepatic Impairment:
Renal Impairment: Usual dosing unless CrCl <30mL/min then dose at 20mg daily and titrate slowly
Dialyzable: Not dialyzed. Dose as in CrCl <30mL/min

Pentazocine (Talwin)
Drug Class & Common Uses: Opioid (Mixed) - Nociceptive Pain
Hepatic Impairment: Reduce dose or avoid use
Renal Impairment: CrCl 10-50mL/min: administer 75% of dose; CrCl < 10mL/min: administer 50% of dose
Dialyzable: No Data

Pentobarbital (Nembutal)
Drug Class & Common Uses: Barbiturate - Delirium, Agitation, Sedation
Hepatic Impairment: Reduce dosage in patients with liver dysfunction
Renal Impairment: Reduce dosage in patients with renal dysfunction
Dialyzable: No Data

Phenazopyridine (Pyridium)
Drug Class & Common Uses: Urinary Analgesic - Urinary Pain
Hepatic Impairment: No Data
Renal Impairment: CrCl 50-80mL/min: administer every 8-16 hours; CrCl < 50mL/min: avoid use
Dialyzable: No Data

Phenobarbital (Luminal)
Drug Class & Common Uses: Barbiturate - Seizures, Delirium, Agitation, Sedation
Hepatic Impairment: Reduce dose in patients with hepatic impairment
Renal Impairment: Dose as in normal renal function unless CrCl 10-20mL/min then avoid very large doses. If CrCl <10mL/min reduce dose by 25-50% and avoid very large single doses
Dialyzable: Dialyzed. Dose as in CrCl <10mL/min

Phenytoin (Dilantin)
Drug Class & Common Uses: Anticonvulsant - Seizures, Hiccups
Hepatic Impairment: Safe in usual doses in mild liver disease; clearance may be substantially reduced in cirrhosis and plasma level monitoring with dose adjustment advisable
Renal Impairment: Dose as in normal renal function
Dialyzable: Not dialyzed. Dose as in normal renal function

Pilocarpine (Salagen)
Drug Class & Common Uses: Cholinergic Agonist - Xerostomia
Hepatic Impairment: Oral: Moderate impairment: 5mg 2 times/day
Renal Impairment: No Data
Dialyzable: No Data

Polycarbophil (Fibercon)
Drug Class & Common Uses: Laxative (Bulk Producing) - Constipation, Diarrhea
Hepatic Impairment: No Data
Renal Impairment: No Data
Dialyzable: No Data

Polyethylene Glycol (Miralax)
Drug Class & Common Uses: Laxative (Osmotic) - Constipation
Hepatic Impairment: No Data
Renal Impairment: Dose as in normal renal function
Dialyzable: Not dialyzed. Dose as in normal renal function

Potassium Chloride (KlorCon, KDur)
Drug Class & Common Uses: Potassium Supplement - Hypokalemia
Hepatic Impairment: No Data
Renal Impairment: Dose according to response
Dialyzable: Dialyzed. Dose according to resonse

Pramipexole (Mirapex)
Drug Class & Common Uses: Dopamine Agonist - Parkinson's, Restless Legs Syndrome
Hepatic Impairment:
Renal Impairment: Initial: 125mcg twice daily, titrate slowly. If CrCl <20mL/min: 125mcg once daily, titrate slowly
Dialyzable: Not dialyzed. Dose as in CrCl <20mL/min

Pramlintide (SymlinPen)
Drug Class & Common Uses: Antidiabetic Agent
Hepatic Impairment: No dosage adjustment necessary
Renal Impairment: No dosage adjustment necessary
Dialyzable: No Data

Prasugrel (Effient)
Drug Class & Common Uses: Antiplatelet (Thienopyridine) - Cardiovascular, Stroke, Thromboembolism
Hepatic Impairment: Mild-to-moderate impairment: no dosage adjustment necessary; Severe: not studied
Renal Impairment: No dosage adjustment necessary
Dialyzable: No Data

Prazosin (Minipress)
Drug Class & Common Uses: Alpha1 Blocker - Hypertension, Urinary hesitancy, BPH
Hepatic Impairment: No Data
Renal Impairment: Dose as in normal renal function
Dialyzable: Not dialyzed. Dose as in normal renal function

Prednisone (Deltasone)
Drug Class & Common Uses: Corticosteroid - Appetite, Bone Pain, Nerve Compression Pain, Respiratory Inflammation, Pruritus, Excessive Sedation, Visceral Pain
Hepatic Impairment: Administer with caution
Renal Impairment: No Data
Dialyzable: Supplemental dose is not necessary

Pregabalin (Lyrica)
Drug Class & Common Uses: Anticonvulsant - Neuropathic Pain, Fibromyalgia, Seizures
Hepatic Impairment:
Renal Impairment: Titrate dose according to patient tolerability and response. For CrCl 30-60mL/min initially dose at 75mg daily. For CrCl 15-30mL/min initially dose at 25-50mg daily. For CrCl <15mL/min initially dose at 25mg daily.
Dialyzable: Dialyzed. Dose as in CrCl <15mL/min

Procainamide
Drug Class & Common Uses: Antiarrhythmic - Cardiovascular
Hepatic Impairment: Reduce dose by 50%
Renal Impairment: Dose as in normal renal function unless CrCl <10mL/min then administer normal loading dose. Maintenance dose according to response, lower doses or longer dosage intervals may be required
Dialyzable: Dialyzed. Dose as in CrCl <10mL/min

Prochlorperazine (Compazine)
Drug Class & Common Uses: Antiemetic (Phenothiazine) - Nausea & Vomiting (Chemoreceptor Trigger Zone)
Hepatic Impairment: No dosage adjustment necessary
Renal Impairment: Dose as in normal renal function unless CrCl <10mL/min then start with small doses.
Dialyzable: Unlikely to be dialyzed. Start with smaller doses.

Promethazine (Phenergan)
Drug Class & Common Uses: Antiemetic (Phenothiazine) - Nausea & Vomiting (Chemoreceptor Trigger Zone)
Hepatic Impairment: Administer with caution in patients with severe hepatic impairment
Renal Impairment: Dose as in normal renal function
Dialyzable: Not dialyzed. Dose as in normal renal function

Propofol (Diprovan)
Drug Class & Common Uses: Anesthetic - Sedation, Delirium, Agitation
Hepatic Impairment: No dosage adjustment necessary
Renal Impairment: Dose as in normal renal function
Dialyzable: Unlikely to be dialyzed. Dose as in normal renal function

Propranolol (Inderal)
Drug Class & Common Uses: Beta Blocker - Hypertension, Essential Tremor, Migraine, Esophageal Varices
Hepatic Impairment: Administer at lower initial dose and regular heart rate monitoring
Renal Impairment: Dose as in normal renal function unless CrCl <20mL/min then start with small doses and titrate according to response
Dialyzable: Not dialyzed. Dose as in CrCl <10mL/min

Pseudoephedrine (Sudafed)
Drug Class & Common Uses: Decongestants - Respiratory
Hepatic Impairment: No Data
Renal Impairment: Dose as in normal renal function. If CrCl <20mL/min use with caution
Dialyzable: Not dialyzed. Dose as in normal renal function

Psyllium (Metamucil)
Drug Class & Common Uses: Laxative (Bulk Producing) - Constipation, Diarrhea
Hepatic Impairment: No Data
Renal Impairment: No Data
Dialyzable: No Data

Quetiapine (Seroquel)
Drug Class & Common Uses: Antipsychotic (Atypical) - Delirium, Agitation, Schizophrenia, Bipolar Disorder
Hepatic Impairment: IR: 25mg/day; ER: 50mg/day; titrate based on clinical response and tolerability to patient
Renal Impairment: For CrCl <50mL/min: administer initial dose at 25mg per day and increase in increments of 25-50mg per day according to response
Dialyzable: Unknown dialyzability. Dose as in CrCl <10mL/min

Quinapril (Accupril)
Drug Class & Common Uses: ACE Inhibitor - Cardiovascular
Hepatic Impairment: Administer with caution
Renal Impairment: Start with low doses and adjust according to response
Dialyzable: 25% dialyzed. Dose as in CrCl <10mL/min

Rabeprazole (Aciphex)
Drug Class & Common Uses: Proton Pump Inhibitor (PPI) - Dyspepsia, GERD, GI Ulcers
Hepatic Impairment: Mild-to-moderate impairment: no dosage adjustment required; severe: use caution
Renal Impairment: Dose as in normal renal function
Dialyzable: Not dialyzed. Dose as in normal renal function

Raloxifene (Evista)
Drug Class & Common Uses: Selective Estrogen Receptor Modulator (SERM) - Osteoporosis
Hepatic Impairment: Mild impairment: not established, use caution
Renal Impairment: Dose as in normal renal function
Dialyzable: Unlikely to be dialyzed. Dose as in normal renal function

Ramelteon (Rozerem)
Drug Class & Common Uses: Hypnotic (Melatonin Agonist) - Insomnia
Hepatic Impairment: Mild-to-moderate impairment: no dosage adjustment required; severe: not recommended
Renal Impairment: No dosage adjustment required
Dialyzable: No Data

Ramipril (Altace)
Drug Class & Common Uses: ACE Inhibitor - Cardiovascular
Hepatic Impairment: No Data
Renal Impairment: Dose as in normal renal function. For CrCl <20mL/min administer initial dose at 1.25mg daily and increase according to response
Dialyzable: Not dialyzed. Dose as in CrCl <20mL/min

Ranitidine (Zantac)
Drug Class & Common Uses: H2 Antagonist (H2RA) - Gastritis, Dyspepsia, GERD
Hepatic Impairment: Dosing adjustments are not necessary; monitor patient
Renal Impairment: Dose as in normal renal function unless CrCl <10mL/min then administer 50-100% of normal dosetion unless CrCl <10mL/min then administer 50-100% of normal dose
Dialyzable: Dialyzed. Dose as in CrCl <10mL/min

Ranolazine (Ranexa)
Drug Class & Common Uses: Antiangina - Cardiovascular
Hepatic Impairment: Contraindicated with any degree of hepatic cirrhosis
Renal Impairment: Use caution, plasma levels increased 50% with renal dysfunction.
Dialyzable: No Data

Rasagaline (Azilect)
Drug Class & Common Uses: MAO-B Inhibitor - Parkinson's
Hepatic Impairment: Mild impairment: 0.5mg/day; Not recommended in moderate to severe liver disease.
Renal Impairment: Dose as in normal renal function
Dialyzable: Unknown dialyzability. Dose as in normal renal function.

Rifaximin (Xifaxan)
Drug Class & Common Uses: Antibiotic - Hepatic Encephalopathy, C. difficile Associated Diarrhea
Hepatic Impairment: No adjustment necessary; use with caution in severe impairment
Renal Impairment: No data
Dialyzable: No Data

Riluzole (Rilutek)
Drug Class & Common Uses: Glutamate Inhibitor - ALS
Hepatic Impairment: Administer with caution
Renal Impairment: Administer with caution
Dialyzable: No Data

Risperidone (Risperdal)
Drug Class & Common Uses: Antipsychotic (Atypical) - Delirium, Agitation, Schizophrenia, Bipolar Disorder
Hepatic Impairment: Oral: 0.5mg twice daily
Renal Impairment: For CrCl <50mL/min initially administer 0.5mg twice daily increasing by 0.5mg BD to 1-2mg twice daily. Use with caution.
Dialyzable: Dialyzed. Dose as in CrCl <50mL/min

Rivaroxaban (Xarelto)
Drug Class & Common Uses: Anticoagulant (Factor Xa Inhibitor) - Thromboembolism, Atrial Fibrillation
Hepatic Impairment: Moderate to severe impairment: Avoid use
Renal Impairment: Avoid use if CrCl < 30mL/min
Dialyzable: Avoid use in ESRD and hemodialysis

Rivastigmine (Exelon)
Drug Class & Common Uses: Acetylcholinesterase Inhibitor - Dementia
Hepatic Impairment: Titrate dose to patient's tolerance
Renal Impairment: Start with low doses and gradually increase
Dialyzable: Likely dialyzable. Start with low doses and gradually increase

Roflumilast (Daliresp)
Drug Class & Common Uses: Phosphodiesterase-4 Enzyme (PDE4) Inhibitor - COPD
Hepatic Impairment: Mild: no dosage adjustment, use with caution; Moderate-to-severe: contraindicated
Renal Impairment: No dosage adjustment is recommended
Dialyzable: No data

Saccharomyces boulardii (Florastor)
Drug Class & Common Uses: Probiotics
Hepatic Impairment: No dosage adjustment necessary
Renal Impairment: Dose as in normal renal function
Dialyzable: Not dialyzable; no oral absorption

Salmeterol (Serevent)
Drug Class & Common Uses: Long Acting Beta2 Agonist (LABA) - Asthma, COPD
Hepatic Impairment: No dosage adjustment required; monitor
Renal Impairment: No Data
Dialyzable: No Data

Salsalate (Disalcid)
Drug Class & Common Uses: Salicylate - Nociceptive Pain, Bone Pain
Hepatic Impairment: Administer with caution
Renal Impairment: Administer with caution
Dialyzable: No Data

Saphris (Asenapine)
Drug Class & Common Uses: Antipsychotic (Atypical) - Schizophrenia, Bipolar Disorder
Hepatic Impairment: Severe hepatic impairment: use is not recommended
Renal Impairment: No dosage adjustment is necessary
Dialyzable: No Data

Saxagliptin (Onglyza)
Drug Class & Common Uses: Antidiabetic Agent (DPP-IV)
Hepatic Impairment: No dosage adjustment necessary
Renal Impairment: CrCl ≤ 50mL/min: 2.5mg once daily
Dialyzable: No data

Scopolamine (Transderm-Scop)
Drug Class & Common Uses: Anticholinergic - Nausea & Vomiting (Vestibular), Bowel Obstruction, Terminal Secretions, Visceral Pain
Hepatic Impairment: Administer with caution
Renal Impairment: Administer with caution
Dialyzable: No Data

Senna (Senokot)
Drug Class & Common Uses: Laxative (Stimulant) - Constipation
Hepatic Impairment: No Data
Renal Impairment: Dose as in normal renal function
Dialyzable: Unknown dialyzability. Dose as in normal renal function.

Sertraline (Zoloft)
Drug Class & Common Uses: Antidepressant (SSRI) - Depression, Anxiety
Hepatic Impairment: Administer with caution; lower dose or less frequent dosing
Renal Impairment: Dose as in normal renal function
Dialyzable: Not dialyzed. Dose as in normal renal function

Sildenafil (Revatio, Viagra)
Drug Class & Common Uses: Phosphodiesterase-5 Enzyme (PDE5) Inhibitor - Pulmonary Hypertension
Hepatic Impairment: No dosage adjustment recommended, consider lower initial dose
Renal Impairment: Dose as in normal renal function
Dialyzable: Unlikely to be dialyzed. Dose as in normal renal function

Silver Sulfadiazine (Silvadene)
Drug Class & Common Uses: Topical Antibiotic - Burns, Skin Infection
Hepatic Impairment: Administer with caution
Renal Impairment: Administer with caution
Dialyzable: No Data

Simethicone (Gas-X, Phazyme)
Drug Class & Common Uses: Antiflatulent - Gas, Hiccups
Hepatic Impairment: No Data
Renal Impairment: No Data
Dialyzable: No Data

Sitagliptan (Januvia)
Drug Class & Common Uses: Antidiabetic Agent (DPP-IV)
Hepatic Impairment: No dosage adjustment necessary. Not studied in severe liver disease.
Renal Impairment: For CrCl 30-50mL/min: 50mg once daily. For CrCl <30mL/min: 25mg once daily
Dialyzable: Not dialyzed. Dose as in CrCl <30mL/min

Sodium Phosphates (Fleet Enema)
Drug Class & Common Uses: Laxative (Osmotic) - Constipation
Hepatic Impairment: No dosage adjustment necessary
Renal Impairment: Administer with caution
Dialyzable: No Data

Solifenacin (Vesicare)
Drug Class & Common Uses: Anticholinergic - Overactive Bladder, Urinary Spasms
Hepatic Impairment: Moderate: 5mg/day. Do not use in severe impairment.
Renal Impairment: Use with caution. CrCl <30mL/min: max 5mg/day
Dialyzable: No Data

Sorbitol 70%
Drug Class & Common Uses: Laxative (Osmotic) - Constipation, Hepatic Encephalopathy
Hepatic Impairment: No Data
Renal Impairment: Administer with caution
Dialyzable: No Data

Spironolactone (Aldactone)
Drug Class & Common Uses: Potassium Sparing Diuretic - Fluid Retention
Hepatic Impairment: No Data
Renal Impairment: For CrCl 10-50mL/min administer 50% of normal dose. For CrCl <10mL/min use with caution
Dialyzable: Not dialyzed. Dose as in CrCl <10mL/min

Statins (Lipitor, Zocor, Crestor)
Drug Class & Common Uses: Antilipemic Agent - Hypercholesterolemia
Hepatic Impairment: Agent dependent; in general, do not use
Renal Impairment: Dose as in normal renal function unless CrCl <10mL/min then administer 10-20mg daily. In severe renal impairment doses above 10mg should be used with caution
Dialyzable: Unlikely to be dialyzed. Dose as in CrCl <10mL/min

Sucralfate (Carafate)
Drug Class & Common Uses: GI Protectant - Gastritis, Stomatitis, GI Ulcers
Hepatic Impairment: No Data
Renal Impairment: For CrCl 20-50mL/min administer 4g daily. For CrCl <20mL/min administer 2-4g daily
Dialyzable: Not dialyzed. Dose as in CrCl <10mL/min

Sulfamethoxazole and Trimethoprim (Bactrim DS, Septra DS)
Drug Class & Common Uses: Antibiotic (Sulfonamide) - Respiratory Infection, Urinary Tract Infection, Skin Infection
Hepatic Impairment: Administer with caution
Renal Impairment: CrCl > 30mL/min: no specific adjustment recommended; CrCl 15-30mL/min: administer 50% of recommended dose; CrCl < 15mL/min: not recommended
Dialyzable: Full daily dose before dialysis and 50% dose after dialysis

Tadalafil (Adcirca, Cialis)
Drug Class & Common Uses: Phosphodiesterase-5 Enzyme (PDE5) Inhibitor - Pulmonary Hypertension
Hepatic Impairment: Mild-to-moderate: use with caution, consider initial dose of 20mg once daily; Severe: avoid
Renal Impairment: Dose as in normal renal function unless CrCl <20mL/min then administer 10mg initially and use with caution
Dialyzable: Not dialyzed. Dose as in CrCl <20mL/min

Tamsulosin (Flomax)
Drug Class & Common Uses: Alpha1 Blocker - BPH, Urinary Hesitancy
Hepatic Impairment: Mild-to-moderate: no dosage adjustment needed; Severe impairment: not studied
Renal Impairment: Dose as in normal renal function. Use with caution if CrCl <10mL/min
Dialyzable: Not dialyzed. Dose as in CrCl <10mL/min

Tapentadol (Nucynta)
Drug Class & Common Uses: Opioid (Misc) - Nociceptive Pain
Hepatic Impairment: Mild: no dosage adjustment necessary; Moderate: IR: 50mg every 8 hours or longer (maximum: 3 doses/24 hours), ER: 50mg every 24 hours or longer (maximum: 100mg once daily); Severe: Avoid
Renal Impairment: Mild-to-moderate: no adjustment necessary; Severe: not recommended
Dialyzable: No Data

Temazepam (Restoril)
Drug Class & Common Uses: Benzodiazepine - Insomnia
Hepatic Impairment: Administer with caution
Renal Impairment: Dose as in normal renal function. If CrCl <20mL/min start with small doses
Dialyzable: Not dialyzed. Dose as in CrCl <20mL/min

Terazosin (Hytrin)
Drug Class & Common Uses: Alpha1 Blocker - Hypertension, Urinary hesitancy, BPH
Hepatic Impairment: No Data
Renal Impairment: Dose as in normal renal function
Dialyzable: Not dialyzed. Dose as in normal renal function

Tetrabenazine (Xenazine)
Drug Class & Common Uses: Central Monoamine-Depleting Agent - Huntington's Disease Chorea
Hepatic Impairment: Contraindicated
Renal Impairment: No Data
Dialyzable: No Data

Theophylline (Theodur)
Drug Class & Common Uses: Methylxanthine Bronchodilator - COPD, Asthma
Hepatic Impairment: No Data
Renal Impairment: Dose as in normal renal function
Dialyzable: Not dialyzed. Dose as in normal renal function

Thymol and Menthol and Glycerin and Calamine (Calmoseptine)
Drug Class & Common Uses: Topical Protectant - Excoriated Skin, Burns
Hepatic Impairment: No Data
Renal Impairment: No Data
Dialyzable: No Data

Ticagrelor (Brilinta)
Drug Class & Common Uses: Antiplatelet- Cardiovascular, Thromboembolism
Hepatic Impairment: Moderate impairment: use caution; Severe impairment: Use is contraindicated
Renal Impairment: No adjustment are recommended
Dialyzable: Use caution (drug is thought to be nondialyzable)

Tiotropium (Spiriva)
Drug Class & Common Uses: Anticholinergic - Long-Acting Bronchodilator
Hepatic Impairment: No Data
Renal Impairment: Dose as in normal renal function. Use caution if CrCl <20mL/min
Dialyzable: Unknown dialyzability. Dose as in normal renal function. Use with caution

Tizanidine (Zanaflex)
Drug Class & Common Uses: Muscle Relaxant - Muscle Spasm
Hepatic Impairment: Avoid use
Renal Impairment: Usual dosing unless CrCl <25mL/min then administer initial dose at 2mg once daily and slowly increase by 2mg increments. Increase daily dose before increasing frequency of administration.
Dialyzable: Unknown dialyzability. Dose as in CrCl <25mL/min

Tolterodine (Detrol)
Drug Class & Common Uses: Anticholinergic - Overactive Bladder, Urinary Spasms
Hepatic Impairment: IR: 1mg twice daily; ER: 2mg once daily
Renal Impairment: Use with caution. Usual dosing unless CrCl <30mL/min then administer 1mg twice daily.
Dialyzable: Unlikely to be dialyzed. Dose as in CrCl <10mL/min

Tolvaptan (Samsca)
Drug Class & Common Uses: Vasopressin Antagonist - Hyponatremia
Hepatic Impairment: Administer with caution
Renal Impairment: CrCl < 10mL/min: not recommended (not studied); contraindicated in anuria
Dialyzable: No Data

Topiramate (Topamax)
Drug Class & Common Uses: Anticonvulsant - Neuropathic Pain, Seizures
Hepatic Impairment: Clearance may be reduced
Renal Impairment: CrCl < 70mL/min: administer 50% dose and titrate more slowly
Dialyzable: Supplemental dose may be needed during hemodialysis

Torsemide (Demadex)
Drug Class & Common Uses: Loop Diuretic - Fluid Retention
Hepatic Impairment: No Data
Renal Impairment: Dose as in normal renal function
Dialyzable: Not dialyzed. Dose as in normal renal function

Tramadol (Ultram)
Drug Class & Common Uses: Opioid (Misc) - Nociceptive Pain
Hepatic Impairment: Cirrhosis: IR: 50mg every 12 hrs; ER: do not use
Renal Impairment: Usual dosing unless CrCl 10-20mL/min then administer 50-100mg every 8 hours initially, and titrate dose as needed. If CrCl <10mL/min administer 50mg every 8 hours initially and titrate dose as tolerated.
Dialyzable: Dialyzed. Dose as in CrCl <10mL/min

Trazodone (Desyrel, Oleptro)
Drug Class & Common Uses: Antidepressant (Serotonin Reuptake Antagonist) - Insomnia
Hepatic Impairment: Administer with caution
Renal Impairment: Usual dosing unless CrCl <20mL/min start with small doses and increase gradually
Dialyzable: Unlikely to be dialyzed. Dose as in CrCl <20mL/min

Triamcinolone (Kenalog)
Drug Class & Common Uses: Topical Corticosteroid - Pruritus, Rash
Hepatic Impairment: No Data
Renal Impairment: Dose as in normal renal function
Dialyzable: Unkown dialyzability. Dose as in normal renal function

Triamcinolone (Nasacort)
Drug Class & Common Uses: Inhaled Corticosteroid - Allergic Rhinitis
Hepatic Impairment: No Data
Renal Impairment: Dose as in normal renal function
Dialyzable: Unkown dialyzability. Dose as in normal renal function

Triamterene and Hydrochlorothiazide (Dyazide)
Drug Class & Common Uses: Potassium Sparing and Thiazide Diuretic - Fluid Retention
Hepatic Impairment: Administer with caution
Renal Impairment: Avoid HCTZ in severe renal disease; triamterene may cause hyperkalemia in renal impairment
Dialyzable: No Data

Trimethobenzamide (Tigan)
Drug Class & Common Uses: Anticholinergic - Nausea & Vomiting (Chemoreceptor Trigger Zone)
Hepatic Impairment: No Data
Renal Impairment: CrCl < 70mL/min: consider dosage reduction or increasing dosing interval
Dialyzable: No Data

Trospium (Sanctura)
Drug Class & Common Uses: Anticholinergic - Overactive Bladder, Urinary Spasms
Hepatic Impairment: No Data
Renal Impairment: Use with caution. CrCl <30mL/min: 20mg/day. Do not use 60mg extended release.
Dialyzable: No Data

Urea (Carmol)
Drug Class & Common Uses: Topical Emollient - Dry Skin
Hepatic Impairment: No Data
Renal Impairment: No Data
Dialyzable: No Data

Ursodiol (Actigall)
Drug Class & Common Uses: Gallstone Dissolver - Pruritus, Jaundice
Hepatic Impairment: Administer with caution in patients with chronic liver disease
Renal Impairment: No Data
Dialyzable: No Data

Valacyclovir (Valtrex)
Drug Class & Common Uses: Antiviral - Herpes Zoster, Herpes Labialis
Hepatic Impairment: No adjustment required
Renal Impairment: Herpes zoster: For CrCl 30-49mL/min: 1g every 12 hours; CrCl 10-29mL/min: 1g every 24 hours; CrCl < 10mL/min: 500mg every 24 hours
Dialyzable: Yes (33%)

Valproic Acid and Derivatives (Depakene, Depakote, Depakote Sprinkles)
Drug Class & Common Uses: Anticonvulsant - Mood Stabilizer, Neuropathic Pain, Hiccups, Seizures
Hepatic Impairment: Dose reduction is required; use is contraindicated in severe impairment
Renal Impairment: Usual dosing unless CrCl <10mL/min Start with a low dose, adjust according to response
Dialyzable: Dialyzed. Dose as in CrCl <10mL/min

Valsartan (Diovan)
Drug Class & Common Uses: Angiotensin II Receptor Blocker - Cardiovascular
Hepatic Impairment: Mild-to-moderate liver disease: no dosage adjustment needed; administer with caution
Renal Impairment: Usual dosing unless CrCl <20mL/min then administer initial dose at 40mg, titrate to response
Dialyzable: Not dialyzed. Dose as in CrCl <20mL/min

Vancomycin (Vancocin)
Drug Class & Common Uses: Antibiotic - C. difficile Associated Diarrhea (CDAD), Enterocolitis
Hepatic Impairment: Degree of hepatic dysfunction does not affect pharmacokinetics of vancomycin
Renal Impairment: CrCl > 50mL/min: 15-20mg/kg/dose every 8-12 hours; CrCl 20-49mL/min: 15-20mg/kg/dose every 24 hours; CrCl < 20mL/min: longer intervals, determined by serum concentration monitoring
Dialyzable: Poorly dialyzable by intermittent hemodialysis (0-5%), generally requires replacement dosing; Intermittent hemodialysis (administer after hemodialysis on dialysis days): following loading dose of 15-25mg/kg, give either 500-100mg or 5-10mg/kg after each dose

Venlafaxine (Effexor)
Drug Class & Common Uses: Antidepressant (SNRI) - Neuropathic Pain, Depression, Anxiety, Fibromyalgia
Hepatic Impairment: Mild-to-moderate impairment: reduce total daily dose by 50%
Renal Impairment: Usual dosing unless CrCl <30mL/min then reduce total dose by 50% and administer daily
Dialyzable: Not dialyzed. Dose as in CrCl <30mL/min

Verapamil (Calan)
Drug Class & Common Uses: Calcium Channel Blocker - Hypertension, Angina, Atrial Fibrillation
Hepatic Impairment: Use 20-50% of normal dose
Renal Impairment: Dose as in normal renal function. Monitor carefully
Dialyzable: Not dialyzed. Dose as in normal renal function. Monitor carefully

Vilazodone (Viibryd)
Drug Class & Common Uses: Antidepressant (SSRI, Partial Serotonin Agonist) - Depression
Hepatic Impairment: Mild-to-moderate impairment: no adjustment needed; Severe: not studied
Renal Impairment: No Data
Dialyzable: No Data

Vitamin A & D
Drug Class & Common Uses: Topical Protectant - Excoriated Skin, Burns
Hepatic Impairment: No Data
Renal Impairment: No Data
Dialyzable: No Data

Warfarin (Coumadin)
Drug Class & Common Uses: Anticoagulant (Vitamin K Antagonist) - Thromboembolism
Hepatic Impairment: Monitor INR; avoid in moderate-severe liver disease
Renal Impairment: Dose as in normal renal function
Dialyzable: Not dialyzed. Dose as in normal renal function

Zafirlukast (Accolate)
Drug Class & Common Uses: Leukotriene Receptor Antagonist - Asthma, Rhinitis
Hepatic Impairment: Use is contraindicated
Renal Impairment: Dose as in normal renal function, but use with care
Dialyzable: Unlikely dialyzable. Dose as in normal renal function, but use with care

Zaleplon (Sonata)
Drug Class & Common Uses: Non-Benzodiazepine Hypnotic - Insomnia
Hepatic Impairment: Mild-to-moderate impairment: 5mg; avoid in patients with severe hepatic impairment
Renal Impairment: Mild-to-moderate impairment: usual dosing; Severe impairment: not adequately studied
Dialyzable: No Data

Ziconotide (Prialt)
Drug Class & Common Uses: Analgesic (Non-Opioid) - Intrathecal, Chronic Pain
Hepatic Impairment: No dosage adjustment necessary
Renal Impairment: Dose as in normal renal function. Use with caution if CrCl <10mL/min
Dialyzable: Unknown dialyzability. Dose as in CrCl <10mL/min

Zinc Oxide (Desitin)
Drug Class & Common Uses: Topical Protectant - Excoriated Skin, Burns
Hepatic Impairment: No Data
Renal Impairment: No Data
Dialyzable: No Data

Ziprasidone (Geodon)
Drug Class & Common Uses: Antipsychotic (Atypical) - Delirium, Agitation, Schizophrenia, Bipolar Disorder
Hepatic Impairment: Administer with caution
Renal Impairment: Oral: No dosage adjustment necessary; IM: administer with caution
Dialyzable: Not removed by hemodialysis

Zolendronic Acid (Zometa)
Drug Class & Common Uses: Bisphosphonate - Osteoporosis, Bone Metastases
Hepatic Impairment: No dose adjustment required. Use in severe impairment has not been studied.
Renal Impairment: Dose as in normal renal function unless CrCl <60mL/min. If CrCl 50-60mL/min administer 3.5mg. For CrCl 40-50mL/min administer 3.3mg. For CrCl 30-39mL/min administer 3mg. If CrCl <29mL/min use 3mg with caution if benefit outweighs risk
Dialyzable: Unknown dialyzability. Dose as in CrCl <29mL/min

Zolpidem (Ambien, Edluar)
Drug Class & Common Uses: Non-Benzodiazepine Hypnotic - Insomnia
Hepatic Impairment: IR: 5mg; ER: 6.25
Renal Impairment: Dose as in normal renal function
Dialyzable: Not dialyzed. Dose as in normal renal function

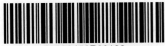

Made in the USA
San Bernardino, CA
14 May 2015